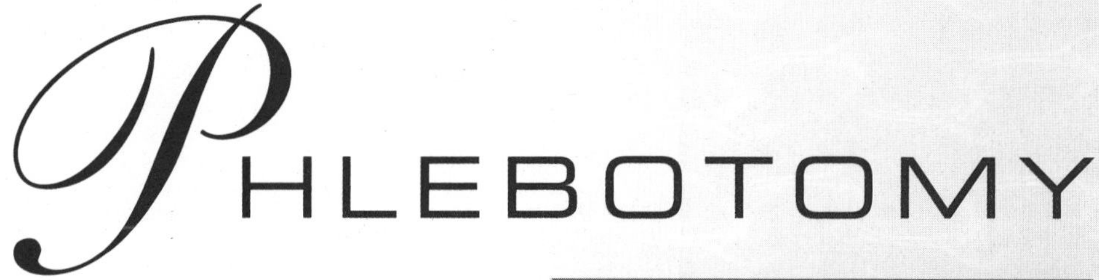

PHLEBOTOMY BASICS

WITH OTHER LABORATORY TECHNIQUES

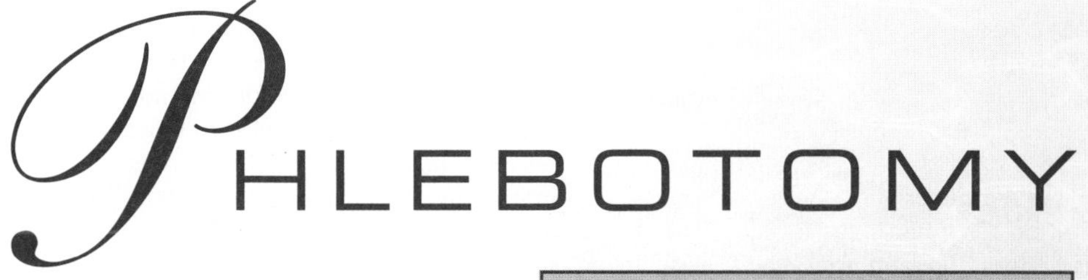

With Other Laboratory Techniques

Bonnie F. Fremgen Ph.D.
University of Notre Dame

Wendy M. Blume Ed.D, MT (ASCP)
Community College of Philadelphia

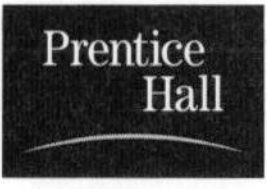

PRENTICE HALL
Upper Saddle River, New Jersey 07458

Library of Congress Cataloging-in-Publication Data
Fremgen, Bonnie F.
Phlebotomy basics with other laboratory techniques / Bonnie Fremgen and Wendy Blume.
p. cm.
Includes bibliographical references and index.
ISBN 0-8359-6164-8
1. Phlebotomy. I. Blume, Wendy. II. Title.
RB45.15 .F74 2001
616.07'561—dc21
00-044109

Publisher: *Julie Alexander*
Executive Editor: *Greg Vis*
Acquisitions Editors: *Barbara Krawiec and Mark Cohen*
Director of Production and Manufacturing: *Bruce Johnson*
Managing Production Editor: *Patrick Walsh*
Production Editor: *Amy Gehl, Carlisle Publishers Services*
Production Liaison: *Danielle Newhouse*
Manufacturing Manager: *Ilene Sanford*
Creative Director: *Marianne Frasco*
Cover Design Coordinator: *Maria Guglielmo*
Cover and Interior Designer: *Jennifer Bergamini, Alamini Design*
Director of Marketing: *Leslie Cavaliere*
Marketing Coordinator: *Cindy Frederick*
Editorial Assistant: *Melissa Kerian*
Composition: *Carlisle Publishers Services*
Printing and Binding: *RR Donnelley & Sons Company*

Prentice-Hall International (UK) Limited, *London*
Prentice-Hall of Australia Pty. Limited, *Sydney*
Prentice-Hall Canada Inc., *Toronto*
Prentice-Hall Hispanoamericana, S.A., *Mexico*
Prentice-Hall of India Private Limited, *New Delhi*
Prentice-Hall of Japan, Inc., *Tokyo*
Prentice-Hall Singapore Pte. Ltd.
Editora Prentice-Hall do Brasil, Ltda., *Rio de Janeiro*

Notice: The authors and the publisher of this volume have taken care that the information and technical recommendations contained herein are based on research and expert consultation, and are accurate and compatible with the standards generally accepted at the time of publication. Nevertheless, as new information becomes available, changes in clinical and technical practices become necessary. The reader is advised to carefully consult manufacturers' instructions and information material for all supplies and equipment before use, and to consult with a health care professional as necessary. This advice is especially important when using new supplies or equipment for clinical purposes. The authors and publisher disclaim all responsibility for any liability, loss, injury, or damage incurred as a consequence, directly or indirectly, of the use and application of any of the contents of this volume.

Cover and Chapter Opener Image: Red blood cells in an arteriole. Courtesy of Photo Researchers, Inc.

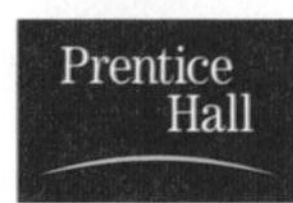

10 9 8 7 6 5 4 3 2 1
ISBN 0-8359-6164-8

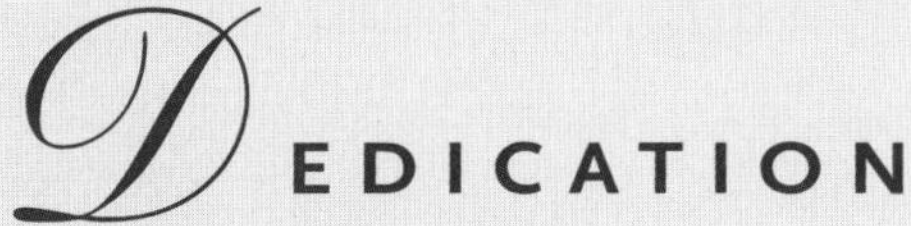

DEDICATION

To our families,

for their support

and encouragement.

Brief Contents

Detailed Contents

Procedures

PREFACE

This book is written for health care students and professionals who collect blood and other specimens as part of their job responsibilities. Practitioners who will benefit from this book include phlebotomists, nurses, respiratory therapists, medical assistants, and clinical laboratory technologists. Given the scope of the text, it can be used to cross-train health care workers in the basics of phlebotomy technique. It is also intended to be used as a reference for practicing phlebotomists who wish to pass a national certification examination.

In this book we provide an explanation, using a step-by-step format, of the clinical procedures that the phlebotomist will use in a variety of settings including the hospital, clinical laboratory, and physician's office laboratory. We present the most current clinical information, including phlebotomy skills, simple laboratory tests, equipment needs, and various specimen collection techniques. In addition, safety measures, infection control, and quality control issues are presented in an easy-to-use format. Current legal and regulatory issues are also discussed as they pertain to the phlebotomist; a chapter relating to the circulatory system is included as a review.

KEY FEATURES OF THE BOOK:

- Objectives and key terms are included for every chapter that can be used by the student as a chapter review.
- Glossary terms are printed in **bold** the first time they are defined in the text.
- Current information is presented on blood-drawing techniques and equipment.
- Procedures are explained using a step-by-step format including a terminal performance competency.
- Med Tips, placed at strategic points in the narrative, provide helpful hints and useful information relating to the discussion within the text.
- Competency review questions at the end of each chapter assist the student with a review of material covered in the chapter.
- Examination review questions at the end of each chapter reflect the type of questions that are asked on a national certification examination.

- Information is included on performing procedures and communicating with patients who have special needs; such as children, the elderly, and hearing-impaired, blind, and difficult patients.
- A chart of laboratory values is contained in appendix A for easy reference.
- Instructions for performing common laboratory math problems are included in appendix B.
- Spanish terms and statements that can be used when working with the Spanish-speaking patient are included in appendix C.
- A four-color format throughout the text to provide clearer illustrations and photos.
- Additional examination review questions for each chapter are in the instructor's manual.

Technology Package

An interactive CD-ROM is packaged with each copy of the book. This powerful tool is designed to enhance learning by offering additional study exercises, an audio glossary, and *Beyond the Basics* features. *Beyond the Basics* takes readers into more detailed or applied material, including interesting facts. Those who have access to the Internet can view the same content by logging onto www.prenhall.com/fremgen.

Ancillary Package

A full instructional support package is included:
Test Manager: 0-13-028612-5
Test Item File: 0-13-028600-1
Instructor's Manual: 0-13-040069-6

Educators may request these items by contacting their local Prentice Hall sales representative or by calling 1-800-947-7700.

ABOUT THE AUTHORS

Bonnie F. Fremgen Ph.D.

Bonnie F. Fremgen is a former associate dean of the allied health program at Robert Morris College. She has taught clinical and administrative topics, as well as phlebotomy, medical terminology, and anatomy and physiology.

Dr. Fremgen holds a nursing degree and a master's degree in health care administration. She received her Ph.D. from the College of Education at the University of Illinois.

She has broad interests and experiences in the health care field, including in physicians' offices, nursing homes, and hospitals.

Dr. Fremgen is currently an associate professional specialist at the University of Notre Dame in South Bend, Indiana.

Wendy M. Blume Ed.D, MT (ASCP)

Wendy M. Blume is the former department head of the clinical laboratory science program at the Community College of Philadelphia. During her tenure as department head, she developed the department's phlebotomy program, and the program was approved by the National Accrediting Agency for Clinical Laboratory Science (NAACLS). In addition to phlebotomy, she has taught many different courses in clinical laboratory science such as clinical hematology, clinical microbiology, and blood banking.

Dr. Blume holds a bachelor's degree in medical technology from Case Western Reserve University and a master's degree in clinical microbiology from Thomas Jefferson University. She is a registered medical technologist in the American Society of Clinical Pathologists (ASCP). She has earned her Ed.D. in health education from Temple University.

In addition to teaching in the allied health field for many years, Dr. Blume has also worked in a clinical environment as a phlebotomist, bench technologist, and laboratory supervisor. Currently she is the acting dean of the Division of Business, Science, and Technology at the Community College of Philadelphia.

ACKNOWLEDGMENTS

This book would not have been possible without the assistance and guidance of many people. We are grateful to the editorial and production staff of Prentice Hall for their skill and patience with this project.

We thank Barbara Krawiec, acquisitions editor, for her leadership throughout this project; Melissa Kerian, editorial assistant, whose courtesy and thoroughness are greatly appreciated; Pat Walsh, managing production editor, whose calm presence is always available; and Danielle Newhouse, production liaison, and Amy Gehl, production editor, whose attention to detail helped move this book along.

The following reviewers provided valuable feedback during the writing process. We thank all these professionals for their contribution and attention to detail.

Virginia Bangert, RN,C
Southern Arkansas University Youth Apprenticeship
Magnolia, Arkansas

K. B. Bello, BSC, M.D.
Instructor/Academic Coordinator
Transworld Academy
Houston, Texas

Mary N. Boyle, MT (ASCP)
Assistant Professor
Phlebotomy Program
New Hampshire Community Technical College
Claremont, New Hampshire

Patricia Bucho, CCMA, A-C, CMA, MT (ASCP)
Medical Assisting Program
Long Beach City College
Long Beach, California

Linda Burke, CMA, CPT
Assistant Director
Star Technical Institute
Lakewood, New Jersey

Karen A. Cassidy, CRRN, B.S.N.
Health Occupations Instructor
United Technology Center
Bangor, Maine

Robin H. Connors
Public Health Laboratory
Santa Cruz Health Services Agency
Santa Cruz, California

Cheri Goretti, M.A., MT (ASCP), CMA
Instructor
Phlebotomy and Medical Assisting Programs
Quinebaug Valley Community Technical College
Danielson, Connecticut

Regina M. Jackson, MT (ASCP)
DeBakey HSHP
Houston, Texas

Robin G. Krefetz, M.Ed., MT (ASCP) CLS (NCA)
Clinical Laboratory Technology Program
Community College of Philadelphia
Philadelphia, Pennsylvania

Stephanie P. Lezniak MT (ASCP)
CLT Clinical Coordinator
Community College of Philadelphia
Philadelphia, Pennsylvania

Donald Richards, M.S., RRT
Health Occupations Specialist
Kansas State Department of Education
Topeka, Kansas

Kimlynne F. Risko, MT (ASCP)
Phlebotomy Technician Program
Harrisburg Area Community College
Harrisburg, Pennsylvania

Linda Williford, MPH, RNC
Continuing Education Health Services Coordinator
Lenoir Community College–Greene County
Snow Hill, North Carolina

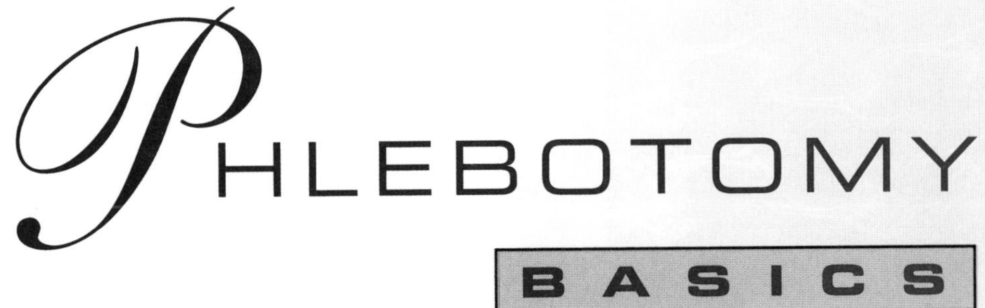

PHLEBOTOMY BASICS

WITH OTHER LABORATORY TECHNIQUES

SECTION I

Phlebotomy and the Health Care Environment

CHAPTER 1

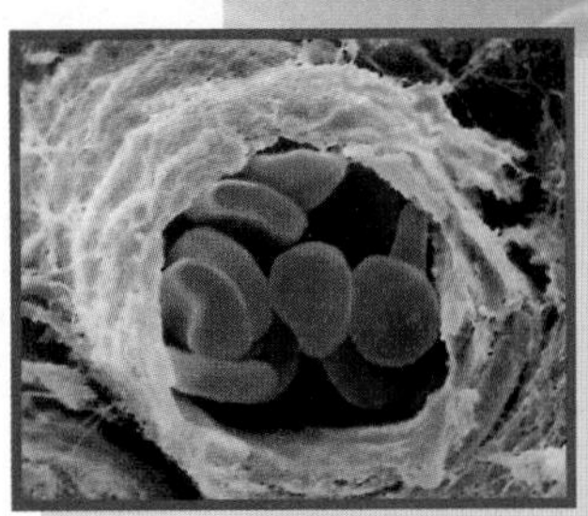

The Role of the Phlebotomist

Chapter Outline

- Introduction
- History of Phlebotomy
- Role of the Phlebotomist
- Personal Characteristics of the Phlebotomist
- Language of Medicine
- Certification
- Licensure
- Program Accreditation
- Regulation of Clinical Laboratories
- Continuing Education
- Employment Opportunities for the Phlebotomist
- Adherence to Legal and Ethical Guidelines
- Summary
- Abbreviations in the Chapter
- Competency Review
- Examination Review Questions
- Bibliography

Learning Objectives

After completing this chapter, you should be able to

1. Define the glossary terms and abbreviations for this chapter.
2. Discuss ten responsibilities and duties of the phlebotomist.
3. Describe five personal characteristics of a professional phlebotomist.
4. Name five organizations that certify phlebotomists.
5. Name three agencies that approve phlebotomy programs.
6. Name four organizations that offer continuing education units (CEUs) to the phlebotomist.
7. Discuss several employment opportunities for the phlebotomist.
8. List five personal qualities you possess that would make you a successful phlebotomist.

GLOSSARY

ACCREDITATION the process in which an institution (school) voluntarily completes an extensive self-study, after which an accrediting association visits the school to verify the self-study statements.

CERTIFICATION the issuance by an official body of a certificate to a person indicating that certain requirements to practice have been met.

CONTINUING EDUCATION UNITS (CEUs) a credit granted to a participant at the completion of a designated program.

EMPATHY the ability to understand the feelings of another person without actually experiencing the pain or distress that person is going through.

LICENSURE the legal permission, granted by the state where the phlebotomist will work, to engage in an occupation or activity.

PHLEBOTOMIST a person trained to perform blood collection procedures using various techniques that include venipuncture and capillary puncture.

PHLEBOTOMY the practice of obtaining blood samples that are used for analysis and diagnostic purposes.

RECIPROCITY agreement in which one state recognizes the licensure granted to a person by another state.

SYMPATHY feeling sorry for or pitying patients.

Introduction

The phlebotomist is an integral member of the health care team and, as such, must be able to function effectively with all patients in a variety of settings. The practice of phlebotomy requires personal characteristics such as integrity, empathy, discretion, diplomacy, confidentiality, and good communication skills. An understanding of medical law and ethics can help to prevent careless decisions. Because blood analysis is a vital diagnostic tool used routinely in medical practice today, phlebotomists must know how to collect, handle, and analyze a blood specimen properly.

History of Phlebotomy

The study of blood goes back to early history, when it was believed that bloodletting, or withdrawing blood from the human body, would help in expelling demons and evil spirits. Evidence of bloodletting goes back to early humans, who left behind various crude instruments used during the Stone Age. Hippocrates (400 B.C.), known as the "Father of Medicine," practiced medicine at a time when little was known of anatomy and physiology or the circulation of blood. During the fifth century B.C., the Greek scientist Empedocles' view that blood is life led to the consideration that the heart was the center of the vascular system. Diogenes (460 B.C.), who was a contemporary of Hippocrates, offered one of the earliest intelligible accounts of the vascular system from his investigation of blood vessels.

Ancient Egyptians used blood baths as a means of resuscitation and for recuperation from illness. Historical records indicate that Mayans used sea-urchin spines to pierce the skin in bloodletting. The Romans were said to have rushed into the gladiatorial arena to drink the blood of dying victims as a method of rejuvenating themselves. Because the blood was all taken in by mouth and not by vein, it had little beneficial effect.

For six centuries in Europe, beginning around 1163, barbers often performed surgery. Ambroise Pare, considered one of the great pioneers of surgery, also gave shaves and haircuts for a living. During that era, doctors considered bloodletting beneath their dignity, so they gladly allowed the barbers to perform bloodletting, lancing of abscesses, and treatment of wounds. The red stripe of the barber pole represents the blood the barber spilled, and the white of the pole represents the bandage.

The circulation of blood was not recognized until 1628, when the English physician William Harvey (1578–1657) published his theory of the movements of the heart and blood. Unfortunately for Harvey, the microscope had not yet been invented and he was never able to view capillaries to complete his understanding of the connections between arteries and veins.

It was not until around the middle of the seventeenth century that authentic references to blood transfusions were made in the literature. References were made to the use of hollow goose quills and metal or silver tubes for transfusions. Many of the first blood recipients died during the process of transfusion. Around 1668 in Paris, Jean Baptiste Denis, using the blood from a lamb, performed the first authentically recorded successful blood transfusion on a human. Incredible as it seems, the patient lived. During the third quarter of the nineteenth century, transfusion was becoming increasingly popular as a means to transfer the blood of a strong person into a weakened individual. One of the major uses of blood transfusion was to prevent the hemorrhaging deaths of women during childbirth.

Bloodletting during the eighteenth century in both Europe and America was popular as a treatment for infection and high fevers. The procedure was done by cupping, which involved affixing small suction cups over a cut in the skin, attaching leeches, and incising for venisection. George Washington's death on December 14, 1799, is attributed to being bled heavily four times in twenty-four hours to treat a quinsy throat (acute laryngitis).

Bloodletting for therapeutic use continued into the beginning of the twentieth century. Today bloodletting is called therapeutic phlebotomy. Although many of the early tools used for bloodletting, such as the lancet, are used in modern-day laboratories, there have been significant advances in their design. **Phlebotomy** is practiced today for the purpose of obtaining blood samples that are analyzed and often form a basis for diagnosis. The word *phlebotomy* can be broken into two parts: *phleb-* (blood vessel) and *-otomy* (incision into).

Role of the Phlebotomist

A **phlebotomist** is a person trained to perform blood collection procedures by using various techniques, including venipuncture and capillary puncture. The skilled phlebotomist requires a thorough theoretical background, excellent manual dexterity for blood-drawing technique, good organizational and communication skills, and accuracy.

Responsibilities and Duties

The responsibilities and duties of the phlebotomist include the following:

- Identifying and preparing patients for blood collection procedures
- Collecting blood specimens using correct venipuncture and capillary puncture technique
- Selecting and labeling the correct specimen containers
- Maintaining aseptic technique
- Processing specimens to maintain stability
- Transporting specimens correctly
- Collecting data and maintaining records
- Practicing quality assurance procedures
- Maintaining records using the computer
- Maintaining a safe working environment
- Complying with all departmental policies and procedures
- Maintaining skills with self-study, in-service, and continuing education programs
- Maintaining patient confidentiality

Personal Characteristics of the Phlebotomist

As a medical professional, the phlebotomist must have certain personal characteristics, including integrity, empathy, discretion, diplomacy, confidentiality, ethics, honesty, communication skills, compassion, dependability, accountability, understanding of the scope of practice, and professional appearance.

Integrity

People with integrity are dedicated to maintaining high standards. For example, integrity means phlebotomists will always wash their hands between patients and use meticulous care to avoid cross-contamination when handling patient specimens even when no one is looking. Phlebotomists must be able to adhere to a code of values, which includes honesty, dependability, punctuality, and dedication to high standards. They should never be late for work or fail to come in when scheduled unless they are ill. Dependability is a key component of integrity.

Empathy

Empathy is the ability to understand the feelings of another person without actually experiencing the pain or distress that person is going through. Acting in a kindly way expresses sensitivity to patients' feelings. For example, phlebotomists can understand the fear that some patients have when they see a needle or blood. Effective phlebotomists are able to demonstrate empathy for their patients but should avoid sympathy. **Sympathy** is feeling sorry for or pitying patients. Patients react better to empathetic listeners than to sympathetic ones.

MED TIP

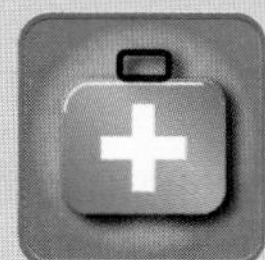

You can acquire the skill of empathetic listening using simple nonverbal techniques such as nodding, leaning toward the patient, positioning yourself at the patient's eye level, and indicating by use of facial expression that you understand what the patient is saying.

Patience is required when working with those who are sick and disabled. For example, even if phlebotomists do not fear needles, being empathetic, they will understand the fear patients might have.

Discretion

The use of good judgment and prudence makes it possible for phlebotomists to offer timely and effective instruction to unwilling patients or to remain calm in emergencies and instill confidence in patients. For example, phlebotomists would not show an alarmed reaction when blood is spilled or there is a negative laboratory report.

Good judgment is required when handling patients' family members. Family members should be asked to wait outside of patients' rooms or laboratory cubicles while a laboratory procedure takes place to provide privacy for patients. The exception to this rule is when the patient is a child. Usually the parents can assist in calming the child or gently restraining the child while the phlebotomist draws the blood.

Diplomacy

Phlebotomists must be able to use tact and understanding when handling patients and their problems. For example, a patient may have to be retested if there is a questionable test result. This message has to be conveyed to the patient so the patient will understand the importance of the retest but not be unduly fearful or angry that the blood needs to be redrawn.

Confidentiality

Confidentiality is the ability to safeguard patient privacy, particularly information in the medical record regarding past or current diseases or illnesses and test results. No information can be disclosed about the patient without the patient's written permission. Violating patient confidentiality is both a legal and ethical issue that carries penalties. The results of blood testing, and even the fact that a patient has had a test, are confidential.

Requisitions bearing the patient's name and the test ordered cannot be left within view of a patient or other persons. Laboratory results are given directly to the physician or the licensed practitioner who ordered the test.

MED TIP

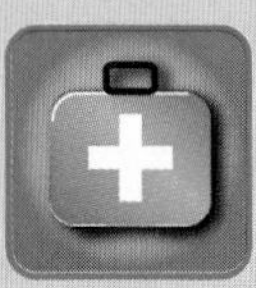

There is an old adage in health care that the walls have ears. All health care workers must avoid discussing any patient information in public areas such as elevators, cafeterias, hallways, and waiting rooms.

Ethics

A moral duty to determine the difference between a right and wrong action and then to always practice the right action is ethical behavior. For example, an error in labeling a specimen must immediately be corrected by admitting the error and taking corrective steps.

Honesty

Ethical phlebotomists will always admit an error. For example, phlebotomists will admit when they are unable to successfully enter a vein and will ask someone else to assist.

Communication Skills

Verbal, nonverbal, and listening skills are needed to communicate with all patients, including persons with disabilities (hard of hearing, blind, sensory deprived, mentally ill, or illiterate). The same skills are used with patients' families, visitors, coworkers, and other health care professionals. Smiling immediately reassures the patient. A considerate, gentle bedside manner, whether in the hospital, laboratory, or medical office, provides an immediate nonverbal communication message to the patient.

MED TIP

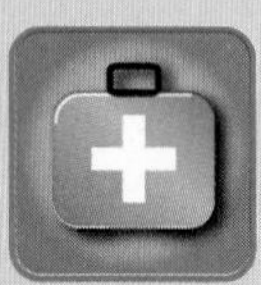

Never forget that the patient is present. No discussion should be held in the patient's presence that does not include the patient. If you are interrupted and it is a matter that needs immediate discussion with another person, then apologize to the patient and step away to hold the conversation.

TABLE 1-1 Messages That Convey Impatience

Interrupting people when they are speaking	Rushing around the laboratory or office
Finishing another person's sentence	Not looking up from work when someone approaches
Rushing the patient	Answering the telephone curtly
Looking at one's watch or the clock	Tapping pencil, pen, or foot
Doing two things at one time	Yawning and sighing

Phlebotomists must always identify themselves to the patient. Handling the inquisitive patient requires every characteristic discussed, but especially diplomacy. If the patient asks a specific question such as "Is this another PT test?" then the phlebotomist can respond with a yes or no. However, the physician must convey any information regarding the type of test and the patient's clinical condition. In most cases the patient will already know this information. Table 1-1 provides examples of messages that carry a negative implication to the patient and imply that the patient is not the first priority.

MED TIP

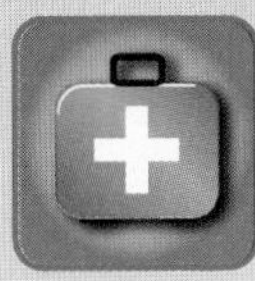

If the patient indicates any confusion during the communication process over the type of test that has been ordered, you must check with the physician who ordered the test *before* drawing the blood.

MED TIP

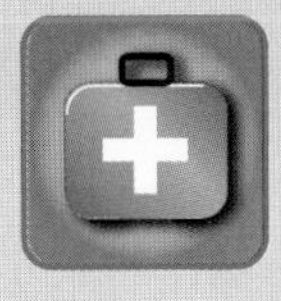

Never argue with the patient! You have an obligation to find an acceptable, calm solution to any situation.

The ability to work and communicate well with others is necessary in the workplace. The phlebotomist is a member of a health care team including people from a variety of disciplines. All of these people, including other health care professionals, maintenance personnel, and cleaning personnel, interact with the patient. Therefore, it is vital that the phlebotomist practice good team-building and communication skills.

Compassion

It is essential to have a gentle, caring attitude toward the frightened and ill patient. Any illness, and in particular a terminal illness, causes a sense of fear and loneliness in many patients.

Dependability

A key requirement for all health care professionals is reliability. A professional must be punctual for work and complete all duties in a timely manner.

Accountability

Phlebotomists are responsible, or accountable, for their actions. They are also working as agents of their employer. The legal concept of *respondeat superior* (discussed further in chapter 3) means "Let the master answer." Therefore, any error or unprofessional behavior is a reflection on the employer as well as the employee.

Understanding the Scope of Practice

Medical professionals must understand and work within the limits of their training. The scope of practice is determined by the certifying agencies for each health care profession. If professionals are licensed, such as nurses and pharmacists, the state issuing the license determines the scope of practice within that state.

MED TIP

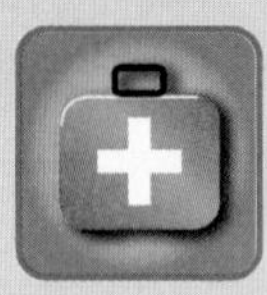

An example of the scope of practice is that the phlebotomist does not interpret test results to patients.

Professional Appearance

In many cases the phlebotomist will be the only health care professional the patient will see during laboratory testing. Therefore, the patient will judge the professionalism of the entire health care team by his or her contact with the phlebotomist. A professional appearance, including good personal hygiene, instills confidence in the patient. For example, the phlebotomist's clothing should be clean at the beginning of every shift, and clothing is always changed immediately if blood is spilled or splashed on it.

Daily habits of good personal hygiene and good grooming are expected in the phlebotomist. Daily bathing or showering and the use of deodorant are expected. The use of strong perfumes can be disturbing to patients who may be ill or allergic. Long fingernails and nail polish should be avoided for sanitary reasons. Nails should be carefully trimmed and scrubbed before beginning work.

Long hair should be pulled back and tied away from the face. All jewelry, except for a single ring and wristwatch, should be avoided since they have small spaces that can harbor bacteria. Men's beards and mustaches must be clean and trimmed.

Protective clothing, such as a laboratory coat, is worn over street clothing and is removed before leaving the laboratory or hospital setting. It serves as a safeguard for the patient and also prevents the phlebotomist from carrying disease-producing microorganisms out of the laboratory setting. Protective clothing must be kept clean and pressed daily. Personal items, such as lipstick and keys, should not be carried in the pockets of protective laboratory coats.

In some laboratories and institutions, such as hospitals, a scrub suit or full white uniform is required. White, well-shined shoes are worn. Open-toed or open-heeled shoes, clogs, sandals, and high-heeled shoes are not appropriate and are against Occupational Safety and Health Administration (OSHA) regulations. Puncture-proof shoes are advisable.

The phlebotomist's identification (ID) badge must be worn within eyesight of the patient. If the phlebotomist is a student, this information should be noted on the badge.

Language of Medicine

The profession of phlebotomy requires a good understanding of medical terminology. The abbreviations used in medicine are a form of communication for people working in the health care field. However, many patients have little understanding of medical terminology. Every effort should be made to avoid using the shorthand abbreviations of medical terminology with patients.

Patients may be reluctant to admit they do not understand a medical term or abbreviation. The phlebotomist might assume patients have been properly instructed when, in reality, they do not have a complete understanding.

MED TIP

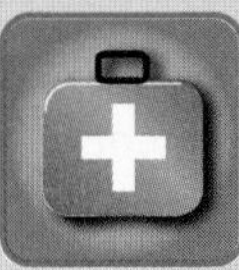

Abbreviations such as NPO, meaning nothing by mouth, are not easily recognized or understood by patients. Always write out clear instructions regarding preparations for laboratory tests.

Certification

Certification is the issuance by an official body of a certificate to a person indicating that he or she has been evaluated and has met certain requirements. National certification usually is an indication that the person has completed a specific academic and training program and attained an acceptable score on a national examination. Many health care facilities require their phlebotomists to be certified by national agencies or be registration eligible. When phlebotomists have met all the certification requirements, they may display the abbreviation of the accrediting agency after their name. Agencies that certify phlebotomists are listed in table 1-2.

Licensure

Licensure is the legal permission, granted by the state where the phlebotomist will work, to engage in an occupation or activity. It is similar to the certification process but is handled at the state or local level. People are licensed in the state in which they practice. Licensed professionals include physicians, dentists,

TABLE 1-2 Phlebotomist Certification	
Certifying Organization	**Title of Award**
American Society of Phlebotomy Technicians (ASPT)	Certified Phlebotomy Technician (CPT)
American Medical Technologists (AMT)	Registered Phlebotomy Technician (RPT)
American Society of Clinical Pathologists (ASCP)	Phlebotomy Technician (PBT)
National Phlebotomy Association (NPA)	Certified Phlebotomy Technician (CPT)
National Credentialing Agency (NCA) for Medical Laboratory Personnel	Clinical Laboratory Phlebotomist (CLPlb)

and nurses. One state may recognize the licensure that is granted by another state. This recognition is referred to as **reciprocity** and may benefit the professional phlebotomist who moves from one state to another and wishes to continue working as a phlebotomist.

Program Accreditation

Accreditation is the process in which an institution (school) voluntarily completes an extensive self-study, after which an accrediting association visits the school to verify the self-study statements. Medical laboratory technician programs and medical technology programs pursue program accreditation.

However, phlebotomy programs seek an approval rather than an accreditation. To be granted approval, a program must meet stringent educational requirements but does not undergo an on-site survey visit. Agencies that provide approval for phlebotomy programs are

- National Phlebotomy Association (NPA)
- National Accrediting Agency for Clinical Laboratory Sciences (NAACLS)
- American Society of Phlebotomy Technicians (ASPT)

Regulation of Clinical Laboratories

All hospital laboratories must follow guidelines and standards for providing patient care. The *National Committee for Clinical Laboratory Standards (NCCLS)* establishes procedural guidelines for all areas of the clinical laboratory. It is a nonprofit agency composed of representatives from the medical laboratory profession, industry, and government.

The *College of American Pathologists (CAP)* is another agency that sets standards for phlebotomy and provides proficiency testing and laboratory inspections. The testing results are compared with results of other laboratory tests conducted throughout the country. If the results are below standard, a plan of correction must be written. CAP sends teams consisting of medical technologists and pathologists to inspect and review laboratories and procedures every two years.

The Joint Commission on Accreditation of Healthcare Organizations (JCAHO) is an accrediting agency for hospitals and nursing homes. To receive a JCAHO accreditation the health care facility must undergo an inspection every three years. Any deficiencies noted must be corrected within a previously established time frame.

MED TIP

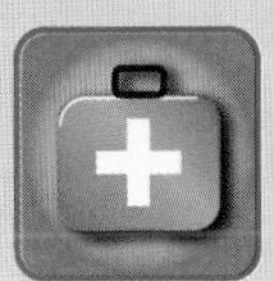

The JCAHO and CAP work jointly to provide laboratory accreditation. If CAP has inspected and awarded accreditation, the JCAHO will grant accreditation to the laboratory through reciprocity.

One of the most recent government regulations affecting medical laboratories is the Clinical Laboratory Improvement Act of 1988 (CLIA 1988). This bill, enacted by Congress, requires the regulation of all laboratories including physician's office laboratories (POLs), hospitals, clinics, health maintenance organizations (HMOs), independent reference laboratories, and government laboratories. The same standards are in effect for all laboratories under CLIA 1988. CLIA 1988 regulations include specific guidelines for quality control, quality assurance, record keeping, and personnel qualifications. A system used by CLIA 1988 classifies laboratories (levels I, II, and III) according to test complexity and risk to the patient if error occurs. These levels are explained in chapter 3.

Continuing Education

Continuing education is a means for phlebotomists to keep current regarding new technologies in the field of laboratory medicine. Continuing education is available through participating in workshops and seminars, viewing videotapes, and attending in-service programs. Phlebotomists must take advantage of every opportunity for self-study, including attending departmental meetings and reading pertinent literature. **Continuing education units (CEUs)** are granted to participants on completion of a designated program. Organizations that offer CEUs are listed in table 1-3.

TABLE 1-3 Organizations Offering CEUs to Phlebotomists
National Phlebotomy Association (NPA)
American Society of Clinical Pathologists (ASCP)
American Society for Medical Technologists (ASMT)
American Society of Phlebotomy Technicians (ASPT)
American Society for Clinical Laboratory Sciences (ASCLS)

TABLE 1-4 Employment Opportunities for Phlebotomists	
Physician Office Laboratories (POLs)	Hospitals
Health Maintenance Organizations (HMOs)	Long-term care facilities
Preferred Provider Organizations (PPOs)	Clinics
Independent Reference Laboratories	Government laboratories

Employment Opportunities for the Phlebotomist

The number and type of employment opportunities increase every year as managed care and the practice of preventive medicine increase in scope. Some of the employment opportunities are listed in table 1-4.

Adherence to Legal and Ethical Guidelines

Phlebotomists have a responsibility to both the patient and the profession to maintain the highest standards of the profession. Because they always have patient contact, they must carefully adhere to professional standards, which include protecting the patient's confidentiality, to avoid legal problems. Phlebotomists practice under the supervision of their employers and, thus, can cause legal problems for the employers when errors are made. Phlebotomists can only perform those procedures for which they have received training and certification.

Phlebotomists must always take immediate action to protect the patient. Examples of protecting the patient are having a fearful or fainting patient recline during a venipuncture and providing a patient's medical report to an outside agency such as an insurance company, only with permission from the patient.

CHAPTER REVIEW

Summary

The role of phlebotomy in medicine has a rich history dating back centuries. The current profession is well regulated, and the contemporary professional needs considerable skill and knowledge.

Abbreviations in the Chapter

AMT	*American Medical Technologists*
ASCP	*American Society of Clinical Pathologists*
ASMT	*American Society for Medical Technologists*
ASPT	*American Society of Phlebotomy Technicians*
CAP	*College of American Pathologists*
CEU	*Continuing Education Unit*
CLIA 1988	*Clinical Laboratory Improvement Act of 1988*
CLPlb	*Clinical Laboratory Phlebotomist*
CPT	*Certified Phlebotomy Technician*
HMO	*Health Maintenance Organization*
JCAHO	*Joint Commission on Accreditation of Healthcare Organizations*
NAACLS	*National Accrediting Agency for Clinical Laboratory Sciences*
NCA	*National Credentialing Agency for Medical Laboratory Personnel*
NCCLS	*National Committee for Clinical Laboratory Standards*
NPA	*National Phlebotomy Association*
NPO	*Nothing by mouth (Latin: nihil per os)*
PBT	*Phlebotomy Technician*
POL	*Physician's Office Laboratory*
PPO	*Preferred Provider Organization*
RPT	*Registered Phlebotomy Technician*

Competency Review

1. Discuss the historical background of phlebotomy.
2. Describe six personal characteristics that you possess that are necessary for a successful career in phlebotomy.
3. Name five organizations that certify phlebotomists.
4. Name four organizations that offer CEUs to phlebotomists.
5. List several health care facilities in your area in which you may choose to work as a phlebotomist.

Examination Review Questions

1. **Adhering to a code of values with honesty, dependability, and dedication is called**
   (A) compassion
   (B) sympathy
   (C) integrity
   (D) the law
   (E) none of the above

2. **Explaining to the patient that another sample will need to be drawn because the first sample was misplaced is an example of**
   (A) confidentiality
   (B) discretion
   (C) diplomacy
   (D) honesty
   (E) dependability

3. **When a person has completed certain requirements and is issued a statement to that effect, he or she is said to be**
   (A) accredited
   (B) certified
   (C) disclosed
   (D) legal
   (E) none of the above

4. **An agency that issues approval for phlebotomy programs is**
   (A) the American Society of Phlebotomy Associations (ASPA)
   (B) the American Society of Clinical Pathologists (ASCP)
   (C) the American Society for Medical Technologists (ASMT)
   (D) the Certified Phlebotomy Technician Program (CPTP)
   (E) none of the above

5. **The association that awards the registered phlebotomy technician (RPT) certificate is the**
   (A) American Society of Phlebotomy Technicians (ASPT)
   (B) American Society of Clinical Pathologists (ASCP)
   (C) National Credentialing Agency (NCA) for Medical Laboratory Personnel
   (D) National Phlebotomy Association (NPA)
   (E) American Medical Technologists (AMT)

6. **Laboratory regulation is handled by**
   (A) the National Committee for Clinical Laboratory Standards (NCCLS)
   (B) the College of American Pathologists (CAP)
   (C) the Joint Commission on Accreditation of Healthcare Organizations (JCAHO)
   (D) the National Phlebotomy Association (NPA)
   (E) a, b, and c only

7. **The federal regulation affecting clinical laboratories is**
   (A) the Clinical Laboratory Improvement Act of 1980
   (B) the Clinical Laboratory Improvement Act of 1988
   (C) the Congressional Laboratory Improvement Act of 1990
   (D) the Congressional Laboratory Improvement Act of 1988
   (E) none of the above

8. **The abbreviation CLPlb after a person's name indicates that he or she is**
   (A) licensed
   (B) accredited
   (C) certified
   (D) illegal
   (E) in training

9. **The discovery of the circulation of the blood is attributed to**
   (A) Hippocrates
   (B) Ambroise Pare
   (C) barbers
   (D) William Harvey
   (E) Diogenes

10. **An early term for phlebotomy was**
    (A) cupping
    (B) venisection
    (C) leeching
    (D) bloodletting
    (E) all of the above

Getting Connected

Multimedia Extension Activities

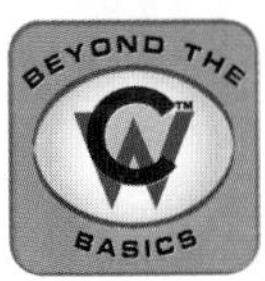

www.prenhall.com/fremgen

Use the address above to access the free, interactive Companion Website created specifically for this textbook. Enhance your studying by answering practice quiz questions, with hints and instant feedback related to chapter 1. If you would like to gain a deeper understanding of selected topics within this chapter, be sure to click on the **Beyond the Basics** feature, which provides more details for further learning. If you do not have a web connection, you may use the CD-ROM enclosed in the back of this book to take advantage of the same features off-line.

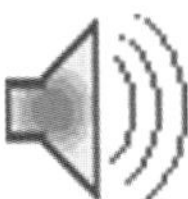

Audio Glossary

Use the CD-ROM enclosed with your textbook to hear the pronunciation of the key terms in the chapter. You may also access this material on the Companion Website www.prenhall.com/fremgen.

Bibliography

American Medical Association. *Current Procedural Terminology.* Chicago: American Medical Association, 1996.

Belsey, R., C. Mulrow, and H. Sox. "How to Handle Baffling Test Results." *Patient Care,* May 30, 1993.

"CDC Summarizes Final Regulations for Implementing CLIA." *American Family Physician,* 45 (1992): 6.

Chernecky, C., R. Krech, and B. Berger. *Laboratory Tests and Diagnostic Procedures.* Philadelphia: W. B. Saunders, 1993.

Encyclopaedia Britannica. Chicago: William Benton, 1990.

Fishbach, F. *A Manual of Laboratory and Diagnostic Tests.* Philadelphia: Lippincott, 1996.

Fremgen, B. *Essentials of Medical Assisting.* Upper Saddle River, N.J.: Brady/Prentice-Hall, 1998.

Marshall, J. *Medical Laboratory Assistant.* Upper Saddle River, N.J.: Brady/Prentice-Hall, 1990.

Palko, T., and H. Palko. *Laboratory Procedures for the Medical Office.* New York: Glencoe, 1996.

Sazama, J. "Licensure of Laboratory Personnel." *Laboratory Medicine,* April, 1993.

Tietz, N. *Clinical Guide to Laboratory Tests,* 2nd ed. Philadelphia: W. B. Saunders, 1992.

Tietz, N., R. Conn, and E. Pruden. *Applied Laboratory Medicine.* Philadelphia: W. B. Saunders, 1992.

Walters, N., B. Estridge, and A. Reynolds. *Basic Medical Laboratory Techniques.* New York: Delmar, 1990.

Contact Information

American Medical Technologists (AMT)
710 Higgins Rd.
Park Ridge, IL 60068
(847) 823-5169
(800) 275-1268

American Society of Phlebotomy Technicians (ASPT)
P.O. Box 1831
Hickory, NC 28603
(704) 322-1334

American Society of Clinical Pathologists (ASCP)
Board of Registry
P.O. Box 12277
Chicago, IL 60612-0277
(312) 738-1336

National Phlebotomy Association (NPA)
1901 Brightfeat Rd.
Landover, MD 20785
(301) 699-3846

National Credentialing Agency (NCA) for Medical Laboratory Personnel
P.O. Box 15945-289
Lenexa, KS 66285
(913) 438-5110

CHAPTER 2

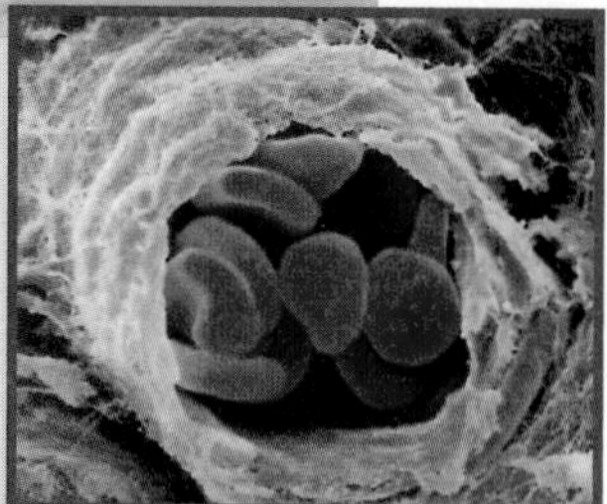

Health Care Facilities and the Clinical Laboratory

Chapter Outline

- Introduction
- Health Care Facilities
- Clinical Laboratory
- Clinical Laboratory Personnel
- Departments within a Clinical Laboratory
- Physician's Office Laboratory
- Clinic
- Independent Laboratories
- Outpatient Testing
- Summary
- Abbreviations in the Chapter
- Competency Review
- Examination Review Questions
- Bibliography

Learning Objectives

After completing this chapter, you should be able to

1. Define all glossary terms and abbreviations in this chapter.
2. Explain the function of various departments within the hospital.
3. Define the medical and surgical specialties discussed in the text.
4. Discuss the role of the laboratory director, laboratory administrator, technical supervisor, medical laboratory technician, laboratory technologist, blood bank technologist, and phlebotomist in the clinical laboratory.
5. Describe the tests run in the clinical chemistry, hematology, microbiology, blood bank, immunology, and cytology laboratories.

GLOSSARY

AUTOPSY tests conducted on the organs and tissues of deceased persons to assist in determining the cause of death.

CYTOLOGY area of surgical pathology that examines bodily fluids and tissues for evidence of abnormality after the histologist has prepared them.

HEMATOLOGY DEPARTMENT department that conducts laboratory analysis testing to identify diseases of the blood and blood-forming tissues.

HISTOLOGY the study of tissues.

IMMUNOLOGY DEPARTMENT department that runs tests on blood samples to determine the presence of an antigen-antibody reaction of the body.

MICROBIOLOGY DEPARTMENT department that analyzes specimens for the presence and identification of type of microorganisms.

INTRODUCTION

The health care environment has been changing rapidly as a result of cost-effective techniques including managed care. As a member of the health care team, the phlebotomist must have an understanding of the health care environment. The hospital is a focal point for much of U.S. health care. Clinical laboratories are located in a variety of settings including the hospital.

Health Care Facilities

Hospital

The hospital is still considered a key resource for health care in America. The patient's primary care is still delivered in the physician's office. However, the hospital treats acute illnesses, provides major surgical procedures, trains and educates health care professionals, conducts research, provides outpatient services, and provides educational resources to the public. A hospital may also be designated as a trauma center for a particular region and, as such, receives accident victims (see figure 2-1). Table 2-1 describes the departments found in most hospitals and medical centers.

Support Services Departments

Support services in the hospital include the accounting or business office, which manages the general business issues in accounting, billing and collections, credit, data processing, and admitting. The central supply department provides equipment and supplies required by patients and departments. Dietary, or food service, provides food for employees and patients, including special dietary requirements. The facilities, grounds, and maintenance department maintains the physical environment of the hospital building and grounds. Housekeeping provides daily cleaning services for patient areas, departments, and office areas. The human resource department interviews and maintains records for all employees.

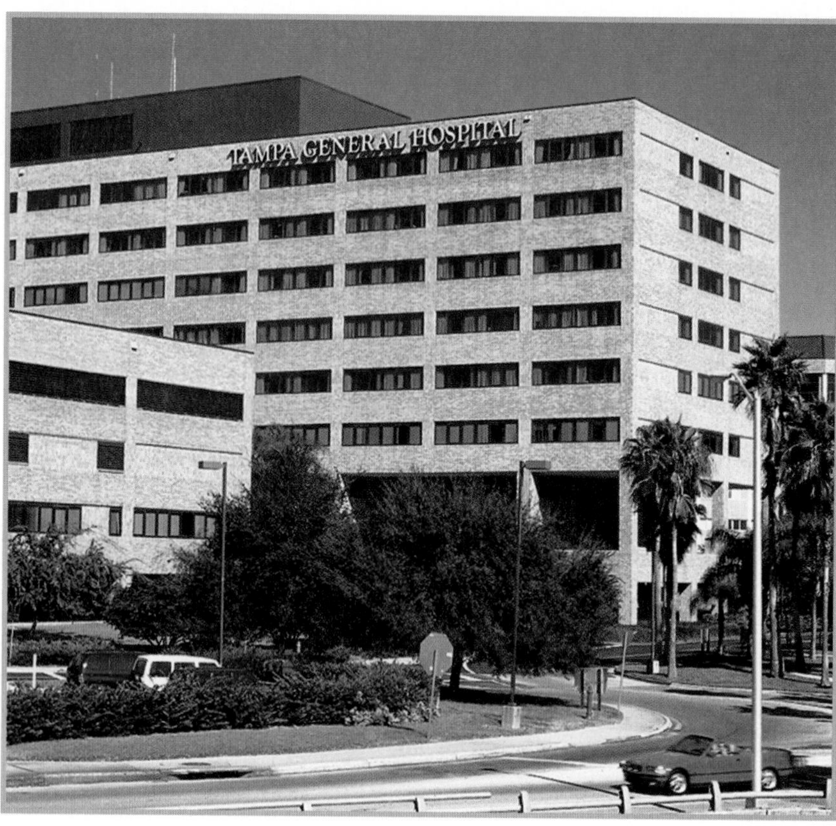

Figure 2-1
A hospital trauma center.

TABLE 2-1 Hospital Departments

Patient Service Departments	Description
Anesthesiology	Administers both local and general drugs to obtain a complete or partial loss of feeling (anesthesia) during an invasive procedure such as surgery
Clinical Laboratory	Performs a variety of tests on blood, tissues, and other body specimens; obtains, processes, preserves, studies, and analyzes specimens, maintains a database of results
Coronary Care Unit or Cardiac Care Unit (CCU)	Treats and provides care for seriously ill heart patients
Diagnostic Imaging	Performs X-ray-related procedures including magnetic resonance imaging (MRI) and computerized axial tomography (CAT) scans
Emergency Room (ER) or Emergency Department (ED)	Provides immediate treatment for seriously ill and injured patients with medical emergencies
Infection Control	Identifies, controls, and educates about infectious diseases
Intensive Care Unit (ICU)	Treats and provides care for seriously ill and injured patients; intensive care units can be found in special areas, such as pediatric ICU, neonatal intensive care (NICU), medical ICU, surgical ICU, and coronary care unit (CCU)
Internal Medicine	Diagnoses and treats patients with general medical conditions such as diabetes, heart disease, and stroke
Labor and Delivery (L&D)	Treats women during the birth process; separate from the nursery and postpartum area
Nuclear Medicine	Uses radioactive isotopes in the diagnosis and treatment of disease
Nursing Services	Provides direct care to ill and injured patients including administering medications
Obstetrics (OB)	Cares for mother and newborn throughout the birth process—labor, delivery, postpartum, and nursery
Occupational Therapy (OT)	Uses techniques to assist mentally and physically disabled or challenged patients to return to activities of daily living
Oncology	Provides care and treatment of cancer patients
Outpatient (OP)	Cares for patients who are not hospitalized

(continued)

TABLE 2-1 Hospital Departments *(continued)*	
Patient Service Departments	**Description**
Pediatrics	Treats and provides health care for infants and children
Pharmacy	Prepares and dispenses patient medications
Physical Therapy (PT)	Provides treatments and therapies to correct disabilities and restore mobility
Pulmonary Medicine	Diagnoses and treats respiratory disorders
Psychiatry	Diagnoses and treats emotional disorders
Radiation Therapy	Uses radioactive substances for the diagnosis and treatment of disease
Radiology	Uses radioactive substances and visualization (X-ray) techniques for the diagnosis and treatment of disease
Respiratory Therapy (RT)	Treats pulmonary (lung) disorders and diseases
Social Service	Assists patients in referrals to other care facilities such as nursing homes and home health care
Surgery	Diagnoses and treats patients using an invasive surgical procedure

The information systems department maintains computerized records for financial, employee, and patient information. Medical Records (also called Health Information Technology) processes reports and dictation relating to patients and maintains permanent patient records. The purchasing department purchases all supplies from selected vendors. Security provides assurance that only approved personnel and visitors are in the facility. Table 2-2 describes members of the health care team.

Allied health professionals include the certified medical assistant (CMA), registered dietitian (RD), electrocardiograph (ECG or EKG) technician, emergency medical technician (EMT) or paramedic, medical records technician, medical transcriptionist, occupational therapist (OT), physical therapist (PT), physician's assistant (PA), respiratory therapist (RT), social worker, ultrasound technologist, psychiatric technician, X-ray technician, medical technologist, and microbiologist.

TABLE 2-2 The Health Care Team

Physician Specializations	Descriptions
Medical Specialties	
Adolescent Medicine	Treats patients from puberty to maturity (ages 11 to 21)
Allergy and Immunology	Treats abnormal responses or acquired hypersensitivity to substances with medical methods including testing and desensitization
Anesthesiology	Administers local and general drugs to induce loss of consciousness and/or sensation during an invasive procedure
Cardiology	Treats cardiovascular (heart and blood vessels) disorders and diseases
Dermatology	Treats injuries and diseases relating to the skin
Family Practice (Primary Medicine)	Treats entire family regardless of members' ages
Geriatric Medicine (Gerontology)	Focuses on care and diseases of the elderly
Hematology	Studies blood and blood-forming tissues
Infection Control	Prevents and treats infectious diseases
Internal Medicine (Primary Care)	Treats adult patients with medical problems such as high blood pressure and heart disease
Nephrology	Treats disorders and diseases of the kidney
Neurology	Treats nonsurgical patients with diseases or disorders of the nervous system
Nuclear Medicine	Uses radioactive substances for diagnosis and treatment of diseases such as cancer
Obstetrics (OB) and Gynecology (GYN)	Treats women through pregnancy and delivery and disorders of the reproductive system
Oncology	Studies cancer and cancer-related tumors
Ophthalmology	Treats disorders of the eye
Orthopedics	Prevents and corrects disorders of the musculoskeletal system
Otorhinolaryngology or Ear, Nose, and Throat (ENT)	Medically and surgically treats ear, nose, and throat diseases
Pathology	Specializes in diagnosing the abnormal changes in tissues that are removed during surgery

(continued)

TABLE 2-2 The Health Care Team *(continued)*

Physician Specializations	Descriptions
Pediatrics	Provides medical care of children from birth to maturity
Physical Medicine or Rehabilitative Medicine	Treats patients after they have suffered an injury or disability
Preventive Medicine	Prevents physical and mental illness or disability
Psychiatry	Treats and diagnoses mental, behavioral, and/or emotional disorders
Radiology	Studies tissue and organs based on X-ray visualization
Rheumatology	Treats disorders and diseases caused by inflammation of the joints
Surgical Specialties	
Cardiovascular	Surgically treats the heart and blood vessels
Colorectal	Surgically treats the lower intestinal tract (colon and rectum)
Cosmetic or Plastic Surgery	Reconstructs underlying tissues to correct defects or remove scars
Neurosurgery	Surgically treats diseases and disorders of the central nervous system
Oral (Periodontics, Orthodontics)	Uses incision and surgery to treat disorders of the teeth, gums, and jaws
Orthopedic	Treats musculoskeletal injuries and disorders, congenital deformities, and spinal curvatures through surgical means
Thoracic	Surgically treats disorders and diseases of the chest
Nursing Services (Direct Patient Care)	
Nurse Practitioner (NP)	Registered nurse (RN) who has received additional training such as in community health or pediatrics
Registered Nurse (RN)	Provides direct patient care, teaches and supervises other staff, receives education and training in a diploma program, a 2-year program, or 4-year program; all states require that a state exam be passed to become licensed
Licensed Practical Nurse (LPN)	Able to perform some of the same tasks as a registered nurse; receives education in a 1- to 2-year program
Certified Nursing Assistant (CNA)	Patient care attendant who can provide patient care such as bathing the patient in bed, checking vital signs, and feeding under the supervision of a nurse

TABLE 2-3 Designations and Abbreviations for Doctors	
Designations	**Abbreviations**
Doctor of Chiropractic	D.C.
Doctor of Dental Medicine	D.M.D.
Doctor of Dental Surgery	D.D.S.
Doctor of Medicine	M.D.
Doctor of Optometry	O.D.
Doctor of Osteopathy	D.O.
Doctor of Philosophy	Ph.D.
Doctor of Podiatric Medicine	D.P.M.

The designation *doctor* is the proper way of addressing—verbally or in writing—someone who holds a doctoral degree of any kind. The abbreviation for doctor is *Dr.* In the medical field, the title *Doctor/Dr.* indicates that a person is qualified to practice medicine within the limits of his or her degree; in other fields, the title means that a person has attained the highest educational degree in his or her field. Several designations for doctor are listed in table 2-3 with the corresponding abbreviations.

Clinical Laboratory

The clinical laboratory is a composite of many health care professionals whose qualifications and job descriptions vary (see figure 2-2). The medical laboratory performs a variety of tests on blood and other body specimens. The laboratory obtains, handles, studies, and analyzes the specimens.

Clinical Laboratory Personnel

Laboratory Director

The laboratory director is usually a pathologist. A pathologist is a physician who has completed a 4- to 5-year residency or period of specialized training in the study of pathology. The pathologist may have a specialty in clinical pathology, which is interpreting test results to diagnose disease, or anatomic pathology, which is the study of tissues in surgical and autopsy specimens.

Laboratory Administrator or Manager

The laboratory administrator is responsible for managing the day-to-day operations within the laboratory, including hiring and supervising personnel and managing the budget. This person acts as a liaison between the laboratory director (pathologist) and the laboratory staff. The laboratory administrator usually has a clinical master's degree and several years of experience as a medical laboratory technologist.

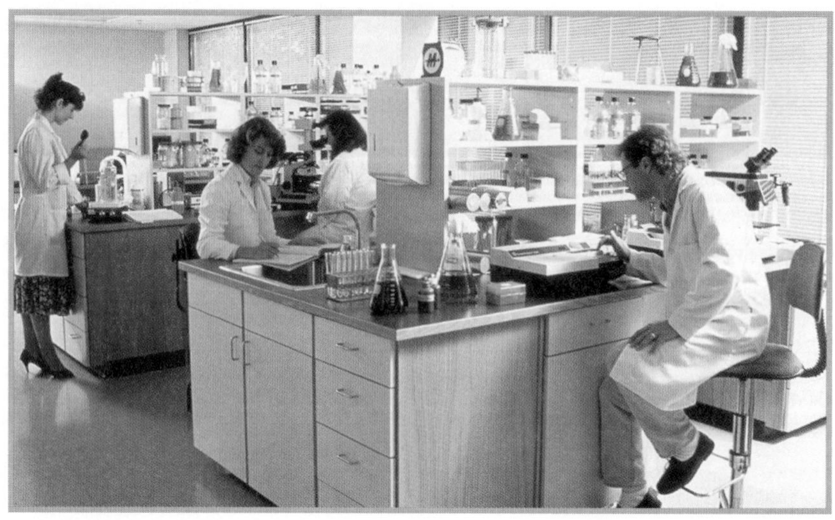

Figure 2-2
Modern hospital laboratory.

Technical Supervisors

Each of the clinical laboratory sections within the laboratory may have its own supervisor. This person has additional experience and education in a particular area such as hematology or microbiology and is responsible for the daily work schedules and staffing.

Medical or Clinical Laboratory Technician

The medical laboratory technician (MLT), or clinical laboratory technician (CLT), is skilled in testing blood, urine, lymph, and blood tissues. The laboratory technician must be able to pay close attention to detail and have an understanding of computer technology and medical terminology. This career requires two years of training in an accredited medical laboratory program and certification by the National Certification Agency for Medical Laboratory Personnel or other certifying agency. Other responsibilities of the MLT include the following:

- Performing routine tests
- Recognizing abnormal test results and reporting them to a supervisor
- Performing quality control procedures
- Preparing specimens to be sent to reference laboratories
- Observing proper safety procedures
- Maintaining records
- Assisting in training new employees and students

Laboratory or Medical Technologist (MT)

A laboratory or medical technologist (MT), whose position is comparable to that of a clinical laboratory scientist (CLS), must complete a four-year medical technology program in a college or university and receive certification as a certified medical technologist (CMT). This person directs the work of other laboratory staff, is responsible for maintaining the quality assurance standards for all equipment, and also performs laboratory analysis. The examination to become certified is prepared by the board of registry of the American Society of Clinical Pathologists (ASCP) or the National Credentialing Agency (NCA) for the Clinical Laboratory Phlebotomist (CLPlb). Other responsibilities of a medical technologist include the following:

- Performing procedures that require judgment and minimal supervision
- Performing and analyzing quality control information
- Evaluating new procedures
- Performing complex laboratory procedures
- Training new employees and students
- Observing proper safety procedures

Blood Bank Technologist

Specialists in blood bank technology perform routine and specialized tests relating to hematology studies. They must be proficient in testing for blood groups, antigens, and antibody identification and compatibility. Technologists must also investigate abnormalities such as hemolytic anemia and diseases of newborns. In addition, they provide support for the physician with transfusion therapy and blood drawing.

Blood bank technologists may work in a blood bank facility, immunohematology department, or independent laboratory. The technologist must use standards that conform to those established by the American Association of Blood Banks. They must be certified in medical technology by the board of registry and receive a baccalaureate degree from a regionally accredited school.

Phlebotomist

See discussion in chapter 1.

Departments within a Clinical Laboratory

The major divisions within the laboratory are clinical analysis and surgical and anatomical pathology, including toxicology, virology, and microbiology. The clinical analysis division includes the areas of chemistry, hematology and coagulation, microbiology, immunology and serology, blood bank, and urinalysis. The surgical and anatomical pathology area includes autopsy tests, surgical biopsy or histology, and cytology.

Computerized equipment can perform multiple tests, or assays, on one sample. The analyzers can perform discrete (individual) tests also.

Chemistry

The chemistry department is one of the largest in the clinical laboratory and performs the majority of tests ordered by physicians. These tests include triglyceride and cholesterol, electrolyte (sodium, potassium, chloride, and CO_2), creatinine, blood urea nitrogen (BUN), uric acid, liver and cardiac enzyme, bilirubin, serum protein, and glucose tests. The chemistry section of the clinical laboratory is now highly automated. Automation has made the analysis more efficient, and quality assurance testing is more accurate.

Hematology and Coagulation

The hematology department conducts laboratory analysis testing to identify diseases of the blood and blood-forming tissues. These test results assist the physician in the diagnosis of such diseases and disorders as leukemia, anemia, infection, and polycythemia. The complete blood count (CBC) is run in this

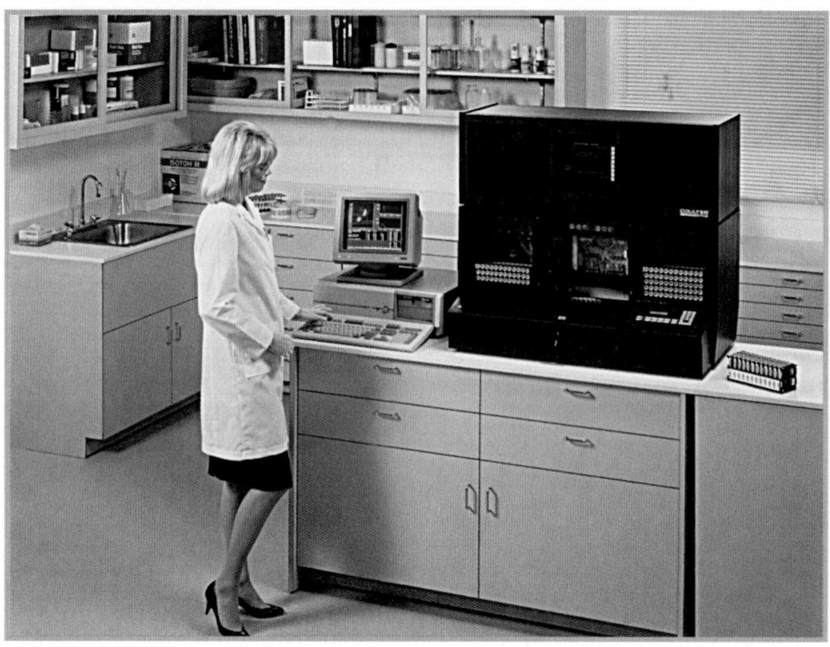

Figure 2-3 An automated hematology analyzer, the Coutler STKS.

laboratory department. See figure 2-3 which shows an automated hematology analyzer, the Coutler STKS. A CBC consists of the following components:

1. Red blood cell (RBC) count
2. White blood cell (WBC) count
3. Hematocrit (crit or Hct)
4. Hemoglobin (Hgb or Hb)
5. Platelet count (not routine as part of CBC in some laboratories)
6. Differential white blood cell count (diff)—either manual or automated

Other assays in the hematology department include erythrocyte sedimentation rate (ESR or Sed rate), fibrinogen, LE preparation, partial thromboplastin time (PTT), prothrombin time (PT), coagulation studies, and reticulocyte count. Microscopic testing, including urine testing and fertility studies, may also be performed in this department.

Microbiology

The microbiology department analyzes a specimen for the presence and type of microorganisms. A culture of the specimen is performed and then a sensitivity test is performed to determine which antibiotic would be effective in killing the organism. The physician would order a culture and sensitivity (C&S) test. Cultures are examined from any body orifice including samples of the urine, stool, blood, nose and throat tissues, body fluids, and wound drainage. Microscopic examination using techniques such as the gram stain is often done directly on a smear of the specimen or after it is cultured.

Bacteriology (study of bacteria), virology (study of viruses), and mycology (study of fungi) are conducted in this department. Acid-fast bacillus (AFB) smears for tuberculosis (TB) may also be performed.

Immunology and Serology

The immunology and serology department runs tests on blood serum (the fluid portion of blood) to determine the antigen-antibody reaction of the body. Technicians in the serology department test for diseases associated with immune disorders and diseases such as mononucleosis, rheumatoid arthritis, AIDS or HIV, and syphilis.

Blood Bank

The blood bank conducts routine testing on red blood cells and serum, including blood typing for compatibility and antibody tests. Blood taken from donors is carefully tested in this department before it is administered to persons who need a blood transfusion.

Urinalysis

Urinalysis may be performed within several departments, depending on the laboratory. The three parts of a urinalysis are physical, chemical, and microscopic. Urine may be examined for its physical appearance, chemical composition to screen for the presence of sugar and proteins in the urine, and/or microscopic appearance to identify other substances such as bacteria, blood cells, and crystals. The urinalysis testing includes specific gravity (S.G.), pH, sugar, protein, ketone, nitrite, urobilinogen, bilirubin, occult blood in stool, and leukocyte tests. Urine pregnancy tests are conducted in this portion of the medical laboratory. A clean-catch urine sample in a sterile container may be cultured to identify any organisms present, but the sample would have to be taken to the microbiology or bacteriology department for this test.

MED TIP

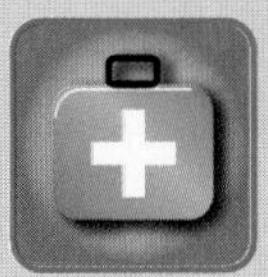

Departments may vary from one laboratory to another. For example, pregnancy tests may be conducted in a chemistry department or a serology department.

Surgical and Anatomical Pathology

The surgical and anatomical pathology departments include

- **Autopsy** tests: Tests are conducted on the organs and tissues of deceased persons to assist in determining the cause of death. An autopsy is performed with the permission of the nearest relative, unless the cause of death appears to be due to violence. The body usually is examined by the coroner or medical examiner.
- Surgical biopsy or histology: **Histology,** or the study of tissues, is conducted on specimens taken during surgical procedures to assist in the diagnosis of disease. The histologist stains sliced tissue samples so the disease cells can be seen more easily.
- **Cytology:** This area of surgical pathology examines body fluids and tissues for evidence of abnormality after the histologist has prepared them. For example, a PAP test to determine if cancer cells are developing in the cervical area of the female is conducted in this department.

A summary of tests performed within these divisions or departments is found in table 2-4.

TABLE 2-4	Subunits of the Clinical Laboratory
Clinical Analysis	**Summary of Tests Performed**
Clinical Chemistry	Total proteins, glucose and glucose tolerance, total cholesterol, triglycerides, hemoglobin high-density lipoprotein (HDL) cholesterol, electrolytes, magnesium, creatinine, uric acid, BUN, blood gases, enzymes, bilirubin and liver function tests, hormone tests, and drug analysis
Hematology and Coagulation	Differential, hemoglobin, eosinophil, hematocrit, CBC, fibrinogen, LE preparation, platelets, RBC, sedimentation rate, PTT, PT, WBC, and reticulocyte count
Microbiology	Gram staining, occult blood in the stool, blood culture, AFB, pinworm test, ova and parasites (O&P), stool culture, strep screen, urine culture, culture and sensitivity (C&S), nose and throat culture
Blood Bank	Blood typing, hepatitis antigen and antibody tests, cross-matching test, and Coombs test
Immunology and Serology	Rubella titer, Venereal Disease Research Laboratory (VDRL), salmonella agglutinins, rheumatoid testing (RA), C-reactive proteins, mononucleosis tests, and ASO titer for *Streptococcus*
Urinalysis	Specific gravity, pH, glucose (sugar), protein, ketones, nitrites, bilirubin, urobilinogen, occult blood, and leukocytes (WBCs)
Surgical and Anatomical Pathology	
Autopsy tests	Examination of tissues and organs to aid in determining cause of death
Surgical Biopsy or Histology	Examination of tissue samples removed during surgery
Cytology	Specimens observed for cancer detection (e.g., PAP test)

Physician's Office Laboratory

The number of physician's office laboratories (POLs) is growing due to the increasing number of physicians entering into a group practice setting. In this type of practice two or more physicians with similar specialties, such as obstetrics and gynecology, enter into practice together. They share one laboratory that is used to test specimens relating to the needs of their patients. In the example given, tests would include pregnancy, hemoglobin, and blood glucose monitoring. These small POLs must follow many of the same Clinical Laboratory Improvement Act of 1988 (CLIA 1988) guidelines as a large laboratory.

Clinic

Clinics, covering many specialty areas such as allergy and immunology, rheumatology, ophthalmology, pediatrics, mental health, sports medicine, and primary health care are established by teaching facilities to serve the general public and some patients who cannot afford to pay for health care. In many cases, the clinic setting is an opportunity for medical students to receive additional training and experience. A growing number of clinics include a medical laboratory that collects and analyzes routine specimens.

Independent Laboratories

A laboratory is a facility equipped for testing of, research on, scientific experimentation with, or clinical studies of materials, fluids, or tissues taken from patients. Medical teaching and research institutions have experimental laboratories on the premises.

Independent laboratories provide routine analysis of a patient's blood, urine, tissue, and other materials. Specimens sent to these laboratories for testing must be packaged carefully in specially designed containers.

Outpatient Testing

Patient services and testing that do not require the patient to stay overnight in a health care facility are referred to as outpatient, or ambulatory care. Laboratory testing once the patient is discharged from the hospital is on an outpatient basis. The term *outpatient* is used even if the test is performed within the hospital facility on a discharged patient.

CHAPTER REVIEW

Summary

There have been dramatic changes in the health care environment, especially concerning managed care, cost containment, and new technology, during the past fifteen years. Trained phlebotomists need a thorough understanding of this work environment to be informed and skilled professionals.

Abbreviations in the Chapter

CCU	*Cardiac Care Unit (Coronary Care Unit)*
CLIA 1988	*Clinical Laboratory Improvement Act of 1988*
CLS	*Clinical Laboratory Scientist*
CLT	*Clinical Laboratory Technician (MLT)*
CMA	*Certified Medical Assistant*
CMT	*Certified Medical Technologist*
CNA	*Certified Nursing Assistant*
D.C.	*Doctor of Chiropractic*
D.D.S.	*Doctor of Dental Surgery*
D.M.D	*Doctor of Dental Medicine*
D.O.	*Doctor of Osteopathy*
D.P.M.	*Doctor of Podiatric Medicine*
ED	*Emergency Department*
ENT	*Ear, Nose, and Throat*
ER	*Emergency Room*
GYN	*Gynecology*
ICU	*Intensive Care Unit*
L&D	*Labor and Delivery*
LPN	*Licensed Practical Nurse*
M.D.	*Doctor of Medicine*
MLT	*Medical Laboratory Technician*
MT	*Medical Technologist*
NP	*Nurse Practitioner*
OB	*Obstetrics*
O.D.	*Doctor of Optometry*
OP	*Outpatient*
OT	*Occupational Therapy*
PA	*Physician's Assistant*
Ph.D.	*Doctor of Philosophy*
PT	*Physical Therapy*
POL	*Physician's Office Laboratory*
RD	*Registered Dietician*
RN	*Registered Nurse*
RT	*Respiratory Therapy*

Competency Review

1. Visit a clinical laboratory or site that contains a clinical laboratory. Ask a phlebotomist to discuss his or her role as a member of the health care team.
2. Explain the roles of all members of the health care team.
3. Design a chart listing the categories of clinical laboratories and the tests conducted in each of the laboratories.
4. Describe the role of the phlebotomist as it relates to other personnel in the medical laboratory.

Examination Review Questions

1. Responsibilities of a medical laboratory technician (MLT) include all of the following *except*

(A) performing quality control procedures
(B) maintaining records
(C) recognizing abnormal test results
(D) reporting test results to patients
(E) assisting in training new employees

2. If a visitor came to you and asked where they could find an elderly parent who was being treated for a serious heart condition, to what department would you send them?

(A) CCU
(B) OR
(C) OP
(D) OT
(E) ENT

3. A clinical laboratory professional comparable to a clinical laboratory scientist (CLS) is a

(A) phlebotomist
(B) medical laboratory technician
(C) medical technologist
(D) laboratory director
(E) none of the above

4. HIV or AIDS testing is conducted in what department of the laboratory?

(A) microbiology
(B) immunology and serology
(C) blood bank
(D) chemistry
(E) hematology

5. The study of tissues in surgical specimens is called

(A) clinical pathology
(B) histology
(C) hematology
(D) chemistry
(E) immunology

6. A nurse specialist who has completed at least a two-year educational training program and is licensed uses the abbreviation

(A) CMA
(B) PA
(C) CNA
(D) RN
(E) LPN

7. Gram-staining procedures are handled in what laboratory department?

(A) hematology
(B) immunology
(C) chemistry
(D) microbiology
(E) histology

8. A laboratory facility located in a doctor's office is called a(n)

(A) independent laboratory
(B) reference laboratory
(C) POL
(D) PPO
(E) DRG

9. **A CBC, RBC, and WBC are performed in what department?**
   (A) chemistry
   (B) hematology
   (C) serology
   (D) microbiology
   (E) histology

10. **What laboratory department handles BUN and cholesterol testing?**
   (A) microbiology
   (B) chemistry
   (C) hematology
   (D) immunology
   (E) serology

Getting Connected

Multimedia Extension Activities

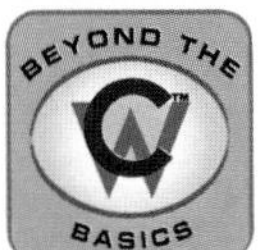

www.prenhall.com/fremgen

Use the address above to access the free, interactive Companion Website created specifically for this textbook. Enhance your studying by answering practice quiz questions, with hints and instant feedback related to Chapter 2. If you would like to gain a deeper understanding of selected topics within this chapter, be sure to click on the **Beyond the Basics** feature, which provides more details for further learning. If you do not have a web connection, you may use the CD-ROM enclosed in the back of this book to take advantage of the same features off-line.

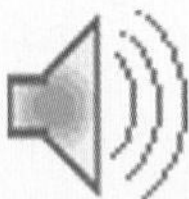

Audio Glossary

Use the CD-ROM enclosed with your textbook to hear the pronunciation of the key terms in the chapter. You may also access this material on the Companion Website www.prenhall.com/fremgen.

Bibliography

American Medical Association. *Current Procedural Terminology.* Chicago: American Medical Association, 1996.

Belsey, R., C. Mulrow, and H. Sox. "How to Handle Baffling Test Results." *Patient Care,* May 30, 1993.

"CDC Summarizes Final Regulations for Implementing CLIA." *American Family Physician* 45 (1992): 6.

Chernecky, C., R. Krech, and B. Berger. *Laboratory Tests and Diagnostic Procedures.* Philadelphia: W. B. Saunders, 1993.

Fishbach, F. *A Manual of Laboratory and Diagnostic Tests.* Philadelphia: Lippincott, 1996.

Marshall, J. *Medical Laboratory Assistant* . Upper Saddle River, N.J.: Brady/Prentice-Hall, 1990.

Palko, T., and H. Palko. *Laboratory Procedures for the Medical Office.* New York: Glencoe, 1996.

Sazama, J. "Licensure of Laboratory Personnel." *Laboratory Medicine,* April 1993.

Tietz, N. *Clinical Guide to Laboratory Tests,* 2nd ed. Philadelphia: W. B. Saunders, 1992.

Tietz, N., R. Conn, and E. Pruden. *Applied Laboratory Medicine.* Philadelphia: W. B. Saunders, 1992.

Walters, N., B. Estridge, and A. Reynolds. *Basic Medical Laboratory Techniques.* New York: Delmar, 1990.

CHAPTER 3

Ethics, Legal Practice, and Regulatory Issues

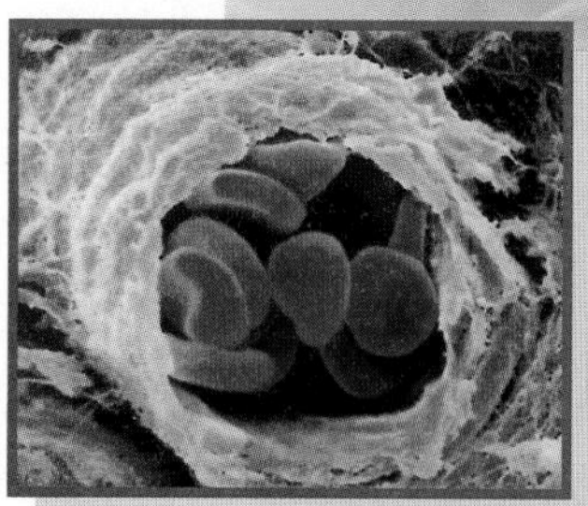

Chapter Outline

- Introduction
- Ethical Considerations
- Legal Considerations
- Drug Abuse Testing
- Federal Regulations
- Summary
- Competency Review
- Examination Review Questions
- Bibliography

Learning Objectives

After completing this chapter, you should be able to

1. Define all glossary terms and discuss their relationship to the health care field.
2. Describe the difference between medical ethics and medical law.
3. Describe the difference between a felony and a misdemeanor.
4. Discuss the six types of intentional torts and give an example of each.
5. List and discuss the four D's of negligence.
6. Define and discuss informed and implied consent.

GLOSSARY

BREACH (NEGLECT) OF DUTY neglect or failure to perform an obligation.

CASE LAW law that is based on precedent.

CONSENT to give permission, permit, or allow.

CONSENT, IMPLIED inference by signs, inaction, or silence that consent has been granted.

CONSENT, INFORMED patient's consent to undergo treatment or surgery based on knowledge and understanding of the potential risks and benefits provided by the physician before the procedure is performed.

CONTRACT agreement between two or more persons that creates an obligation to perform or not perform some action or service.

CRIMINAL LAW court action brought by the state against persons or groups of people accused of committing a crime, resulting in a fine or imprisonment if found guilty.

DAMAGES compensation for a loss or injury.

DEFENDANT person or group of persons who are accused in a court of law.

DUTY obligation or responsibility as a result of the physician-client relationship.

EMANCIPATED MINORS persons under the age of 18 who are free of parental care and financially responsible for themselves.

ETHICS principles and guides for moral behavior.

FELONY a crime more serious than a misdemeanor; it carries a penalty of death or imprisonment.

GUARDIAN AD LITEM court-appointed guardian to represent a minor or unborn child in litigation.

LAW rules of conduct established and enforced by an authority such as the legislature.

LIBEL false statements placed in writing about another person.

MALPRACTICE "bad practice"; also called professional negligence.

MATURE MINOR person, usually under 18 years of age, who possesses an understanding of the nature and consequences of proposed treatment.

MINOR person under the age of 18.

Misdemeanor crime that is less serious than a felony; it carries a penalty of up to one year imprisonment and/or a fine.

Negligence failure to perform professional duties in an accepted standard of care.

Plaintiff person or group of persons who bring an action to litigation (lawsuit).

Precedent law that is established in a prior case.

Proximate cause natural continuous sequence of events, without an intervening cause, that produces an injury. Also referred to as the direct cause.

Res ipsa loquitur Latin phrase that means "the thing speaks for itself." This is a doctrine of negligence law.

Respondeat superior Latin phrase that means "let the master answer." This means the physician or employer is responsible for the acts of the employee.

Rule of discovery the statute of limitations begins to run at the time the injury is discovered or when the patient should have known of the injury.

Slander false, malicious spoken words about another person.

Standard of care the ordinary skill and care that medical practitioners such as physicians, nurses, and phlebotomists must use that is commonly used by other medical practitioners when caring for patients.

Statute of limitations maximum time set by federal and state governments during which certain legal actions can be brought forward.

Statutes acts of a federal, state, or county legislature.

Subpoena court order for a person to appear in court. Both documents and persons may be subpoenaed.

Tort wrongful act (other than a breach of contract) committed against another person or property.

Introduction

Patients have become more knowledgeable regarding the quality of their health care and their rights as patients. Today's health care consumers expect to be part of the decision-making process regarding their care and treatment. Lawsuits have been brought against physicians and other medical practitioners, including laboratory personnel, when patients believe their treatment is not satisfactory.

Ethics is a branch of philosophy relating to morals or moral principles. Medical ethics refers to the moral conduct of people in the medical profession. The moral conduct of medical professionals is governed by the principles and standards that these professionals set for themselves and willingly choose to follow through personal dedication. Medical law, on the other hand, refers to the regulations and standards set by federal, state, and local governments. Medical ethics and law overlap sometimes, making it difficult to tell the difference between the two.

Law refers to rules of conduct that are established and enforced by an authority such as the legislature. All citizens must obey the standards or rules established by the government.

MED TIP

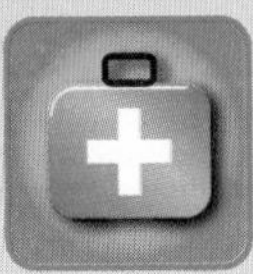

An illegal act, or one that is against the law, is always unethical. However, an unethical act may not be illegal. For instance, when an employee looks at a neighbor's medical record out of curiosity, it is not necessarily against the law, but it is unethical.

Ethical Considerations

Patient Confidentiality

All patients have the right to have their personal privacy respected and their medical records handled with confidentiality. Any information such as test results and even the fact that a patient is having a laboratory test cannot be told to another patient, friend, or family. No information can be given over the telephone or by fax without the patient's permission. No patient records can be given to another person or physician without the patient's written permission (consent) or unless the court has subpoenaed it. A **subpoena** is a court order for a person or documents to appear in court.

The Patient's Bill of Rights, developed by the American Hospital Association, describes the physician-patient relationship. This statement discusses rights that every patient has while undergoing treatment and procedures. These rights include the right to confidentiality, the right to consent or decline to participate in research studies, the right to make decisions about care, including the right to decline treatment, the right to privacy, and, above all, the right to considerate and respectful care.

Legal Considerations

Three branches of government control laws: legislative, executive, and judicial. Written laws are the result of **statutes** (legislative), administrative (executive) laws, and **case** (judicial) **law,** which is based on **precedent.** Statutes are acts of legislative bodies at the federal, state, and county levels. Precedent refers to law established in a prior case. Two major classifications of law are criminal and civil law.

Criminal Law

Criminal laws are made to protect the public from the harmful acts of others. A violation of a state or federal law means that the government will bring criminal charges against the person who committed the crime. If found guilty, the defendant, or person or group of persons who are accused of a criminal action, can be fined and/or imprisoned. Federal offenses include kidnapping, illegal transport of drugs, and actions that affect national security. State criminal offenses include practicing medicine without a license, murder, robbery, rape, and burglary.

Criminal acts fall into two categories: felony and misdemeanor. A **felony** carries a punishment of death or imprisonment in a state or federal prison. These crimes include practicing medicine without a license, murder, rape, robbery, and tax evasion. A **misdemeanor** carries a punishment of fines or imprisonment in jail for up to a year. Misdemeanors are less serious offenses. They include traffic violations, theft, and disturbing the peace.

MED TIP

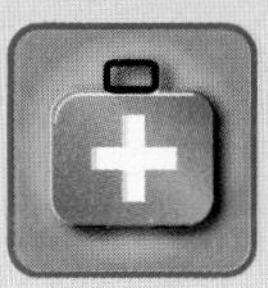

Remember that practicing medicine without a license is a state criminal offense. The phlebotomist cannot order blood tests or discuss the results with the patient. According to the law, only the physician may perform these actions.

CIVIL LAW

Civil law concerns the relationship between individuals and the government. It generally does not involve the same crimes that are handled by criminal law. (An exception would be murder, which can be tried under both criminal and civil law.) An individual can sue another person, a business, or the government. Civil law cases include slander, libel, auto accidents, child support, and trespassing.

The branch of civil law includes contract law, administrative law, and tort law. **Contract law** includes enforceable promises and agreements between two or more persons to do or not do a particular thing. **Administrative law** covers regulations that are set by governmental agencies. **Tort law** covers acts that are committed against another person or property that result in harm. These harmful acts may be intentional or unintentional. Health care employees are most frequently involved in cases of civil law, particularly tort and contract law. To meet the definition of a tort, there must be damage or injury to the patient that was caused by the action of the health care professional and/or his or her employee. This action, or tort, can be either unintentional (accidental) or intentional.

Unintentional torts, such as negligence, occur when the patient is injured as a result of the health care professional not exercising the ordinary standard of care. **Standard of care** refers to the ordinary skill and care that medical practitioners such as physicians, nurses, and phlebotomists must use and that is commonly used by other medical practitioners when caring for patients.

Intentional torts include assault, battery, false imprisonment, defamation of character, fraud, and invasion of privacy. Table 3-1 provides a description and example of each of these torts.

NEGLIGENCE

Negligence is the failure to perform professional duties in an accepted standard of care. For example, a phlebotomist is negligent when he or she fails to have a patient lie down when the patient states he or she has fainted in the past during a blood collection procedure. **Malpractice** can be described as "bad practice," whereas negligence is described as failure to give care that can normally be expected in a similar situation, with a resulting injury to the patient. However, generally speaking, the terms *negligence* and *malpractice* mean the same thing and, thus, are interchangeable.

MED TIP

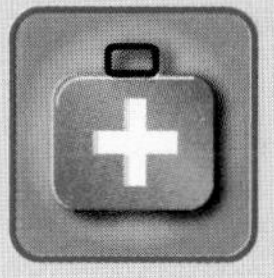

It is easier to prevent negligence than it is to defend yourself against charges of it in court.

TABLE 3-1 Intentional Torts

Tort	Description	Example
Assault	The threat of bodily harm to another; there does not have to be actual touching (battery) for assault to take place	Threatening to harm patients or to perform a laboratory procedure (such as HIV or AIDS testing) for which they do not consent
Battery	Offensive or harmful contact to another person without permission; this is referred to as unlawful touching or touching without consent	Performing a procedure such as venipuncture without the informed consent (permission) of the patient
False imprisonment	A violation of the personal liberty of another person through unlawful restraint	Refusing to allow a patient to leave a medical laboratory or facility when he or she requests to do so
Defamation of character	Damage caused to a person's reputation through spoken or written word; **slander** is false or malicious spoken words, and **libel** is false statements in writing	Making a negative statement about a physician's ability or discussing a patient's laboratory tests outside of the laboratory
Fraud	Deceitful practice	Promising a miracle cure or test
Invasion of privacy	The unauthorized statements or publication of information about a patient	Allowing personal information, such as test results for HIV or pregnancy to become public without the patient's consent

To obtain a judgment of negligence against a physician (the **defendant** in this case) or other health care professional, the patient (the **plaintiff** in this case) must be able to show what is referred to as the "four D's"—duty, dereliction of duty, direct cause, and damages. The four D's of negligence are as follows:

1. **Duty** refers to the physician-client (patient) relationship. The patient must prove that this relationship has been established. When the patient has an appointment and has been seen by the physician, then a relationship has been established. The physician may then order laboratory testing, and the phlebotomist will carry out the order. The physician-patient relationship then becomes a **contract,** or agreement between two persons to perform some service or action.
2. Dereliction, or neglect **(breach) of duty,** refers to a physician or health care professional's failure to act as an ordinary and prudent professional would act in a similar circumstance when treating a patient. The patient would have to prove that the care given did not comply with an established standard of care, as, for example, if a phlebotomist did not wash his or her hands between patients when drawing blood samples from two patients.

3. Direct cause requires the patient to prove that the physician's or health care professional's derelict or breach of duty was the direct cause of the injury that resulted. The plaintiff must prove **proximate cause** in a case of negligence. This means that the plaintiff must prove that there was a continuous, natural sequence of events without interruption that produced an injury. For example, if a patient has blood drawn and then sustains a break in that same arm from a fall, any subsequent nerve damage could have resulted from the broken arm rather than the venipuncture. However, if a patient suffers nerve damage during or immediately following a venipuncture, he or she may have a case based on proximate cause.
4. **Damages** refers to any injuries to the patient. The court may award compensatory (monetary) damages to pay for the patient's injuries.

Although most discussions concerning lawsuits refer to medical care and treatment provided by the physician, it is important to note that according to the doctrine of ***respondeat superior,*** a Latin phrase meaning "let the master answer," the employer is responsible for the acts of the employee. Thus, the phlebotomist's employer is responsible for the negligent actions of anyone working for him or her.

Res Ipsa Loquitur

The doctrine of ***res ipsa loquitur*** applies to the law of negligence. This Latin phrase means "the thing speaks for itself." This doctrine states that a breach of duty is so obvious that it does not need further explanation, or "it speaks for itself." For example, if a patient faints while having blood drawn and hits his or her head during the fall, the injury to the head can be seen as a direct result of the fall. If a lawsuit results, the patient (plaintiff) would have to prove that the phlebotomist was negligent in not preventing the fall.

Consent

Patients have the right to approve or give **consent,** or permission, for all treatment and procedures. In addition, they can expect to receive information concerning the advantages and potential risks of all treatments. This is called **informed consent.** Patients should be informed by the physician of the possible consequences of both having and not having certain procedures and treatments. In some cases the treatment may even make a patient's condition worse, and the physician should fully explain this possibility. Patients are asked to sign a consent form for invasive procedures such as surgery after they indicate that they understand the risks. It is the physician's responsibility to explain the risks and obtain consent.

Implied consent means that patients grant consent by means of signs, inaction, or silence. In this case patients would not necessarily have signed a consent form. For example, when patients roll up their sleeves to have a blood sample taken, they are giving implied consent for the procedure.

MED TIP

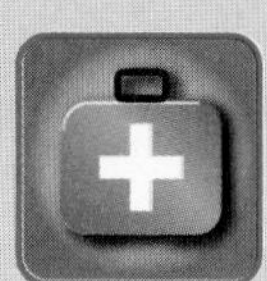

Consent is an important concept to understand. Touching a patient without consent is referred to as battery. If the patient has clearly implied consent for the treatment or procedure, then there would be no battery.

Patients have the right to refuse treatment. Some members of religious groups do not wish to receive blood transfusions or certain types of medical treatments. Adults would not receive treatment against their wishes. In the case of a minor child, the court may appoint a **guardian ad litem** who can give consent for the treatment.

Statute of Limitations

The **statute of limitations** refers to the period after the incident that a patient has to file a lawsuit. The court will not hear a case after the time limit has run out. The time limit varies from state to state; in some states it is two years.

The statute of limitations does not always begin when the treatment is administered. It may begin when the problem is discovered, which may be some time after the actual treatment. This is referred to as the **rule of discovery.** For example, if a patient is infected by a contaminated needle, the problem may not be found until symptoms of the infection occur.

Rights of Minors

A **minor** is a person who has not reached the age of maturity or majority, which in most states is eighteen. In most states minors are unable to give consent for treatment. Exceptions are special cases involving testing and treatment for sexually transmitted diseases, pregnancy, request for birth control information, abortion, and problems with substance abuse. There are two types of minors who can give consent for treatment: mature minors and emancipated minors.

A **mature minor** is a young person generally under the age of 18 who possesses a maturity to understand the nature and consequences of the treatment in spite of his or her young age. **Emancipated minors** actually have the same legal capacity as adults under any of the following five conditions:

1. Living on their own
2. Married
3. Self-supporting
4. In the armed forces
5. Any combination of the preceding conditions

MED TIP

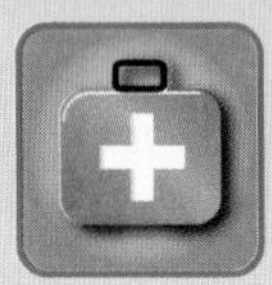

Because not all states recognize the categories of mature and emancipated minors, it is wise to handle consent on a case-by-case basis.

Drug Abuse Testing

A chain-of-custody form is required when collecting blood specimens for drug abuse testing. The use of this form helps to ensure that the specimen has been obtained from the person whose name is listed on the label. The chain-of-custody form must include the following information:

- Name of subject
- Subject's Social Security number
- Type of specimen (blood, urine, or other)
- Amount of specimen in milliliters (mL)
- Name of person who collected sample
- Signature of collector

- Date, time, and location of the collection
- Name of witness or witnesses to the collection
- Signature of person transporting the specimen
- Name of person receiving the specimen in the laboratory
- Date and time specimen was received
- Condition of the seals on the outside and inside containers

A specimen to determine drug abuse must be handled carefully. It is placed in a specimen transfer bag with a special seal that is only opened when the specimen is analyzed.

Federal Regulations

The federal government now mandates that all clinical laboratories that test human specimens be controlled. The Clinical Laboratory Improvement Act of 1988 (CLIA 1988) divides laboratories into three categories. Simple testing or waivered tests are simple, stable tests that require a minimum of judgment or interpretation, as for example, dipstick urinalysis and visual color comparison pregnancy tests. Moderate (intermediate) testing consists of tests of moderate complexity, which comprise about 75 percent of all laboratory tests. High-complexity tests are highly sophisticated tests that are generally performed by pathologists and/or doctors in a specific field of medicine. These three categories are described in table 3-2.

Provider-performed microscopy procedure (PPMP) is another limited level (e.g. level III) in which licensed providers, such as physicians and pathologists, may perform a limited list of microscopic lab procedures.

CLIA 1988 regulations include specific guidelines for quality control, quality assurance, record keeping, and personnel qualifications. The Health Care Financing Administration (HCFA) and Centers for Disease Control and Prevention (CDC) regulate CLIA 1988 standards at the federal level, but states can seek to implement their own standards provided that the state standards are equivalent to the federal standards.

TABLE 3-2 Clinical Laboratory Improvement Act of 1988 (CLIA 1988)

Category	Explanation
1. Waivered (Level I)	Incorrect test results pose little risk for the patient Laboratory is subject to random inspections only Some physician laboratories fall in this category
2. Moderate (Intermediate) complexity (Level II)	Risk to patient if there is an incorrect test result Must be certified by approved accrediting agency Must be staffed by credentialed personnel; requires an MLT or higher discipline to perform Must meet quality assurance standards
3. High complexity (Level III)	High risk to patient if there is an incorrect test result Must be certified by approved accrediting agency Must be staffed by credentialed personnel; requires an MT or higher to perform Must meet quality assurance standards.

Chapter Review

Summary

Even though today's health care consumers are more informed, medical costs and the state of medical technology pose new financial, moral, ethical, and legal problems for consumers. Today, more than previously, court cases and rulings have a greater impact on the way health care professionals practice. Careful concern for medical ethics and medical law is a right that patients can expect from the phlebotomist.

Competency Review

1. Interview a phlebotomist to discover how he or she protects patient confidentiality.
2. Describe the three categories of laboratories as developed by CLIA 1988.
3. Discuss the concepts of informed consent and implied consent and their importance for the phlebotomist.
4. Why should a phlebotomist be familiar with the four D's of negligence?
5. Give two examples of intentional torts that might occur in the clinical laboratory.

Examination Review Questions

1. A patient is told that he or she has to remain still during a laboratory procedure or be restrained. This is an example of which intentional tort?

(A) assault
(B) battery
(C) false imprisonment
(D) fraud
(E) A and C

2. *Res ipsa loquitur* is a Latin phrase meaning

(A) let the master answer
(B) let the master beware
(C) the thing speaks for itself
(D) proximate cause
(E) libel

3. The patient's permission to undergo treatment after he or she understands the risks and benefits is called

(A) implied consent
(B) informed consent
(C) case law
(D) precedent
(E) subpoena

4. The period of time during which a patient has to file a lawsuit is known as

(A) standard of care
(B) respondeat superior
(C) res ipsa loquitur
(D) statute of limitations
(E) tort

5. To be considered emancipated, a minor child must be

(A) married
(B) self-supporting
(C) in the armed forces
(D) living on his or her own
(E) any combination of the preceding conditions

6. The regulation of laboratories is mandated by

(A) CLIA 1998
(B) CLIA 1988
(C) CLIA 1987
(D) the individual laboratory
(E) no agency

7. The ordinary skill and care that medical practitioners must use is referred to as

(A) statute of limitations
(B) standard of care
(C) precedent
(D) breach of duty
(E) proximate cause

8. **A law that has already been established in a prior case is called**
   (A) statute of limitations
   (B) standard of care
   (C) precedent
   (D) breach of duty
   (E) proximate cause

9. **Practicing medicine without a license is called a**
   (A) felony
   (B) misdemeanor
   (C) precedent
   (D) statute
   (E) rule of discovery

10. **A court-appointed person to represent an unborn child or minor in litigation is a**
   (A) mature minor
   (B) emancipated minor
   (C) guardian ad litem
   (D) plaintiff
   (E) defendant

Getting Connected

Multimedia Extension Activities

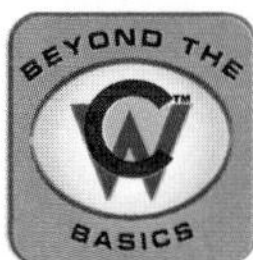

www.prenhall.com/fremgen

Use the address above to access the free, interactive Companion Website created specifically for this textbook. Enhance your studying by answering practice quiz questions, with hints and instant feedback related to chapter 3. If you would like to gain a deeper understanding of selected topics within this chapter, be sure to click on the **Beyond the Basics** feature, which provides more details for further learning. If you do not have a web connection, you may use the CD-ROM enclosed in the back of this book to take advantage of the same features off-line.

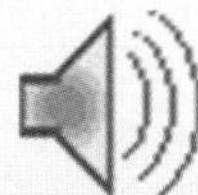

Audio Glossary

Use the CD-ROM enclosed with your textbook to hear the pronunciation of the key terms in the chapter. You may also access this material on the Companion Website www.prenhall.com/fremgen.

Bibliography

American Hospital Association. *A Patient's Bill of Rights.* Chicago: American Hospital Association, 1992.

Black, H. *Black's Law Dictionary.* St. Paul, Minn.: West, 1991.

Code on Medical Ethics: Current Opinions and Annotations. Chicago: Council on Ethical and Judicial Affairs of the American Medical Association, 1997.

Dubler, N., and D. Nimmons. *Ethics on Call.* New York: Harmony Books, 1992.

Fremgen, B. *Essentials of Medical Assisting.* Upper Saddle River, N.J.: Brady/Prentice-Hall, 1998.

Garrett, T., H. Baillie, and R. Garrett. *Health Care Ethics.* Upper Saddle River, N.J.: Brady/Prentice-Hall, 1993.

Hall, M., and I. Ellman. *Health Care Law and Ethics in a Nutshell.* St. Paul, Minn.: West, 1990.

Judson, K., and S. Blesie. *Law and Ethics for Health Care Occupations.* New York: Macmillan/McGraw, 1994.

Lewis, M., and C. Tamparo. *Medical Law, Ethics, and Bioethics in the Medical Office.* Philadelphia: F. A. Davis, 1993.

Lipman, M. *Medical Law and Ethics.* Upper Saddle River, N.J.: Brady/Prentice-Hall, 1994.

McConnell, T. *Moral Issues in Health Care.* New York: Wadsworth, 1997.

Munson, R. *Intervention and Reflection: Basic Issues in Medical Ethics.* New York: Wadsworth, 1996.

Snell, M. *Bioethical Dilemmas in Health Occupations.* New York: Macmillan/McGraw, 1991.

Taber's Cyclopedic Medical Dictionary, 18th ed. Philadelphia: F. A. Davis, 1997.

CHAPTER 4

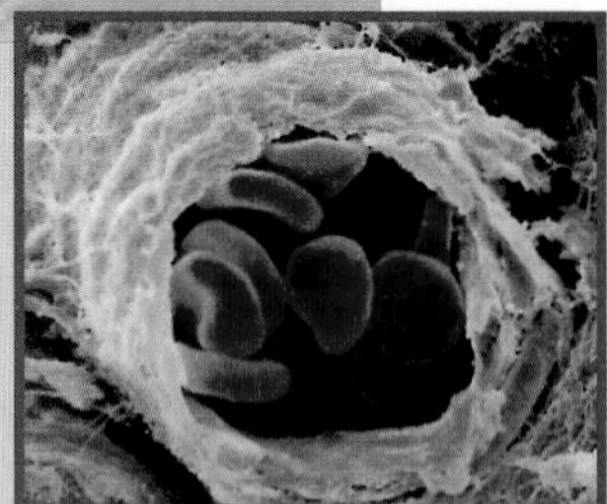

Infection Control, Safety, and Quality Control

Chapter Outline

Learning Objectives

After completing this chapter, you should be able to

1. Define and spell all glossary terms.
2. Discuss the differences between Universal Precautions and Standard Precautions.
3. Describe a floor book.
4. Discuss a delta check.
5. Explain the various types of isolation.
6. Describe the four types of physical safety hazards in the laboratory.
7. Describe the four types of biological hazards in the laboratory.

GLOSSARY

ACQUIRED IMMUNODEFICIENCY SYNDROME (AIDS) a series of infections and disorders that occur as a result of infection by the human immunodeficiency virus (HIV), which causes the immune system to break down.

AEROBIC microorganism that is able to live only in the presence of oxygen.

ANAEROBIC microorganism that thrives best or lives without oxygen.

ASEPSIS germ free.

BIOLOGICAL SAFETY HOOD a protective cabinet that should be used when in contact with aerosols (airborne particles) to draw the particles away from the laboratory worker.

BLOODBORNE PATHOGENS disease-producing microorganisms transmitted by means of blood and bodily fluids containing blood.

CARRIER a person who is unaware that he or she has a disease but who is capable of transmitting it to someone else.

CAUSTIC capable of burning or eating away tissue.

CONTACT ISOLATION a form of isolation in which anyone entering the patient's room and having direct contact with the patient wears gloves and a gown.

CRITERIA standards against which something is compared to make a decision or judgment.

CUMULATIVE having an effect that builds over time.

DATA statistics, figures, or information.

DELTA TEST a comparison between the current results of a laboratory test and the previous test results for the same patient.

ENTERIC ISOLATION isolation used for persons with infections of the intestinal tract.

FLOOR BOOK a laboratory reference manual; also referred to as a procedure, reference, or test manual.

HUMAN IMMUNODEFICIENCY VIRUS (HIV) virus that causes AIDS.

INCIDENT REPORT a formal written description of an unusual occurrence.

MEDICAL ASEPSIS killing organisms after they leave the body.

MICROORGANISMS small living organisms that are capable of causing disease. Also called microbes.

Nonpathogenic non-disease-producing.

Norm standard, criterion, or the ideal measure for a specific group.

Nosocomial infection infection that is acquired after a person has entered the hospital. It is caused by the spread of an infection from one person to another.

Occurrence any event or incident outside of the norm.

Pathogens disease-producing microorganisms.

Procedure manual a collection of policies and procedures for carrying out day-to-day operations in the laboratory.

Quality assurance gathering and evaluating information and data about the services or tests provided as well as the results achieved compared with an acceptable standard.

Quality assurance program a program in which laboratories and hospitals evaluate the services and/or tests they provide by comparing their services and/or tests with accepted standards.

Reservoir source of the infectious pathogen.

Respiratory isolation used for patients with diseases that can be spread by droplet infection. Anyone entering the patient's room must wear a mask.

Reverse isolation isolation procedure put into effect to protect the patient from infection. Also called protective isolation.

Strict isolation isolation required for patients with highly contagious diseases.

Surgical asepsis a technique practiced to maintain a sterile environment.

Wound or skin isolation isolation used to protect the medical worker when a patient has an open wound.

Introduction

Just as in any workplace, general infection control measures, employee safety, and quality assurance are critical to maintaining the safety and comfort of the patient and laboratory staff. In the laboratory additional safety issues may arise, including chemical hazards, bloodborne pathogens, biological hazards, and the improper handling of laboratory specimens. Constant surveillance to control and monitor infections, especially in high-risk populations such as the elderly and children, is the duty of all health care professionals.

Infection Control

Microorganisms

Microorganisms, also called microbes, are small, living organisms capable of causing disease that can only be seen with a microscope. Some microorganisms are normally found on the skin, in the urinary and gastrointestinal tract, and in the respiratory tract.

Microorganisms are either bacteria, fungi, protozoa, or viruses. The sizes of microorganisms can be expressed in micrometers. (A micrometer [μm] is one-millionth of a meter, or one-thousandth of a millimeter.) Examples of microorganisms are listed in table 4-1.

TABLE 4-1 Microorganisms

Microorganism	Description	Examples
Bacteria	Most numerous of all microorganisms Unicellular Many are pathogenic to humans Identified by shape and appearance	(See cocci, bacilli, and spirilla)
Cocci	Three types of spherical bacteria	
Staphylococci	Form grapelike clusters of pus-producing organisms	Boils, pimples, acne, and osteomyelitis
Streptococci	Form chains of cells or cocci	Rheumatic heart disease, scarlet fever, and strep throat
Diplococci	Form pairs of cells	Pneumonia, gonorrhea, and meningitis
Bacilli	Rod-shaped bacteria	Gram-positive bacilli: tuberculosis, tetanus, diphtheria, and gas gangrene Gram-negative bacilli: *Escherichia coli* (urinary tract infection) and *Bordetella pertussis* (whooping cough)
Spirilla	Spiral-shaped organisms	Syphilis and cholera
Fungi	Parasitic and some nonparasitic plants and molds Reproduction method is budding Depend on other life forms for their nutrition, such as dead or decaying organic material Yeast is a typical fungus Fungus means "mushroom" in Latin Feed on antibiotics and flourish on antibiotic therapy	*Histoplasma capsulatum* (histoplasmosis), tinea pedis (athlete's foot), candidiasis (yeast infection), and ringworm

(continued)

TABLE 4-1 Microorganisms *(continued)*

Microorganism	Description	Examples
Protozoa	One-celled organisms Typically 2 to 200 mm in size Both parasitic and nonparasitic Can move with cilia or false feet	Amebic dysentery, malaria, and *Trichomonas vaginitis*
Rickettsia	Visible under a standard microscope Transmitted by insects (ticks and fleas) Susceptible to antibiotics	Rocky Mountain spotted fever and Lyme disease
Virus	Smallest of all microorganisms Can only be seen with electron microscope Can only multiply within a living cell (host) Difficult to kill with chemotherapy because they become resistant to the drug Can be destroyed by heat (autoclave sterilization) but generally not by chemical disinfection More viruses than any other category of microbial agents Feed on antibiotics and flourish on antibiotic therapy	Herpes virus (oral and genital), HIV, AIDS-related complex (ARC), AIDS, common cold, influenza virus, hepatitis A, hepatitis B, rabies, chicken pox, mumps, and shingles

How Microorganisms Grow

Microorganisms occur everywhere in nature and have several requirements to grow: food, moisture, darkness, and a suitable temperature. In addition, some bacteria require oxygen (**aerobic**) or the absence of oxygen (**anaerobic**) to live. Table 4-2 presents the four conditions necessary for the growth of bacteria.

Some microorganisms, such as certain types of fungi and bacteria, are necessary for normal body function. For example, normal flora within the digestive system breaks down food and converts unused food into waste products. In some cases the normal flora (or **nonpathogenic**) invade areas of the body where they do not belong and, thus, convert to **pathogens,** which are disease-producing microorganisms. For example, *Escherichia coli* (*E. coli*) is a normal bacterium within the colon, where it aids in food digestion. When *E. coli* contaminates the bladder or bloodstream, through improper hygiene habits such as improper hand washing, it can cause urinary and blood infections.

Transmission of Infection

Scientists have determined that certain germs can multiply every 12 minutes. If not controlled, germs may spread infection rapidly from one person to another. The principles of **asepsis,** or a germ-free con-

TABLE 4-2 Conditions Required for Bacterial Growth

Condition	Explanation
Moisture	Bacteria grow best in moist areas: skin, mucous membranes, wet dressings, wounds, dirty instruments and needles
Temperature	Bacteria thrive best at body temperature (98.6°F or 37°C); low temperatures (32°F or 0°C and below) retard, but do not kill, bacterial growth, and temperatures of 107°F (42°C) and above will kill most bacteria
Oxygen	Aerobic bacteria require an oxygen supply to live; anaerobic bacteria can survive without oxygen
Light	Darkness favors the growth of bacteria; bacteria will die if exposed to direct sunlight or ultraviolet light

dition, are applied in the hospital setting to prevent the spread of **nosocomial** (hospital-acquired) **infection.** The same emphasis on halting the spread of infection exists in the laboratory.

The presence of a pathogenic organism, or microorganism, is not enough to cause an infection. Several factors, known as the "chain of infection," must be in place for infection to occur. These factors are described in table 4-3.

The chain of infection is illustrated in figure 4-1.

TABLE 4-3 Chain of Infection

1. The presence of a *pathogen*
2. A *reservoir*, or source, of disease including individuals who are ill with a disease and human *carriers* of disease who are unaware they have the disease but can still spread it
3. A *portal of exit,* or means of escape, from the reservoir (e.g., through respiratory tract secretions, intestinal waste products, reproductive tract secretions, blood and blood products, and across the placental barrier)
4. A *means of transmission* for the pathogen to pass directly from the reservoir to the new host (e.g., milk or water can harbor the pathogen until it is transmitted to a human)
5. A *portal of entry,* or means of entry, such as the respiratory tract, skin and mucous membranes, reproductive and urinary tracts, blood, and across the placental barrier, for the pathogen to enter into the new host
6. A *susceptible host* that cannot fight off the pathogen; an example is an elderly patient whose health is already compromised by poor nutrition or reduced immunity

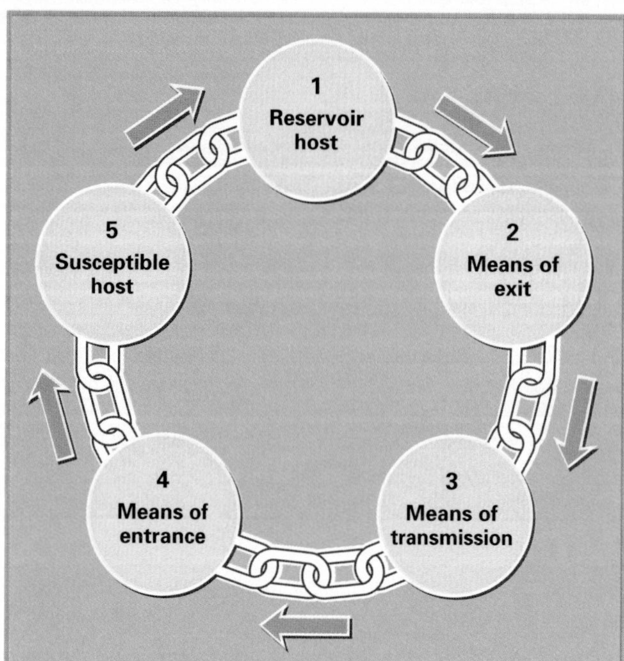

Figure 4-1
The chain of infection.

MED TIP

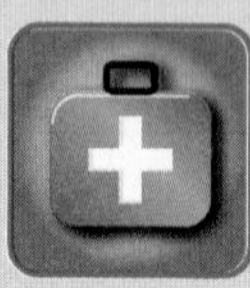

A missing link in the chain of infection will prevent infection from occurring. For example, even if a pathogen, a reservoir, and means of transmission are present, an infection cannot be transmitted if there is not a portal of entry. Protective barriers, such as masks and gloves, can prevent pathogens from entering a host.

The Infection Control System

An infection control system is meant to break the chain of infection. The body has several natural barriers to infection, including the skin, mucous membranes, gastrointestinal tract, and lymphoid and blood systems. The largest natural barrier to infection is the intact skin because the low pH of the skin inhibits bacterial action. Mucous membranes lining the body's orifices and the respiratory, digestive, reproductive, and urinary tracts also assist in repelling microorganisms. The gastrointestinal tract (GI), which contains hydrochloric acid (HCl), causes a bactericidal action that destroys disease-producing bacteria. A notable exception is *Helicobacter pylori,* which can survive in the gastrointestinal tract and is the causative agent of ulcers.

MED TIP

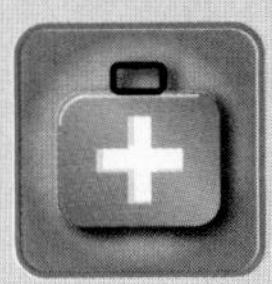

The use of so many over-the-counter medications that prevent gastric juice production is eliminating the gastrointestinal body defense in many people.

Asepsis

Medical asepsis refers to the destruction of organisms after they leave the body. Techniques such as hand washing, using disposable equipment, and wearing gloves can help reduce the number and transfer of pathogens. **Surgical asepsis** is a technique used to establish a sterile environment. Surgical hand-washing technique, sterile gloves, and equipment are used.

Hand Washing

Hand washing, the single best step in preventing the spread of infection, provides the first defense against the spread of disease and should be done often. See procedure 4-1 for a description of proper hand-washing technique.

Isolation Procedures

Isolation procedures are implemented to protect both the patient and the health care worker. Personal protective equipment (PPE), such as eye shields, and clothing, such as gloves, masks, and gowns, are worn by anyone coming into the presence of a patient.

MED TIP

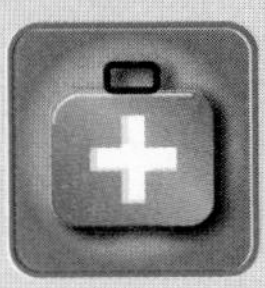

Remember that isolation can have very disturbing psychological effects on patients. Always treat patients who are in isolation in a caring, professional manner.

The types of isolation include strict, enteric, contact, respiratory, wound or skin, and reverse.

Strict isolation, or complete isolation, is used when patients have a highly contagious disease such as bacterial pneumonia, smallpox, diphtheria, or chicken pox. Patients must be placed in a private, closed room. Anyone entering the room must wear a gown, mask, and gloves. All items taken into the room, such as tube holders, needles, and syringes, must be disposed of in special containers in the room.

Enteric isolation is used for patients who have intestinal infections, such as *Salmonella, Shigella,* and hepatitis A and E, which usually result in diarrhea or dysentery. Anyone entering the room must wear a gown and gloves. All waste material is disposed of in special containers in the room.

Contact isolation is used for patients who have diseases, such as influenza, that can be transmitted to another person by means of direct contact. Anyone entering the room should wear gloves and add a gown and mask if there is close contact with patients. Strict isolation is not necessary for contact isolation.

PROCEDURE 4•1

HANDWASHING TECHNIQUE

Purpose:

Careful handwashing can provide an effective barrier to infection as the first defense against the spread of disease.

Terminal Performance Competency:

Perform handwashing procedure without error.

Equipment:

Soap in liquid soap dispenser, nail brush, hot running water, paper towels, and waste container.

Procedure:

1. Remove jewelry (include rings with the exception of a plain wedding band and watch). *Rationale: Jewelry has crevices and grooves that can harbor bacteria and dirt.*
2. Stand at sink without allowing clothes to touch sink. Turn water on and, using paper towel, adjust temperature. Discard paper towel. *Rationale: Avoid direct contact with contaminated faucets. Sinks are also considered contaminated. Paper towel is considered contaminated after touching the faucet(s).*
3. Wet hands under running water and place liquid soap (about a teaspoon or size of nickel) into palm of hand. Work soap into lather by moving it over palms, sides, and backs—the entire surface—of both hands for 2 minutes. Use a circular motion and friction. Interlace fingers and move soapy water between them. *Rationale: Friction assists in removing organisms and dirt.*
4. Keep hands pointed downward with hands and forearms at elbow level or below during the entire hand-washing procedure. *Rationale: Water will run off hands and not back up onto arms for further contamination.*
5. Use hand brush to clean under fingernails. Thoroughly scrub wedding band if present. *Rationale: Running water and soap may not be sufficient to remove dirt particles under nails.*
6. Rinse hands under running water with fingers pointed down, using care not to touch the sinks or faucets. *Rationale: The sink is not sterile (only clean) and may have contaminants present. Running water will wash away soap and organisms.*
7. Reapply soap and wash wrists and forearms for 1 more minute using circular motions.
8. Rinse hands under running water.
9. Dry hands thoroughly with paper towel. Discard paper towel.
10. Using a dry paper towel, turn off faucets. *Rationale: Paper towel will protect clean hands from coming into contact with contaminated faucet handles.*

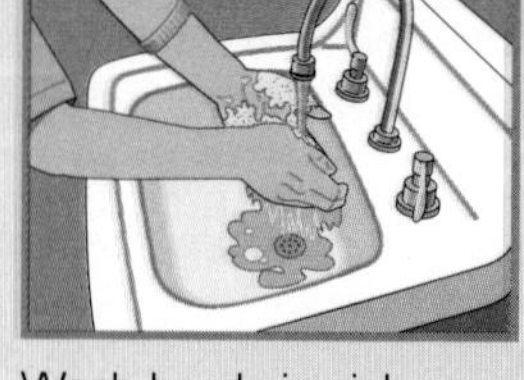

Wash hands in sink.

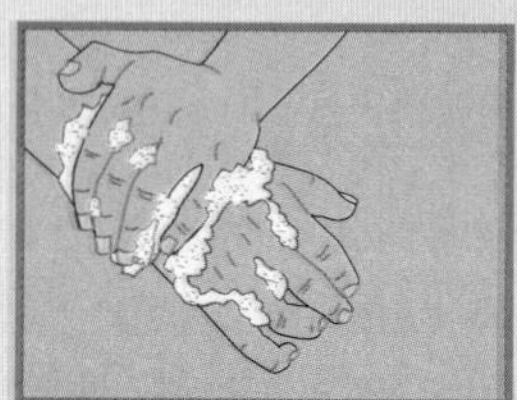

Scrub wrists.

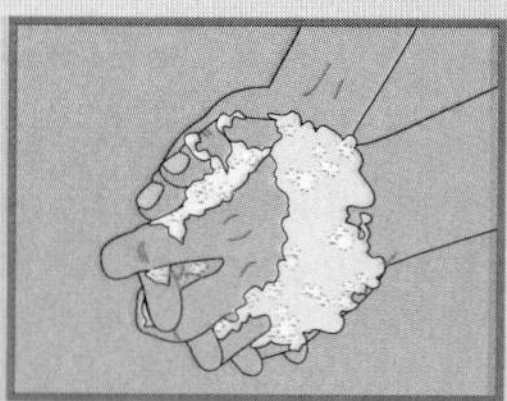

Scrub hands.

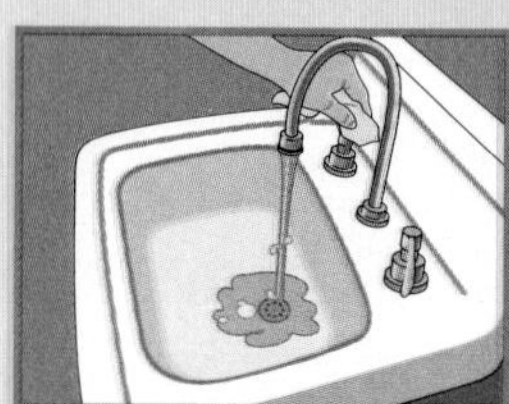

Turn off faucet with towel.

Respiratory isolation is used for patients who have diseases that can be spread by droplet infection such as *Haemophilus influenza,* meningococcal meningitis, tuberculosis (acid-fast bacilli), or measles. Anyone entering the room should wear a mask. Affected patients should have private rooms with closed doors.

Wound or skin isolation is used for patients who have an open wound, sore, or skin infection. Anyone entering affected patients' rooms should wear a gown and gloves.

Reverse isolation, or protective isolation, is used to protect noninfectious patients who may be susceptible to disease or infection. In these cases anyone entering the patients' rooms or vicinity must wear a mask and sterile gloves and gown. Anything brought into the room or used on the patients must be sterile. Examples would include patients with immunodeficiency diseases, dialysis treatments, tissue transplants, burns, or chemotherapy and newborn nurseries.

Occupational Safety and Health Administration (OSHA)

The Occupational Safety and Health Administration (OSHA) was established by the U.S. Congress in the Occupational Safety and Health Act of 1970 to assure, as far as possible, every working man and woman in the nation a safe and healthful working condition. This act covers every employer whose business affects interstate commerce. OSHA is a federal agency that has the power to enforce regulations concerning the health and safety of employees. Every laboratory must be aware of OSHA recommendations and carefully monitor potential violations. OSHA, in cooperation with other agencies, carries out research to establish basic safety standards. For instance, the Centers for Disease Control and Prevention (CDC) has issued recommendations for a set of universal precautions that all health care workers must follow when dealing with hazardous materials. The CDC has authorized OSHA to enforce these precautions.

OSHA inspectors carry out frequent, surprise inspections of workplaces to see that standards are met. OSHA visits are commonly associated with employee complaints. OSHA safety regulations include standards for exposure to toxic chemicals, fumes, lead, pesticides, noise, and asbestos. Violators of OSHA standards must pay fines if found guilty.

OSHA Bloodborne Pathogens Standards

Laboratories must follow the OSHA guidelines for handling contaminated materials. These guidelines are available from the U.S. Department of Labor in Washington, D.C.

In December 1991, OSHA released a set of regulations that was designed to reduce the risk of medical employees to infectious diseases. The OSHA standards went into effect on July 6, 1992, and are formally known as OSHA Occupational Exposure to Bloodborne Pathogens Standards. There is a severe penalty of up to $7,000 for each violation of the standards by employers.

Employer responsibilities under OSHA standards mandate that all health care employers provide a means for protecting their employees from potential exposure to hepatitis B. Every employee must be given the choice to elect or refuse immunization. If refused, the employee has the right to change his or her mind and receive immunization at no charge. The employer must cover all costs associated with this immunization.

Employee responsibilities mandate that any employee who has occupational exposure adhere to the OSHA standards. Occupational exposure is defined as a reasonable anticipation that the employee's duties will result in skin, mucous membrane, eye, or parenteral contact with **bloodborne pathogens** or other potentially infectious material. Examples of employees who have occupational exposure are laboratory workers, housekeeping personnel, physicians, and nurses.

MED TIP

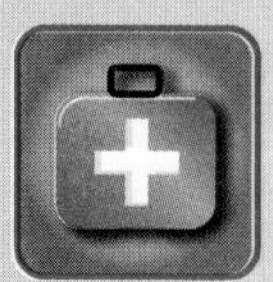

The OSHA standards refer to urine, stool, sputum, nasal secretions, vomitus, and sweat only if there is visible evidence of blood present.

Exposure Control Plan

OSHA requires that each laboratory have a written Exposure Control Plan to assist in minimizing employee exposure to dangerous infectious material. This exposure plan must be reviewed by all laboratory personnel and updated annually. An OSHA record for each employee must be kept on file, including documentation of the employee's review of the Exposure Control Plan. In addition, records must be maintained on each employee regarding hepatitis B vaccination and an exposure incident report. These report records must be maintained for the duration of employment plus 30 years. Records of all training sessions must be maintained for 3 years. General safety and housekeeping procedures from OSHA are described in table 4-4.

Centers for Disease Control and Prevention (CDC)

The Centers for Disease Control and Prevention (CDC), a federal agency established in 1946 with headquarters in Atlanta, Georgia, is part of the U.S. Public Health Service. The CDC is a governmental agency that employs more than 400 people with the purpose of preventing and controlling disease. The CDC seeks information about causes of disease to find cures and acts as a resource for the medical profession. This agency alerts the medical profession to potential outbreaks of disease, such as influenza; describes the group most at risk during an outbreak of disease, such as the aged; and recommends the proper treatment. Laboratories play an important role as fact finders for the CDC because often the first objective knowledge about an outbreak is as a result of laboratory tests.

The CDC's work has included a determination of the nature and cause of Legionnaires' disease and of toxic shock syndrome. The agency is currently engaged in a study of **acquired immune deficiency syndrome (AIDS).** AIDS is a series of infections that occur as a result of infection by the **human immunodeficiency virus (HIV),** which causes the immune system to break down.

Prior to the implementation of OSHA standards, the CDC issued recommendations that became known as Universal Precautions. According to Universal Precautions, *all* blood and body fluid is to be treated as if it contains the HIV, hepatitis B virus (HBV), or other bloodborne pathogens. OSHA standards state that Universal Precautions must be maintained at all times when there is a potential for contamination by bloodborne pathogens. Using Universal Precautions means that one must consider all blood and certain body fluids potentially infectious for all individuals.

The CDC issued new isolation guidelines in 1994 that emphasize two tiers of approach to infection control. The first and most important tier, or level, contains precautions designed to care for all patients in a health care setting regardless of their diagnosis or risk of infection. This tier contains precautions designed to decrease the risk of transmission of disease through body fluids. It is referred to as Standard Precautions and is used regardless of the patient's diagnosis or whether the patient has a known infectious disease. It uses the major features of universal precautions and body substance isolation, which alert those in the health care field to handle *all* materials as if they are contaminated.

TABLE 4-4 Safety and Housekeeping Procedures from OSHA

1. Immediately clean and disinfect surfaces exposed to infectious materials. All surfaces must be decontaminated on a regular schedule that is posted, signed, and kept with OSHA records. Figure 4-3 shows one type of single-use cleanup kit.
2. Never pick up broken glass with hands. Use a dust pan or other mechanical device.
3. Properly bag contaminated clothing and laundry in leak-proof, labeled bags. Contaminated laundry should not be handled or washed at the laboratory facility or with other noncontaminated clothing.
4. Handle regulated waste (highly infectious material such as contaminated needles and surgical waste) by placing in clearly labeled biohazard waste containers. Waste must be removed by a licensed waste disposal service and incinerated or autoclaved before placing in a designated landfill area.
5. Replace a damaged biohazard bag by placing a second bag around the first. Do not remove infectious material from the damaged bag.
6. Use puncture-proof, sealable, biohazard sharps containers for all needles and sharps, such as glass pipettes and razors.
   - Place the container close to the work area.
   - Keep the sharps container upright.
   - Never reach into the sharps container or push sharps further into the container.
   - Replace the sharps container when two-thirds full.
   - Seal and label sharps containers before placing with biohazard waste for removal by disposal service.
7. Wash hands both before and after using gloves.
8. Personal protective equipment (PPE) may not be worn out of the laboratory areas. Failure to observe this precaution may result in an OSHA citation.

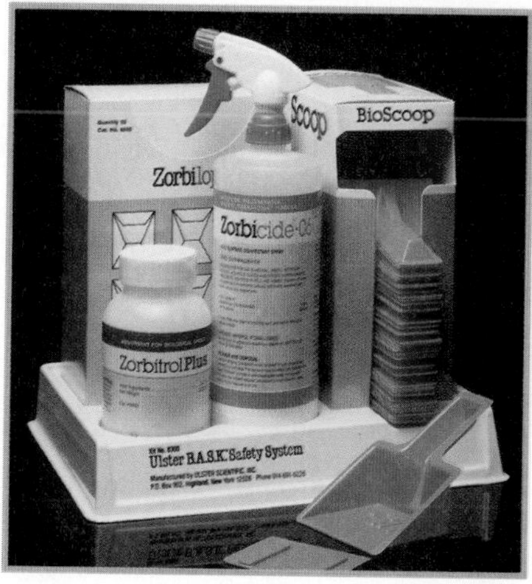

Figure 4-3
A type of single-use cleanup kit.

Standard Precautions apply to (1) blood, (2) all body fluids (except sweat) regardless of whether they contain blood, (3) nonintact skin, and (4) mucous membranes. Body fluids include the following:

Blood	*Cerebrospinal fluid*
Body fluids containing blood	*Pleural fluid*
Tissue specimens	*Pericardial fluid*
Semen	*Peritoneal fluid*
Vaginal secretions	*Interstitial fluid*
Amniotic fluid	

Also included are feces, nasal secretions, sputum, tears, urine, vomitus, saliva, and breast milk that contain visible blood.

Standard Precautions promote hand washing and the use of gloves, masks, eye protection, or gowns when appropriate for patient contact. Masks, protective eyewear, gowns, and gloves are referred to as a barrier type of protection, or personal protective equipment. Standard Precautions equipment, or personal protective equipment (PPE), is described in table 4-5.

The second tier of the CDC guidelines is focused on patients who are either suspected of carrying an infectious disease or are already infected. This second tier, which requires extra precautions in addition to the Standard Precautions, is known as Transmission-based Precautions. It includes three types of categories: Airborne Precautions, Droplet Precautions, and Contact Precautions.

Airborne Precautions are designed to reduce the transmission of certain diseases, such as tuberculosis (TB), measles (rubeola), or chicken pox. In addition to practicing Standard Precautions, Airborne Precautions are used when collecting a specimen from patients who are known to be infected with microorganisms that are transmitted via airborne droplet nuclei (smaller than 5 μm) that can remain suspended in the air and widely dispersed throughout a room by air currents. Airborne Precautions include isolation of the patient in a private room if hospitalized and use of a mask, gloves, and protective gown by the laboratory worker.

Droplet Precautions are used for patients known or suspected to be infected with microorganisms transmitted by droplets generated by a patient during sneezing, coughing, talking, or performance of procedures that induce coughing, such as a sputum specimen. Examples include invasive *Haemophilus influenzae* type b (HIB) disease (meningitis and pneumonia), invasive Neisseria meningitis disease (meningitis, pneumonia, and sepsis), diphtheria, pertussis, streptococcal pneumonia, scarlet fever, mumps, and rubella. Precautions include isolation of the patient in a private room if hospitalized. Gloves, gowns, and a mask should be worn.

Contact Precautions are used for patients known to be infected with a microorganism that is not easily treated with antibiotics and that can be transmitted easily by direct contact between the patient and phlebotomist, from patient to patient, or by indirect contact with items touched by the patient. Examples of these illnesses include enteric (intestinal), gastrointestinal, respiratory, skin, or wound infections; diphtheria; herpes simplex virus; impetigo; hepatitis A; scabies; pediculosis; and herpes zoster.

TABLE 4-5 Standard Precautions: Equipment and Situations

Precaution	Description
Gloves	Gloves must be worn when in contact with blood, all body fluids, secretions, excretions (except sweat) regardless of whether they contain visible blood, mucous membranes, nonintact skin, or contaminated articles (see figure 4-4 for illustration of glove removal) Examples: Venipuncture, capillary stick, injections, wound care, and cleaning contaminated equipment
Gowns	Gowns must be worn during procedures (or situations) in which there may be exposure to blood, body fluids, mucous membranes, or draining wounds; wash hands after removing gown Example: Laboratory procedures and minor surgery
Mask and protective eyewear (goggles or shield)	Masks and protective eyewear must be worn during procedures that are likely to generate droplets of blood or body fluids (splashes or sprays), such as when a patient is coughing excessively Example: Performing blood smear
Hand-washing	Hands must be washed both before applying gloves and after gloves are removed; hands must be washed immediately if contaminated with blood or body fluids, between patient contact, and when indicated to prevent transfer of microorganisms between other patients and the environment
Multiple-use	Common multiple-use equipment, such as blood pressure cuffs or stethoscopes, must be cleaned and disinfected after use or when they become soiled with body fluids or blood; single-use items are discarded
Needles and sharp instruments	Needles and sharp instruments must be discarded into a puncture-proof container; needles should not be recapped.

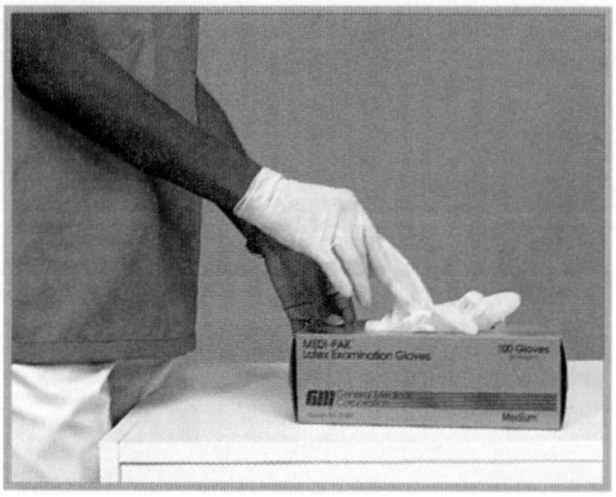

A

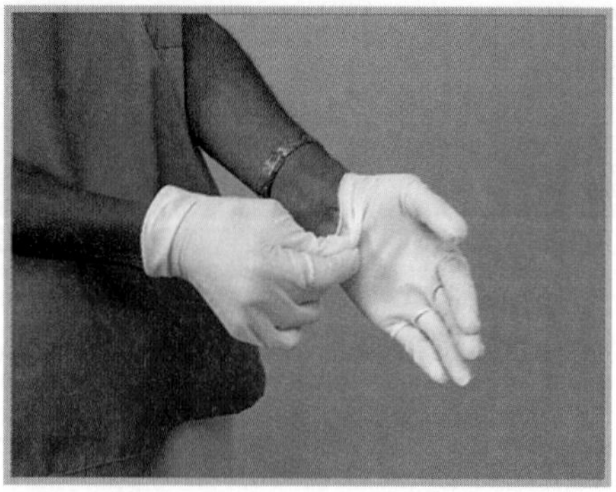

C

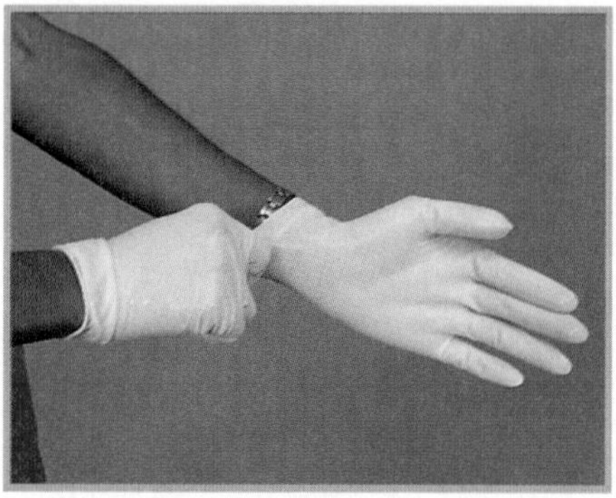

B

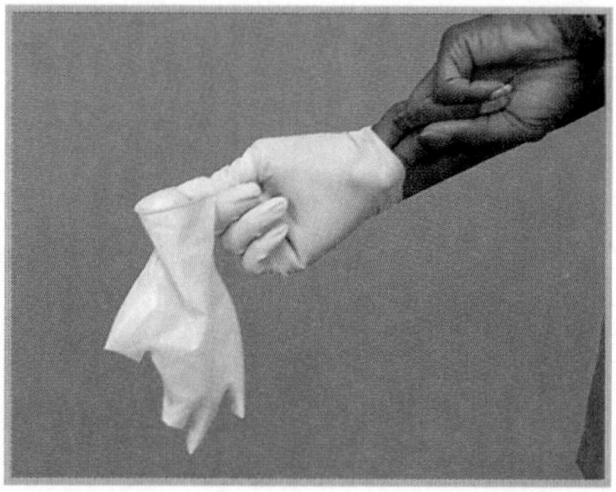

D

Figure 4-4
Removing gloves. (A) Use a clean pair of gloves for each patient contact. (B) Grasp the glove just below the cuff. (C) Pull the glove over your hand while turning the glove inside out. (D) Place the ungloved index finger and middle finger inside cuff of the glove, turning the cuff downward. (E) Pull the cuff and glove inside out as you remove your hand from the glove.

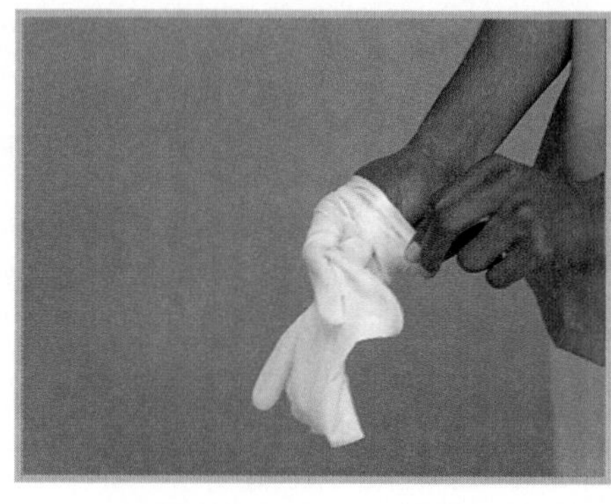

E

Precautions include isolation of the patient in a private room if hospitalized. Gloves, gown, and mask should be worn. Standard Precautions are summarized in table 4-6.

TABLE 4-6 Summary of Standard Precautions

1. Wear protective barrier equipment (e.g., face mask, eye shield, or goggles) when there is any risk of splashing, splattering, or aerosolization (becoming airborne in small particles) of potentially infectious body fluids.
2. Wear gloves when there is any potential for exposure to blood or body fluids, secretions, excretions, and contaminated items, including handling tissue and clinical specimens and touching the nonintact skin of patients.
3. Wear gloves when drawing blood, including finger and heel sticks on infants, and during preparation of blood smears.
4. Change gloves after each patient. Wash hands before putting on gloves and after removing them.
5. Change gloves if they become contaminated with blood or other body fluids and dispose of properly in biohazard waste container.
6. Wash hands or other skin surfaces if they become contaminated with potentially infectious blood or body fluids.
7. Care for equipment and linens that are contaminated with blood, blood products, body fluids, excretions, and secretions in a manner that avoids contact with your skin and mucous membranes or cross-contamination to another person.
8. Wear a gown or other protective clothing when there is a risk of splashing, splattering, or other means of exposure to a patient's body fluids.
9. Wear a mask if a patient has an airborne disease. A special mask is recommended if a patient has an active case of tuberculosis (TB).
10. Use care with needles, scalpels, and other sharp instruments to avoid unintentional injury.
11. Dispose of needles and other sharp items in a rigid, puncture-resistant sharps container.
12. Do not recap or handle used needles.
13. Store reusable sharp instruments and needles in a puncture-resistant container.
14. Avoid mouth-to-mouth breathing in all but life-threatening situations. Use a mechanical device or mask barrier instead.
15. Use a solution of household bleach (1:10 dilution) to disinfect environmental surfaces and reusable equipment.
16. Use hazardous waste containers for contaminated materials.

MED TIP

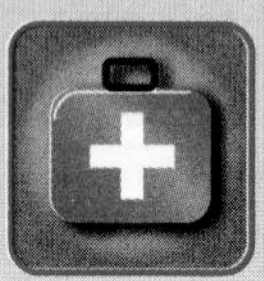

The CDC's Standard Precautions are similar to Universal Precautions, because both are directed at body fluids that are blood, blood related, or contain blood. However, Standard Precautions are broader and include precautions for any moist body substance. Both precautions were established to protect everyone from any infectious disease.

General Laboratory Safety

General safety rules throughout the laboratory protect the staff and the patients. General guidelines to observe when working in a laboratory include the following:

1. Walk, never run, in a laboratory. In emergencies, move quickly without running.
2. Never carry uncapped syringes, needles, or sharp instruments when walking in the laboratory or hallways.
3. Keep floors clear. Immediately wipe up spills using the accepted procedure or call specially trained housekeeping personnel to assist. Never pick up broken glass with bare hands. Use OSHA standards when cleaning up glass, spilled specimens, and spilled liquids.
4. Open doors carefully to avoid injuring someone on the other side.
5. Report all unsafe conditions, such as burned-out lightbulbs over exit signs, at once.
6. Wear long hair pulled back and tied to prevent it from coming into contact with hazardous materials and falling into the patient's face.
7. Never eat, drink, or smoke in the laboratory.
8. Never store any personal items such as food or drink in the laboratory refrigerator.
9. Never apply lipstick, makeup, or contact lenses while in the laboratory.
10. Never place anything in your mouth, such as a pen or pencil, when in the laboratory.
11. Wear personal protective equipment (PPE) (e.g., masks, eye shields, laboratory coats, and gloves) as required.
12. Wear shoes that cover the entire foot. Open-toed, open-heel shoes are not recommended due to the danger of slipping, dropping specimens directly on the skin, and other injuries.
13. Keep all chemicals below eye level to avoid damaging eyes if a spill occurs.
14. Have frequent fire and disaster drills for employees.
15. Avoid wearing loose clothing, such as scarves, which can become tangled in equipment such as the centrifuge.

A disaster is anything that can cause injury or damage to a group of people. Disasters in the laboratory include fire, flood, smoke, fumes, or explosions. The guidelines for handling a disaster are

1. Remain calm. Try to count to ten quickly and assess the situation.
2. Remove all patients from the area.

3. Remove all other staff and employees who are in immediate danger if it is safe to do so.
4. Make sure that the fire department has been notified in the event of a fire.
5. Notify others of the emergency according to the policy of the laboratory or institution.
6. Use stairs, never the elevator.

All medical facilities and laboratories must have a disaster plan. This plan should include the following information:

- The floor plan of the facility
- The nearest exit
- The location of alarms and fire extinguishers
- How to use the fire equipment such as extinguishers and hoses
- The role of each employee when a disaster strikes

Physical Hazards: Fire, Electrical, Radiation, and Mechanical Safety

Fire Safety

Because there is a potential for fire in the laboratory, fire extinguishers should be attached on laboratory walls in several locations. Each employee should be instructed on the proper use of fire equipment including all extinguishers. Fire hoses enclosed in glass are generally reserved for fire personnel since the high-water pressure requires two people to hold the hose.

Fires need oxygen, heat, and fuel to start. All three are present in the laboratory. In addition, medical facilities such as hospitals have an additional oxygen supply or portable oxygen tanks that support combustion.

In the event of a fire, after notifying the fire department, the most important function during a fire is to see that all patients and employees are safely out of danger.

The National Fire Protection Association (NFPA) classifies fires in the following four categories:

1. Class A: Fires from ordinary combustible materials such as paper, cloth, wood, and plastics
2. Class B: Fires resulting from flammable solvents such as gases, oil, paints, and grease and an interaction with air and vapors
3. Class C: Fires taking place in or near electrical equipment
4. Class D: Fires occurring from combustible metals such as lithium and magnesium

The NFPA classifies fire extinguishers that are used to control the four classifications of fires:

1. Class A extinguishers contain soda and water or acid; they are used for ordinary combustible fires
2. Class B extinguishers contain foam, dry chemicals, or CO_2 and are used for fires resulting from solvents and air-vapor mixes
3. Class C extinguishers contain dry chemicals and are used to fight electrical fires
4. An ABC fire extinguisher is a multipurpose or all-purpose extinguisher; it is often used in laboratories and health care facilities to avoid confusion over which extinguisher is appropriate

The acronym RACE should be kept in mind when confronted with a fire in the laboratory.

R = *R*emove the patients from the vicinity of the fire

A = *A*ctivate the alarm and alert other staff members

C = *C*ontain or confine the fire by closing all doors

E = *E*xtinguish the fire if it is safe to do so

The use of the fire extinguisher is easier to remember by recalling the acronym PASS.

P = *P*ull the pin on the extinguisher

A = *A*im the nozzle just above the base of the fire

S = *S*queeze the trigger of the extinguisher

S = *S*weep the nozzle of the extinguisher over the fire

Electrical Safety

Electrical shock is a hazard in the laboratory due to the equipment being used. All equipment should be grounded, or connected to the ground, according to the manufacturer's instructions. All plugs should be three pronged and not frayed.

The circuit breakers in the laboratory should be clearly marked so they can be located during an electrical fire or shock. If an employee or patient is being shocked, he or she should not be touched. The main source of power should be turned off immediately. A call for help should be made if the victim is unresponsive after the power is turned off. Cardiopulmonary resuscitation (CPR) will have to be administered if the victim is not breathing.

Radiation Safety

In most laboratories the exposure level of radiation is well below the safe limits that have been established by federal and state regulations. However, hospital laboratory personnel may work in close proximity to X-ray equipment that is found in other departments. All employees must pay close attention to signs near radiology rooms and equipment indicating that there is a danger due to radiation. Employees who work around X-ray equipment on a regular basis must wear small radiation badges that indicate the level of radiation they are receiving. Medical personnel must wear a lead apron and gloves if they are in close proximity to a patient receiving X rays.

Exposure to radiation has a **cumulative** effect, which means that the effect builds over time. Thus continued exposure and buildup of radiation are dangerous. Laboratory personnel have the potential for exposure to radiation when collecting specimens from patients in the X-ray or nuclear medicine department.

The chance for exposure to radiation is greater if the phlebotomist must collect a specimen from a patient with a radium implant in the pelvic area. The blood specimen should be drawn in a minimal amount of time. There will be a radiation sign on the patient's door. The phlebotomist should always go to the nursing station for directions before entering the radiation patient's room.

Mechanical Safety

Many pieces of equipment in the laboratory can cause harm if they are not used properly. Some of these pieces of equipment include the centrifuge, autoclave, sterilizers, and oxygen equipment. All equipment comes with detailed operating instructions. In most cases the equipment must be grounded with a three-prong plug and will require a particular type of loading technique.

Improper loading and sealing of the centrifuge can result in blood-filled glass tubes cracking or breaking as well as being expelled from the centrifuge while it is in motion. This is a very dangerous hazard. Laboratory personnel should always double-check that the lid is properly fastened on the centrifuge.

MED TIP

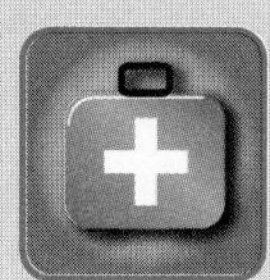

Remember to ask for instructions when using unfamiliar equipment. It is better to admit ignorance than to make a disastrous mistake.

Chemical Hazards

Laboratories contain chemicals, such as hydrochloric acid (HCl) and sodium hydroxide (NaOH), which are highly **caustic** and can cause severe burns. Any caustic chemical or material that comes into contact with the skin or eyes should be washed away immediately. The skin should be washed under cold running water for at least 5 minutes; the eyes should be rinsed for a minimum of 15 minutes.

MED TIP

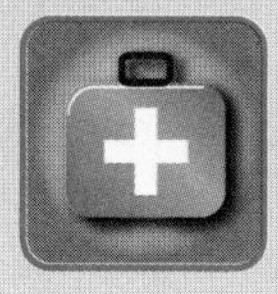

When working with an acid, always add acid to water (instead of water to acid) to prevent a violent chemical reaction that could cause injury.

Laboratory workers should carefully read all labels for instructions when disposing of chemicals. All chemical spills should be carefully cleaned up, using a spill-cleanup kit containing absorbents and neutralizers. Signs indicating chemical hazards, such as poison, should be placed in clear view.

MED TIP

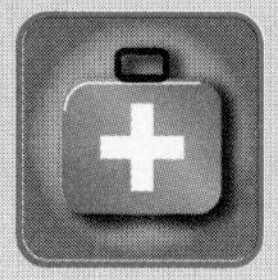

Eyewash stations should be easily accessible in all laboratories. Anyone experiencing a splash of chemicals into the eyes should rinse his or her face and eyes under running water for a minimum of 15 minutes.

Material Safety Data Sheets (MSDSs)

Material safety data sheets (MSDSs) are required for all hazardous materials and drugs. They should be maintained in a prominent place so that all employees can enter data on them. Chemical manufacturers are required to supply MSDSs for their chemicals.

Biological Hazards and Wastes

Laboratories, hospitals, physicians' offices, dental practices, and other health care facilities generate 3.2 million tons of hazardous medical waste each year. Much of this waste is dangerous, especially when it is potentially infectious or radioactive. There are four types of medical waste:

- Solid
- Chemical
- Radioactive
- Infectious

Solid Waste

Solid waste is generated in every aspect of medicine, including laboratories, patient rooms, cafeterias, and administration. It includes trash such as paper goods, bottles, cardboard, and cans. Solid waste is not considered hazardous but can cause pollution of the environment. Mandatory recycling programs have assisted in reducing solid waste in many health care facilities and laboratories.

Chemical Waste

Chemical wastes include substances such as germicides, cleaning solvents, and pharmaceuticals (drugs). This waste can create a hazardous situation such as a fire or explosion. It can also cause harm if ingested, inhaled, or absorbed through the skin or a mucous membrane. Toxic, inflammable, foul-smelling, or irritating chemicals should not be poured down the drain. These chemicals are generally placed in sturdy containers such as buckets. The Material Safety Data Sheet (MSDS) gives information on handling chemicals safely and should include specific disposal information.

Radioactive Waste

Radioactive wastes have increased with recent advances in nuclear medicine and include iodine 123, iodine 131, and thallium 201. Radioactive waste is any waste that contains or is contaminated with liquid or solid radioactive material. It is not generated by X rays or other external beam therapy procedures. Radioactive waste must be clearly labeled as such and never placed in an incinerator, down the drain, or in public areas. These waste products must be removed by a licensed facility.

Infectious Waste

Infectious waste is any waste material that has the potential to carry disease. Between 10 and 15 percent of all medical waste is considered infectious. Infectious waste, which is handled every day, includes laboratory cultures, blood, and blood products from blood banks, operating rooms, emergency rooms, doctor and dentist offices, autopsy suites, and patient rooms.

The three most dangerous types of infectious pathogens (microorganisms) found in medical waste are hepatitis A virus (HAV), hepatitis C, and human immunodeficiency virus (HIV), which causes acquired immune deficiency syndrome (AIDS).

Hepatitis, a virulent, potentially life-threatening infection of the liver, is transmitted directly or indirectly from blood and feces. AIDS is a virus that attacks the immune system and is considered a terminal (life-ending) disease.

Infectious waste must be separated from other solid and chemical waste at the point of origin (laboratory). Infectious waste must be labeled, decontaminated on-site, or removed by a licensed removal facility for decontamination. Methods for treating infectious waste include

1. Steam sterilization
2. Incineration
3. Thermal inactivation
4. Gas or vapor sterilization
5. Irradiation sterilization
6. Chemical disinfectant

Steam sterilization, which saturates waste with high-temperature steam in an autoclave, and incineration using a crematory are the most commonly recommended treatments for most infectious waste, including

- Blood cultures
- Sharps (such as needles and scalpels)
- Isolation wastes
- Pathology waste
- Dialysis unit waste

Guidelines for handling biological specimens include the following:

- Gloves and other protective clothing (e.g., laboratory coat, eye shield, and protective facial shield) must always be worn when handling and processing blood.
- A **biological safety hood** or protective cabinet should be used when in contact with aerosols (airborne particles) to draw the particles away from the laboratory worker.
- Mouth pipetting should not be used.
- All bacteriological specimens must be handled as if they carry disease.
- All biological waste must be autoclaved before disposal.
- The workstation must be disinfected both before and after use with a 1:10 bleach solution.

Laboratory Security

There are unique security issues in laboratories. Laboratories make an attractive target for a thief or drug addict, who can sell stolen needles and syringes. Doors and windows need to have secure locks. Only authorized persons should be allowed to enter a laboratory and carry keys to the laboratory. If a key is missing, the locks should be changed.

Figure 4-5
An example of quality control testing materials.

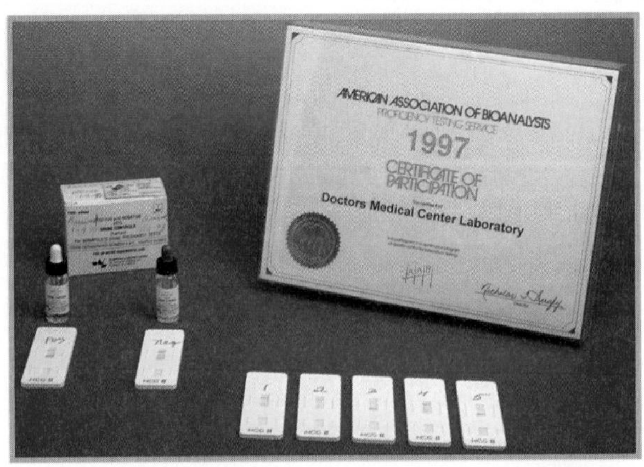

Quality Control

In the early 1960s, the health care industry began to feel an increasing demand from the public for accountable quality care. **Quality assurance** is gathering and evaluating information and data about the services or tests provided as well as the results achieved compared with an acceptable standard. A **quality assurance program** is one in which laboratories and hospitals evaluate the services and/or tests they provide by comparing their services and/or tests with accepted standards or **criteria.** The actual program will have as a goal a desired degree, or level, of care or service. **Data,** which include statistics, facts, or information, are gathered for evaluation and comparison to an acceptable standard.

The results of an evaluation when compared with standard results pinpoint deficiencies and offer recommendations for improvement. For example, the number of successful needle stick attempts compared with a **norm,** or the ideal measurement for a group, would be examined. The overall goal is to effect quality improvement, including accuracy and precision, in the care or service provided. Figure 4-5 illustrates an example of quality control testing materials.

Joint Commission on Accreditation of Healthcare Organizations (JCAHO)

The Joint Commission on Accreditation of Healthcare Organizations (JCAHO), headquartered in Chicago, Illinois, is a private, nongovernmental agency that establishes guidelines for hospitals and health care agencies to follow regarding quality of care. The JCAHO has developed a ten-step process for quality assessment of health care performance (see table 4-7).

MED TIP

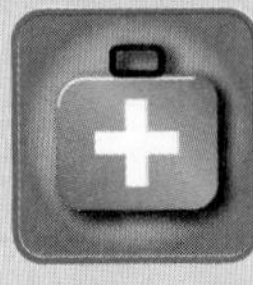

One of the most common errors when collecting blood specimens is to incorrectly identify the patient. Rather than having the patient answer yes or no to a question about the name, such as "Are you Mr. Smith?" it is better to ask the patient to tell you his or her name. Then carefully match that name, with the correct spelling, to the name on the requisition form.

TABLE 4-7	JCAHO's Ten-Step Process for Quality Assessment
1.	Assign responsibility for monitoring and evaluating service quality.
2.	Determine the scope of care for all major sections of the medical facility or laboratory.
3.	Identify the key or major aspects of care that would include high-risk and high-volume procedures.
4.	Construct indicators that specify which activities and/or outcomes to monitor.
5.	Define the thresholds of evaluation that specify the lowest limits for acceptable quality.
6.	Collect and organize the data.
7.	Evaluate the data gathered by comparing it with standards. Also analyze any trends or patterns and causes for deviation from the standard.
8.	Develop a corrective action plan that shows what actions should be taken and details who or what needs to change. A date when the corrective action should take place is included.
9.	Make an assessment of the actions and document all improvements.
10.	Communicate the relevant information through a formal reporting structure, preferably in writing.

A Delta Test

If possible, a **delta test** should be conducted on all blood tests. A delta test consists of a comparison between the current results of a laboratory test and the previous test results for the same patient. There may normally be a slight difference between two of the same tests that are taken at different intervals (or dates) for the same patient. However, a wide variation in results is a red flag that could indicate an error.

The Floor Book

A **floor book,** also referred to as a procedure, reference, or test manual, consists of a series of charts that list the name of each test or procedure. It is a useful tool to aid in consistency of testing for quality assurance purposes. A log book would include the following information:

- The type of specimen to be obtained (e.g., urine, blood, fasting blood, or semen)
- The minimum amount of sample required to run the test
- Reference (normal) values for the test
- Any special handling of the specimen (e.g., refrigerating and keeping out of direct light)
- Normal turnaround time for the specific test

Monitoring Quality Control in the Laboratory

Effective quality control begins in the laboratory even before the specimen is collected. The patient needs to receive effective instructions regarding preparation for the test, such as fasting or abstaining from medications for a period of time before the blood specimen is drawn. The correct laboratory tube or specimen container must be selected and prepared with a label. Laboratory equipment must be recalibrated and tested for accuracy on a prescribed basis. Quality control is a part of a quality assurance (QA) program in all medical laboratories. Some of the areas and issues that need quality monitoring in the laboratory are described in table 4-8.

Documentation on Logs

One of the most effective means for continually monitoring quality assurance in the laboratory is with the use of logs for documentation purposes. A log is a record or history of data such as instrument maintenance, laboratory requisitions, and specimens entering and leaving the laboratory. The logs are examined in quality assurance meetings to determine any problem areas. Logs must be maintained meticulously and kept in a secured storage area. The length of time a log is kept on file will vary depending on individual laboratory policy. In some cases a federal act, such as the Clinical Laboratory Improvement Act of 1988 (CLIA 1988), will establish the length of time a log must be kept.

Incident Reports

One means of documenting problem areas within the laboratory is through the incident report. An **incident report** is a formal written description of an incident or unusual occurrence, such as a patient injury resulting from fainting while having a venipuncture procedure performed. The report should be completed whenever there is an unusual occurrence such as a fall, inability to perform a venipuncture, or patient complaint. The

TABLE 4-8 Issues Requiring Quality Monitoring in the Laboratory

Failure to correctly identify the patient	Needle stick incidents of staff
Long waiting time for patient	Adverse reactions to procedures
Patient complaints	Errors in labeling laboratory specimens
Patient falls and/or fainting	Turnaround time between the ordering of the test and the reporting of a test result
Inability to obtain venous blood on the first attempt	Any delay in the collection of a timed test
Failed blood collection attempts (with no more than two attempts)	Improper disposal of needles
Redraw due to lack of sufficient blood sample	Incorrect calibration of instruments
Hematomas (number and size)	Improper preparation and use of test control substances
Specimens gathered in incorrect tubes	Incorrect or lack of documentation of all instrument checks and maintenance
Errors in patient identification	Failure to notify physician of all patient samples with values that enter the "panic range" or "critical range"
Lack of correct patient instruction	
Incomplete documentation on requisitions	

purpose of the report is to objectively document exactly what happened, with the goal of preventing another episode. Incident reports are generally designed to meet the needs of the individual facility or laboratory.

Details on completing the incident report are usually included in every facility's policy and **procedure manual**—a collection of policies and procedures for carrying out the day-to-day operations in the laboratory. In addition, a laboratory procedure manual should describe the standards, equipment, supplies, step-by-step instructions, and normal values for all tests and procedures. The procedure manual should also contain the panic or critical range for all tests. Any test result that falls within this panic range must be immediately reported to the physician.

An **occurrence** is any incident outside of the norm. Some incidents that require documentation and/or an incident report are

- Fire
- Theft
- Computer crash
- Improper needle stick
- Needle stick accident for patient or staff
- Patient fall
- Fire
- Patient complaint
- Syringes and needles missing from supply area
- Patient faints while having blood drawn
- Administration of an incorrect test on a patient
- Misplaced or lost specimen

MED TIP

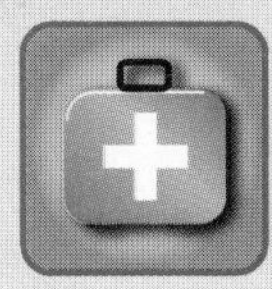

The incident report, like all other information relating to the patient, is subject to subpoena in litigation. Therefore, documentation must be accurate and timely.

CHAPTER REVIEW

Summary

Infection control, safety, and quality control are vital to successful laboratory operation. No matter how well a laboratory test is performed, it is useless if the specimen is taken from the wrong patient or somehow mishandled. When errors of any type occur, they affect the reputation of the laboratory. In some cases, an error can adversely affect the life of the patient. A quality assurance program can help to determine where potential errors might occur and how to prevent them.

Competency Review

1. Correctly perform hand washing.
2. Be able to demonstrate the use of a fire extinguisher.
3. Name six types of isolation and discuss their purposes.
4. Describe quality assurance as it applies to the laboratory.
5. Demonstrate correct gloving and ungloving technique.

Examination Review Questions

1. **A fire that takes place in or near electrical equipment is what classification?**
   (A) Class A
   (B) Class B
   (C) Class C
   (D) Class D
   (E) Class ABC

2. **PPE includes all of the following *except***
   (A) gown
   (B) street clothing
   (C) laboratory coat
   (D) mask
   (E) eye shield

3. **The proper method for disposing of radioactive waste is to**
   (A) burn it in a special incinerator
   (B) treat it with disinfectant and then discard it with other hazardous wastes
   (C) pour it down a designated drain
   (D) have it removed by a licensed facility
   (E) all of the above are acceptable

4. **Universal Precautions must be maintained when there is a potential for contamination by**
   (A) semen
   (B) saliva
   (C) sweat
   (D) bloodborne pathogens
   (E) all of the above

5. **When using a fire extinguisher it is helpful to remember the acronym**
   (A) RACE
   (B) PASS
   (C) OSHA
   (D) JCAHO
   (E) CDC

6. **Hepatitis B virus (HBV) is transmitted through**
   (A) blood only
   (B) blood and feces
   (C) feces only
   (D) mucous membranes
   (E) none of the above

7. **An infection acquired after a person enters the hospital is referred to as**
   (A) nonpathogenic
   (B) universal
   (C) opportunistic
   (D) nosocomial
   (E) aerobic

8. **The type of isolation used for persons with infections of the intestinal tract is**
   (A) reverse
   (B) enteric
   (C) protective
   (D) strict
   (E) none of the above

9. **A solution of bleach used for cleaning a workstation is what concentration?**
   (A) 1:1
   (B) 1:2
   (C) 1:5
   (D) 1:10
   (E) 1:100

10. **OSHA reports for employee hepatitis B vaccine records must be maintained for at least**
   (A) 30 years or duration of employment
   (B) 3 years
   (C) 1 year
   (D) forever
   (E) none of the above is correct

Getting Connected

Multimedia Extension Activities

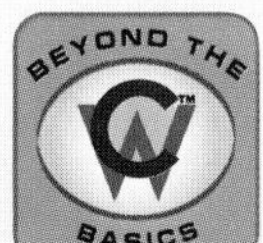

www.prenhall.com/fremgen

Use the address above to access the free, interactive Companion Website created specifically for this textbook. Enhance your studying by answering practice quiz questions, with hints and instant feedback related to chapter 4. If you would like to gain a deeper understanding of selected topics within this chapter, be sure to click on the **Beyond the Basics** feature, which provides more details for further learning. If you do not have a web connection, you may use the CD-ROM enclosed in the back of this book to take advantage of the same features off-line.

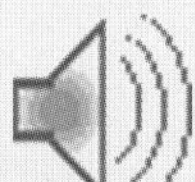

Audio Glossary

Use the CD-ROM enclosed with your textbook to hear the pronunciation of the key terms in the chapter. You may also access this material on the Companion Website www.prenhall.com/fremgen.

Bibliography

Caring for Someone with AIDS. Washington, D.C.: U.S. Department of Health and Human Services, 1994.

CDC National AIDS Clearinghouse. Rockville, Md.: Centers for Disease Control National AIDS Clearinghouse, 1996.

"CDC Summarizes Final Regulations for Implementing CLIA." *American Family Physician* 45:6, 1992.

Decker, M. "The OSHA Bloodborne Hazard Standard." *Infection Control and Hospital Epidemiology* 12:7, 1992.

Gerberding, L. "Reducing Occupational Risk of HIV Infection." *Hospital Practice,* June 1991.

HIV/AIDS Prevention. Atlanta: Centers for Disease Control and Prevention, October 1994.

HIV/AIDS Surveillance Reports. Rockville, Md.: Centers for Disease Control National AIDS Clearinghouse, 1996.

Kelsey, M. "Understanding OSHA's Bloodborne Pathogens Standard." *PMA,* July–August 1992.

Limmer, D. *Emergency Care.* Upper Saddle River, N.J.: Brady/Prentice-Hall, 1995.

Michels, K. "Final OSHA Bloodborne Standard Released." *AANA Journal* 60:1, 1992.

Richardson, D. "OSHA Releases Final Standard on HIV, Hepatitis B Exposures." *American Nurse* 24:1, 1992.

Rodriques, P. "Handling and Disposal of Infectious Waste in the Office Setting." *Orthopedic Nursing* 10:5, 1991.

Sazama, J. "Licensure of Laboratory Personnel." *Laboratory Medicine,* April 1993.

Stutz, D., and S. Janusz. *Hazardous Materials Injuries: A Handbook for Prehospital Care,* 2nd ed. Beltsville, Md.: Bradford Communications, 1988.

Taber's Cyclopedic Medical Dictionary, 18th ed. Philadelphia: F. A. Davis, 1997.

TB/HIV—The Connection: What Health Care Workers Should Know. Atlanta: Centers for Disease Control and Prevention, September 1993.

U.S. Department of Health and Human Services, Centers for Disease Control and Prevention. "Draft Guidelines for Isolation Precautions for Hospitals." *Federal Register,* November 7, 1994.

Welding, M., and S. Toenjes. *Medical Laboratory Procedures.* Philadelphia: F. A. Davis, 1992.

Contact Information

Centers for Disease Control and Prevention (CDC)
1600 Clifton Rd., NE
Atlanta, GA 30333
(404) 639-3883

Joint Commission on Accreditation of Healthcare Organizations (JCAHO)
One Renaissance
Oakbrook Terrace, IL 60181
(630) 792-5000

National Committee for Clinical Laboratory Standards (NCCLS)
940 W. Valley Rd., S-1400
Wayne, PA 19087-1898
(610) 525-2435

Occupational Safety and Health Administration (OSHA)
U.S. Department of Labor
200 Constitution Ave., NW
Washington, DC 20210
(202) 523-8148

Section I

Case Study for End of Part I

DENNIS BROWN IS A phlebotomist working in the office laboratory of Dr. Williams. Dennis is a graduate of an accredited phlebotomy program and has successfully completed his certification examination. He is a trusted employee who has been working in Dr. Williams's office laboratory for 2 years.

He has just finished taking a blood sample from Jay White to test for the immunodeficiency virus HIV. Dennis is now drawing blood for a CBC from another patient of Dr. Williams, Marge Allan. Marge says to Dennis, "That man looked so sick. What blood test was he having? Was it for AIDS?" How should Dennis respond?

How should Dennis respond?

1. What, if anything, should Dennis say to Marge?
2. Dr. Williams has telephoned Dennis to say she was behind schedule and would be late arriving in the office. Dr. Williams asked Dennis as a favor to call one of their patients, Josephine Moore, who was very worried about the results of a recent blood test and tell her the test was negative. Given the scope of Dennis's education and experience, would this favor fall within his responsibilities?

SECTION 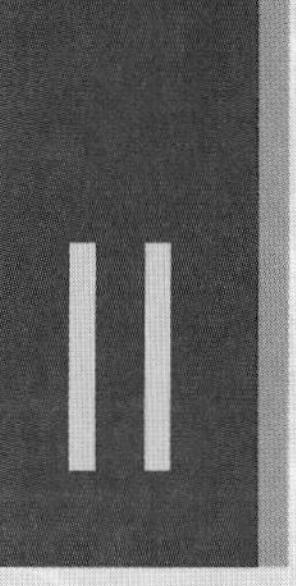

Phlebotomy Procedures and Equipment

CHAPTER 5

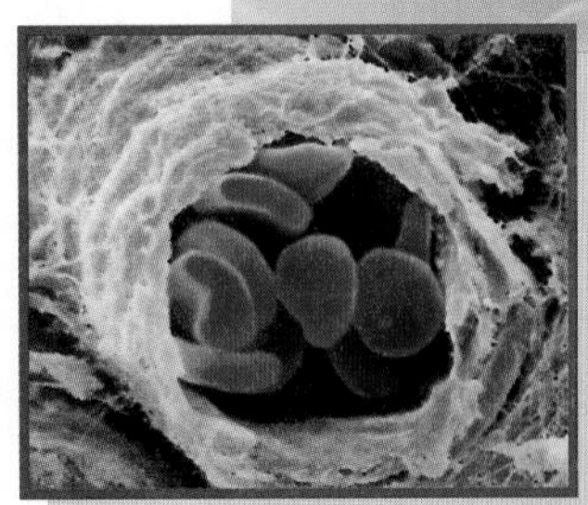

Patient Preparation for Blood Collection

Chapter Outline

Learning Objectives

After completing this chapter, you should be able to

1. Define and spell the glossary terms listed in this chapter.
2. Discuss why it is necessary to draw a blood specimen.
3. Identify the information required on a requisition.
4. Discuss the importance of correct patient identification.
5. Define proper patient identification for both inpatients and outpatients.
6. Discuss the importance of gaining the patient's confidence subsequent to performing specimen collection.

GLOSSARY

INPATIENT hospitalized patient.

OUTPATIENT patient who is not staying in a hospital but comes to the hospital for treatment.

REQUISITION physician's order to obtain a specimen for testing.

INTRODUCTION

In this chapter we discuss the most important aspect of the blood collection process—the patient. The patient should always be the phlebotomist's number-one priority. A competent phlebotomist must learn to interact in a competent, professional manner with patients in a wide variety of settings.

Why Do We Need to Draw Blood?

Blood acts as the primary means of transporting nutrients and other substances throughout the body. As blood circulates throughout the body, it carries oxygen and carbon dioxide to and from the lungs, digested food products from the intestines to tissues, waste products to the kidneys for excretion, and hormones from the endocrine glands. In addition to acting as a transportation conduit, blood helps to fight infections, regulates body temperature, and maintains body pH.

Because blood provides a needed role in many body functions, a great deal of information can be obtained from the analysis of blood. For example, blood can be analyzed to determine the number and types of cells that are present or to quantitate the amount of various carbohydrates or electrolytes that are found in blood serum. The patient's physician uses this information to determine the state of the patient's health and to aid in the diagnoses of various disease states.

Although blood is analyzed in the clinical laboratory, the quality of that work and the information derived from testing in the laboratory is only as good as the blood specimen the laboratory receives; therefore, it is crucial that the phlebotomist use the utmost care in drawing the specimen and always follow the proper protocol.

MED TIP

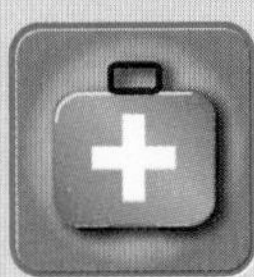

As a phlebotomist, you are responsible for providing the clinical laboratory with a properly collected blood specimen and transporting the specimen to the laboratory within the allotted time frame and under the proper conditions.

Requisitions

The process of blood collection always begins with a physician's order, also called a **requisition,** to draw a blood sample for a laboratory test or tests. Blood should never be drawn without a requisition. Requisitions vary a great deal from one health care institution to another. They may be handwritten, preprinted, or computer generated. Computer-generated requisitions may come with preprinted specimen labels. These labels have all of the needed patient information and are placed by the phlebotomist on the tube of blood after it is drawn but before leaving the patient's side. Preprinted labels save the phlebotomist from having to write patient information on each patient specimen. An example of the special patient identification number is illustrated in figure 5-1.

MED TIP

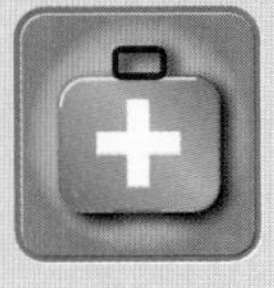

As a phlebotomist, you should *never* collect a blood specimen without a requisition.

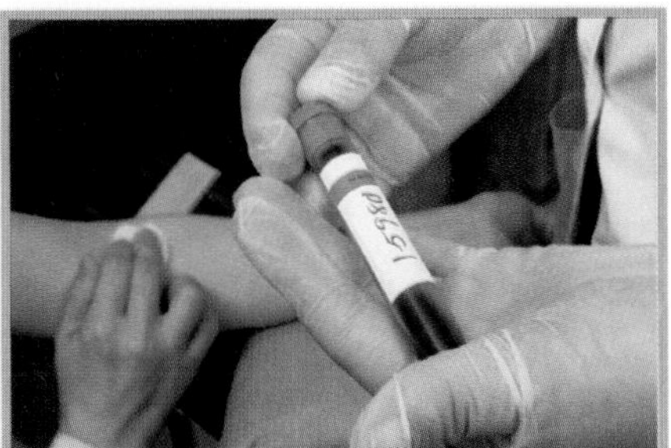

Figure 5-1
An example of the special patient identification number.

Although the type of requisition varies from one institution to another, all requisitions must contain the same basic information:

- Patient's name
- Patient's identification number: A specific identification number is issued to each patient upon entering the hospital and is used to identify all hospital work associated with that patient; in many clinics and outpatient settings, the identification number is the patient's Social Security number
- Patient's location: Room number for inpatients or patient address for outpatients
- Name(s) of test(s) ordered
- Physician's name
- Date and time of specimen collection

Other information that is not required but may be found on the requisition includes the following:

- Patient diagnosis
- Patient date of birth
- Patient gender
- Phlebotomist's identification such as name or initials (this information is necessary if the laboratory has questions about the blood sample)

In addition to the listed information, the requisition also provides the phlebotomist with the information needed to collect the proper specimen. The type of tests ordered by the physician determines the equipment the phlebotomist will use to draw the blood specimen. Before beginning the specimen collection process, the phlebotomist should carefully check the requisition to make certain that all needed equipment is available. This equipment check is necessary to ensure that all of the blood required for the ordered tests can be completed with one collection.

Identification of the Patient

The most important task a phlebotomist has is to properly identify the patient. If the wrong name is placed on a blood specimen, the consequences to the patient may be catastrophic. If a patient specimen is mislabeled, the patient may receive a transfusion of the wrong blood type or be given the incorrect medication. In addition, all of the effort the phlebotomist has expended in obtaining the proper specimen and all of the time and expense the laboratory personnel have spent in analyzing the specimen will be wasted if the specimen is identified with the wrong name. If at any time during the specimen collection process, specimen transportation, and specimen processing or testing phase the identification of the specimen is in doubt, that specimen should be discarded and another blood specimen should be drawn.

MED TIP

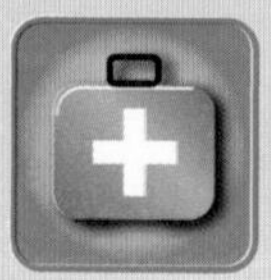

Correct identification of the patient is your single most important task as a phlebotomist.

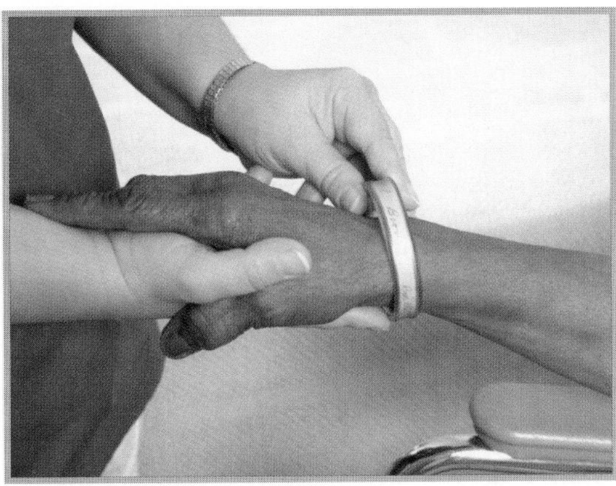

Figure 5-2
The patient's identification band.

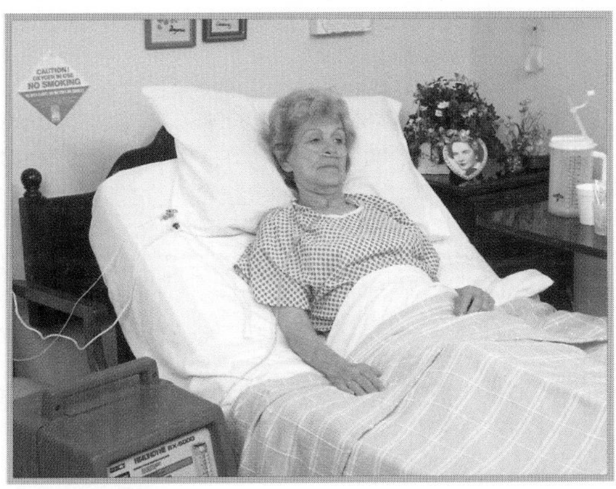

Figure 5-3
Match the patient information on the requisition with the information on the patient's identification band.

Inpatient Identification

Correct **inpatient** identification is so critical that it is normally a two-step process. The first part of the process is to ask the patient some personal information such as his or her name or date of birth. Then the phlebotomist confirms the patient's answer with the information on the requisition. The second part of the identification process is to match the patient information on the requisition with the information on the patient's identification band. The identification band as shown in figure 5-2 contains the patient's name, hospital room number and unique identification number. All hospitalized patients should have an identification band. See figure 5-3.

MED TIP

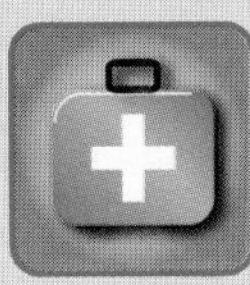

Never draw blood on a patient who is not wearing an ID band. Have the problem corrected before drawing the specimen.

Outpatient Identification

Proper **outpatient** identification is more difficult because outpatients do not have identification bands as shown in figure 5-4. An outpatient is a patient who is not staying in a hospital but comes to the hospital for treatment. Each facility has its own protocol for establishing the identification of an outpatient. In some facilities, patients may bring the requisition with them to the specimen collection area. In that situation, it is sufficient to ask patients to spell their name or state their date of birth or Social Security number and compare it with the information on the requisition. Other facilities may ask to see picture identification such as a driver's license. Remember, it is just as important to correctly identify an outpatient as an inpatient and to correctly identify the specimen.

Figure 5-4
Proper outpatient identification is more difficult because outpatients do not have identification bands.

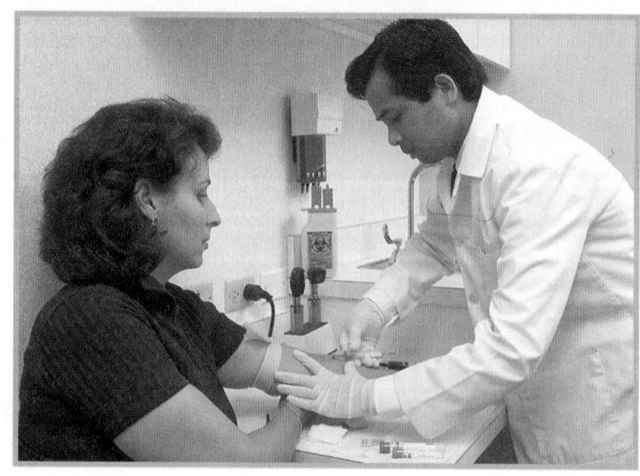

Preparing the Patient

Many patients are very unhappy to learn that they must have their blood drawn. For a few patients, this news may be terrifying. The phlebotomist is the individual who represents both the hospital and the laboratory to the patient. It is essential for the phlebotomist to gain the patient's confidence to reduce anxiety and to ensure patient cooperation during the blood collection process. Patient confidence can be gained by appearing and acting in a professional and courteous manner at all times. The impression that the phlebotomist makes on the patient is the impression that the patient will have of the health care facility.

The phlebotomist should only enter the patient's room after knocking and warmly greeting the patient. He or she should then offer a simple introduction such as "I am from the laboratory and I am here to draw your blood." It is extremely important for the phlebotomist to identify himself or herself as coming from the laboratory. Many hospital personnel are dressed alike, and in many cases patients are unable to identify hospital personnel by their appearance. The patient has a right to know the identity and function of every person entering his or her room. The phlebotomist should then describe the upcoming procedure to the patient in simple terms. He or she should also attempt to carry on a conversation with the patient while performing the blood collection. Hopefully, this conversation will distract the patient from the blood collection process. Conversation usually helps a nervous patient relax. When the venipuncture is complete, the phlebotomist should make certain that no materials have been left on the patient's bed or table. When the procedure is completed, the phlebotomist should thank the patient before leaving the room.

Many patients are apprehensive about the blood collection process and have questions for the phlebotomist. The phlebotomist should answer all questions as truthfully as possible while at the same time minimizing patients' fears. If patients ask if the collection process will hurt, the phlebotomist should tell the truth and say they may feel slight discomfort. If patients ask why their blood is being drawn, the proper response is that their physician ordered the test(s) as part of the patients' treatment. If patients desire more information, they should be instructed to speak to their doctor.

Special Situations

Occasionally a phlebotomist may encounter a patient situation that is out of the ordinary. The phlebotomist must be prepared to handle these situations without jeopardizing the patient or the integrity of the specimen. The following discussion highlights some common special situations that a phlebotomist might encounter.

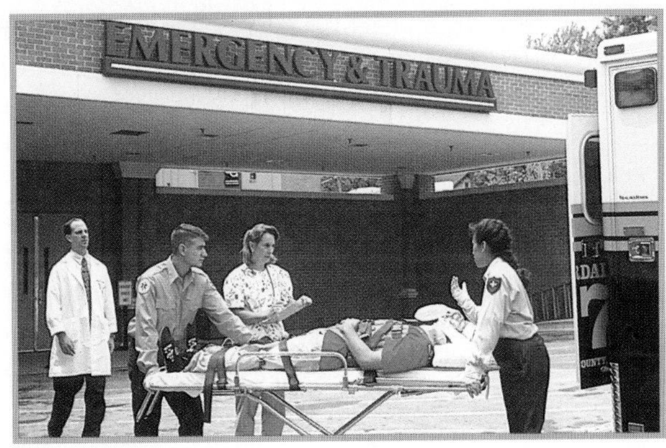

Figure 5-5
While performing a venipuncture on a patient in the emergency room, the phlebotomist may encounter many problems.

No Identification Band on Inpatient

A phlebotomist must never draw blood from an inpatient without an identification band. If the ID band is missing, the phlebotomist should find the nurse to identify the patient and have an ID band placed on the patient prior to drawing the specimen. If it is not possible to attach the identification band to the patient, a nurse can identify the patient. The phlebotomist should write the nurse's name and the fact that the patient was identified by the nurse on the requisition.

Unconscious Patient

If the patient is unconscious, the phlebotomist should check the ID band and compare it with the requisition. The phlebotomist should never rely on the patient name posted on the room door or bed frame, because that information is often incorrect. Unconscious patients should be treated in the same manner as conscious patients. The phlebotomist greets the unconscious patient and describes the blood collection process in the normal manner. Unconscious patients may be aware of their surroundings even if they do not appear to be.

Patient in the Emergency Room

While performing a venipuncture on a patient in the emergency room, the phlebotomist may encounter many problems (see figure 5-5). The patient may be unconscious and not have an identification band. In addition, the identity of the patient may be unknown to emergency room personnel. Each facility has its own protocol for identifying unknown emergency room patients. Many hospitals rely on a temporary ID band. The temporary ID band usually has a number on it. That number should appear on the requisition and all patient specimens. In addition, emergency rooms may be extremely chaotic at times. Phlebotomists who work in emergency rooms must be able to perform their duties quickly and accurately while many times working under extremely stressful conditions.

The Sleeping Patient

The phlebotomist should gently wake the sleeping patient before beginning the blood collection process; blood collection should never be attempted on a sleeping patient as shown in figure 5-6. The patient may wake with a sudden movement and could harm himself or herself or the phlebotomist. The patient will need a few minutes to orient himself or herself before the phlebotomist begins the collection process.

Patient out of the Room

If the blood specimen does not have to be drawn at a specific time, the phlebotomist may return later to collect the specimen. If it is important that the specimen be drawn at a specific time, the phlebotomist should check with the floor secretary to determine the location of the patient. Many patients receive therapy in other hospital areas, such as physical therapy or radiology, as part of their treatment plan. The phlebotomist may have to go to these areas to find the patient. It may be possible to perform the specimen collection there. If it is not possible to collect the specimen, the phlebotomist must note that on the requisition.

Visitor with the Patient

If a patient has a visitor, the phlebotomist must use his or her best judgment to decide if the visitor should remain in the room. If the phlebotomist senses that the visitor will make the patient more nervous or apprehensive, then it is appropriate to politely ask the visitor to wait outside the room. If, however, it appears that the visitor's presence calms the patient, the visitor may remain in the room during the procedure. If the patient is a child, it is usually helpful to have the visitor remain in the room with the child.

Pediatric Patient

The child's age determines how the phlebotomist will handle the situation. If the child is old enough to understand the procedure, the phlebotomist should briefly explain the procedure in simple terms to the child and the accompanying adult as shown in figure 5-7. Proper preparation of the child should help reduce the child's anxiety and increase cooperation. More information on the pediatric patient can be found in chapter 9.

Patient Refusal

A phlebotomist occasionally encounters patients who refuse to have a venipuncture. The phlebotomist should try to determine the reason for the patients' resistance to the procedure and attempt to relieve their fears about blood collection. If the patients state that they do not want their blood drawn, the phlebotomist may gently remind them that the laboratory tests were ordered by their physician as part of their care. The phlebotomist must never force a patient to undergo a venipuncture but should report this development to the nursing staff and write on the requisition that the patient refused to consent. The phlebotomist must never draw blood against a patient's wishes. (See the Patient's Bill of Rights in chapter 3.)

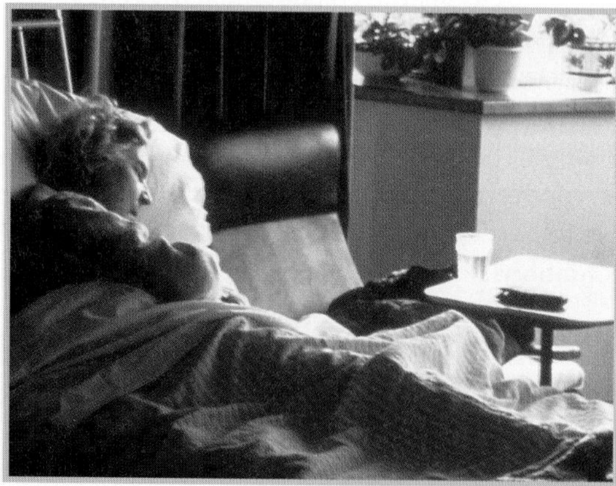

Figure 5-6
The phlebotomist should gently wake the sleeping patient before beginning the blood collection process; blood collection should never be attempted on a sleeping patient.

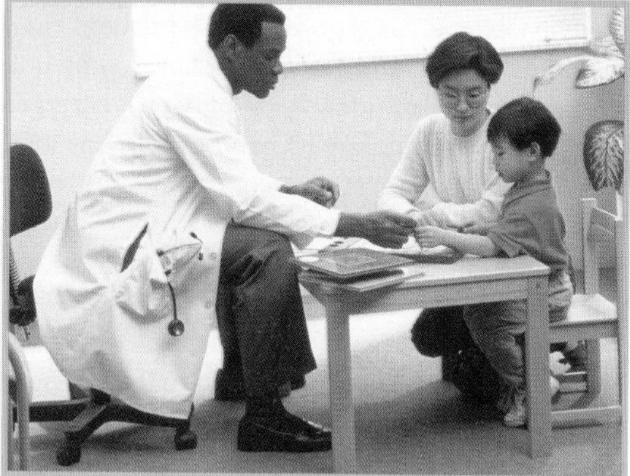

Figure 5-7
If the child is old enough to understand the procedure, the phlebotomist should briefly explain the procedure in simple terms.

CHAPTER REVIEW

Summary

There is much more to being a phlebotomist than perfecting the technique of performing venipunctures. A phlebotomist must follow the proper protocol to ensure that the appropriate specimen is drawn and identified correctly. The patient should be informed about the impending venipuncture not only to ensure their cooperation but also to ease their concerns. In addition, a phlebotomist must be prepared to deal in a professional manner with situations that are out of the ordinary.

Competency Review

1. What is the proper procedure if the requisition and the patient identification band do not match?
2. Why is it necessary to know the name of the phlebotomist who drew the blood specimen?
3. Discuss one procedure for labeling specimens from an unidentified patient in the emergency room.
4. Why is it important to correctly identify a patient's specimen?
5. How can a phlebotomist gain a patient's trust?

Examination Review Questions

1. **Which of the following is not required on a requisition?**
   (A) patient identification number
   (B) date of specimen
   (C) address of patient
   (D) physician's name
   (E) ordered tests

2. **If the requisition and the patient identification band do not match exactly, the phlebotomist should**
   (A) rely on the requisition
   (B) rely on the identification band
   (C) rectify the problem before drawing the specimen
   (D) refuse to draw the specimen and return the next day
   (E) change either requisition so it matches the patient identification band

3. **If a phlebotomist finds the patient sleeping, the proper procedure is to**
   (A) wake the patient before drawing the sample
   (B) return when the patient awakes
   (C) draw the sample as quietly as possible without waking the patient
   (D) note on the requisition that the patient was sleeping and return the next day
   (E) stay in the patient's room until the patient wakes up

4. **Blood is the most common specimen analyzed in the clinical laboratory because**
   (A) blood is easily collected
   (B) everyone has excess blood for testing
   (C) laboratory instruments are based on analyzing blood
   (D) analysis of blood can give the patient's physician a great deal of information
   (E) it is inexpensive to analyze blood

5. **If a patient does not have an identification band**
   (A) ask the patient his or her name
   (B) rely on the name posted on the bed
   (C) rely on the name posted outside the patient room
   (D) seek assistance from the floor nurse
   (E) use the name on the requisition

6. **The patient's identification number is**
   (A) his or her location in the hospital
   (B) always the same as his or her Social Security number
   (C) his or her date of birth
   (D) a unique number the hospital assigns to each patient
   (E) a number the patient selects

7. **If a phlebotomist misidentifies a patient**
   (A) the specimen will only be discarded if it was difficult to obtain
   (B) the specimen will be relabeled
   (C) the consequences can be very serious
   (D) the patient probably gave the phlebotomist the wrong name
   (E) the phlebotomist should tell the floor nurse

8. **Outpatient identification can be established by all of the following except**
   (A) looking at the identification band
   (B) asking the patient for his or her requisition
   (C) asking the patient to spell his or her name
   (D) asking the patient for his or her birth date
   (E) asking the patient for his or her Social Security number

9. **If a patient asks the phlebotomist a question about the procedure, the phlebotomist should**
   (A) always lie to the patient
   (B) answer truthfully
   (C) tell the patient to ask the nurse
   (D) demonstrate the procedure
   (E) pretend not to know the answer

10. **If a patient refuses to have his or her blood drawn, the first thing a phlebotomist should do is to**
   (A) tell the patient's physician
   (B) tell the floor nurse
   (C) leave the patient's room and write "patient refused" on the requisition
   (D) try to alleviate the patient's fear
   (E) draw the specimen anyway

Getting Connected

Multimedia Extension Activities

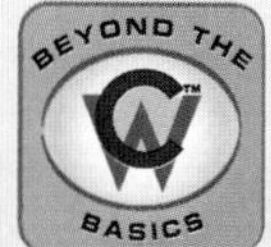

www.prenhall.com/fremgen

Use the address above to access the free, interactive Companion Website created specifically for this textbook. Enhance your studying by answering practice quiz questions, with hints and instant feedback related to chapter 5. If you would like to gain a deeper understanding of selected topics within this chapter, be sure to click on the **Beyond the Basics** feature, which provides more details for further learning. If you do not have a web connection, you may use the CD-ROM enclosed in the back of this book to take advantage of the same features off-line.

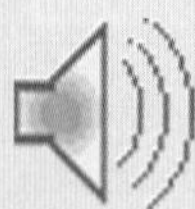

Audio Glossary

Use the CD-ROM enclosed with your textbook to hear the pronunciation of the key terms in the chapter. You may also access this material on the Companion Website www.prenhall.com/fremgen.

Bibliography

Farber, V. "Pediatric Phlebotomy." *Advance for Medical Laboratory Professionals,* January 27, 1997, 5–8.

Henry, J. B. *Clinical Diagnosis and Management by Laboratory Methods,* 19th ed. Philadelphia: W. B. Saunders, 1996.

National Committee for Clinical Laboratory Standards. *Procedures for the Collection of Diagnostic Blood Specimens by Venipuncture,* 3rd ed. (document H3-A3). Villanova, Pa.: National Committee for Clinical Laboratory Standards, July 1991.

CHAPTER 6

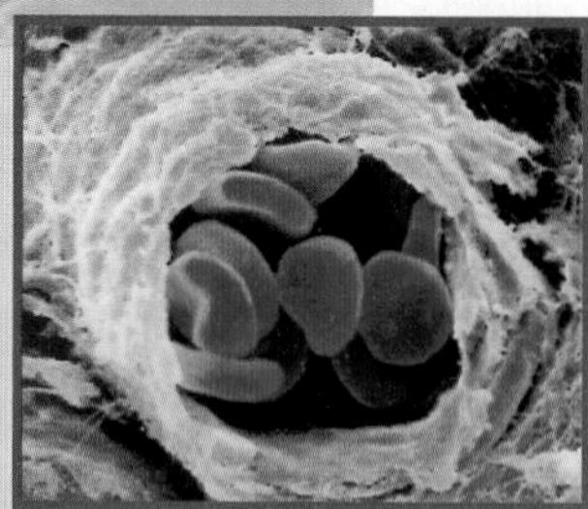

Venipuncture

Chapter Outline

- Introduction
- Equipment
- Evacuated Tube Method
- Winged Infusion (Butterfly) Method
- Syringe Method
- Prepuncture Procedure
- Procedures for Puncturing the Vein
- Postpuncture Procedure
- Multiple Sample Collection
- Summary
- Competency Review
- Examination Review Questions
- Bibliography

Learning Objectives

After completing this chapter, you should be able to

1. Define and spell the glossary terms listed in this chapter.
2. List the supplies usually found on a phlebotomist's blood collection tray.
3. Identify the most common venipuncture sites.
4. Identify alternative sites for venipuncture and describe when they would be used.
5. Explain the decontamination process and the reasons for it.
6. Describe the procedure for venipuncture using the evacuated tube method.
7. List the reasons for using the butterfly method of venipuncture and describe the procedure.
8. List the reasons for using the syringe method of venipuncture and describe the procedure.
9. Describe the procedure for proper disposal of the equipment and supplies used in a venipuncture.
10. Describe the order for filling the evacuated tubes in a multisample collection when using the evacuated tube method and the syringe method.

GLOSSARY

ANTECUBITAL FOSSA area formed at the inside bend of the elbow.

ANTISEPTIC substance used to reduce the bacterial population of the skin.

CANNULA temporary surgical connection between an artery and a vein.

EDEMA an accumulation of fluid in tissues.

EVACUATED TUBE collection tube with a vacuum used in blood collection.

FISTULA an artificial connection between an artery and a vein.

GAUGE diameter or internal size of a needle.

HEMATOMA collection of blood underneath the skin (i.e., bruise).

HEMOCONCENTRATION a condition in which plasma enters the tissues, resulting in a higher than normal concentration of the cellular components of blood.

HEMOLYSIS the destruction of red blood cells.

LANCET sterile, disposable, sharp instrument used in dermal puncture.

LUER ADAPTER a device that tightly connects the syringe to the needle.

LYMPHOSTASIS obstruction of the normal flow of lymph.

PALPATION to examine by touching.

SCLEROSED hard and gnarled.

SUPINE a reclining position on the back with face looking upward.

SYNCOPE sudden loss of consciousness (i.e., fainting).

TOURNIQUET a strap or beltlike device applied to the upper arm to reduce the speed of venous blood flow.

Introduction

In this chapter we take the reader step by step through three different methods of venipuncture. It is important to follow the procedural steps in the proper sequence. Personal protective equipment (PPE) should be used whenever taking a blood sample and working with blood or other body fluids.

Equipment

There are three primary methods of performing a venipuncture:

- Evacuated tube method
- Butterfly method
- Syringe method

The primary drawing equipment varies depending on which method is used. Some general equipment is common to all three methods: disposable gloves, needles, puncture-resistant disposable container (sharps container), **tourniquets** (a strap or beltlike device applied to the upper arm to reduce the speed of venous blood flow), **antiseptic** (substance used to reduce the bacterial population of the skin), sterile gauze pads, and bandages. The evacuated tube method uses vacuum tubes with rubber stoppers and holders for the tubes and needles. The butterfly method requires the use of a winged infusion set, and the syringe method requires a disposable plastic or glass sterile syringe (disposable syringes are commonly used) and needles.

Disposable Gloves

The Centers for Disease Control and Prevention (CDC) strongly recommends that gloves be worn when a health care worker risks coming in contact with any body fluid. Disposable, nonsterile latex gloves are recommended for phlebotomists. Latex appears to offer better protection against bloodborne pathogens than vinyl. For individuals who are sensitive to latex, liners made of cotton or nylon are available. Gloves must always be changed between patients.

Needles

Venipuncture needles have a beveled point, shaft, lumen, and hub. Needles penetrate the skin very easily due to the beveled point and the silicon-coated shaft. The bevel of the needle should be visually inspected for any irregularities before use. The lumen of the needle is the internal core of the needle, and the hub is the end that attaches to the collection system. Venipuncture needles are disposable and come wrapped in sterile, single-unit containers. The containers are sealed and will remain sterile as long as the seal is not broken. Single-sample and multisample needles are available. Single-sample needles are to be used when only one evacuated tube is to be drawn. Multisample needles should be used when more than one evacuated tube is required. They have a rubber sleeve that covers the short end of the needle when the tube is being changed and prevents blood from leaking into the needle holder.

Needles are identified by their length and their **gauge** (diameter or internal bore). The higher the gauge number, the smaller the diameter of the needle. For example, a 21- to 23-gauge needle is used for children with small veins, and a 17-gauge needle is used to draw a unit of blood for transfusion. The typical needle for venipuncture on an adult is a 20- to 22-gauge needle that is 1 to 1 1/2 inches long.

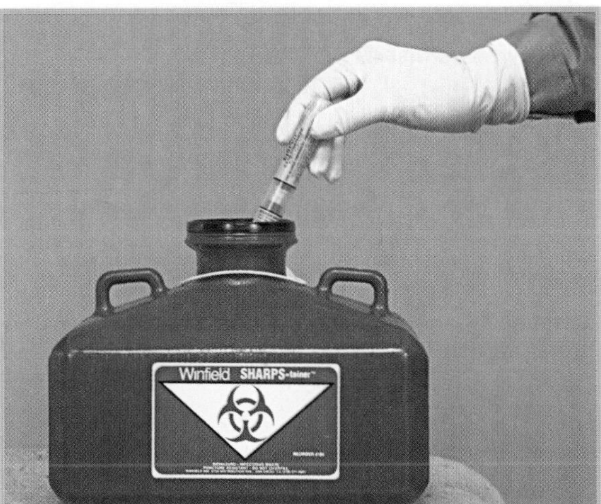

Figure 6-1
An example of a sharps container.

Recently, manufacturers have developed safety needles that protect the phlebotomist from needle stick injuries. One example is a needle that automatically covers after the completion of the venipuncture. Some states are requiring that only these needles be used in an effort to reduce the number of needle stick injuries to health care personnel.

Disposable needles, **lancets** (sterile, disposable sharp instrument used in dermal puncture), and any other sharp objects must always be disposed of in a sharps container. A sharps container is a leak-proof, puncture-resistant container for safe disposal of sharp objects. The top of a sharps container has a device in which the needle can be safely unscrewed from the holder. Sharps containers are usually made of bright orange or red plastic and are identified with a biohazard label. See figure 6-1 for an example of a sharps container. Before beginning a venipuncture, the phlebotomist should note the location of the sharps container. Sharps containers may be carried on the phlebotomist's tray, attached to the wall of the patient's room, or placed on the counter with the venipuncture equipment in a drawing station.

MED TIP

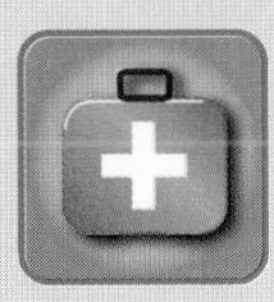

Needles should never be cut, bent, or manually recapped before disposal.

Tourniquets

Tourniquets are straps or beltlike devices that are applied tightly to the upper arm during venipuncture. The tourniquet should be tight enough to reduce the speed of venous blood flow but have no effect on arterial blood flow. As the venous blood flow is slowed, the veins become more prominent and easier to **palpate.** Palpation is the process of examination by touch. Tourniquets are applied 3 to 4 inches above the **antecubital fossa.** The antecubital fossa is the area formed at the inside bend of the elbow. Several types of tourniquets are available, each with advantages and disadvantages. Simple latex straps are frequently used. These flat straps are inexpensive and disposable but may be difficult to apply while wearing gloves. Velcro straps are easier to apply than the latex straps but are more expensive. If they become contaminated with blood, they are extremely difficult to clean and usually must be discarded. A new type of tourniquet has a buckle similar to a seat belt buckle. When using this type of tourniquet, the phlebotomist can slowly release the pressure or quickly reapply pressure; however, it is also difficult to clean if it becomes contaminated with blood. A blood pressure cuff may also be used as a tourniquet. The pressure should be maintained midway between the patient's systolic and diastolic reading.

Antiseptics

Antiseptics are substances that are used to reduce the bacterial population of (disinfect) the skin. Antiseptics are used for two reasons:

1. To reduce the risk of skin bacteria causing an infection at the puncture site
2. To prevent skin bacteria from contaminating the blood sample

The most commonly used antiseptics are 70 percent isopropyl alcohol, usually found as prepackaged single-use wipes, and povidone-iodine.

Sterile Gauze Pads and Bandages

Sterile gauze pads and bandages are also used in blood collection. Sterile 2 × 2 gauze pads can be folded and used to apply pressure to puncture sites. Once bleeding has stopped, a bandage is applied to the site. Many times the bandage is placed over the folded gauze pad to form a pressure bandage. Sometimes sterile cotton is used in place of the gauze pad, but many phlebotomists find that the tiny cotton fibers may interfere with the adhesion of the bandage.

Venipuncture usually takes place at a blood-drawing station or in a hospital room. A blood-drawing station may be a freestanding center not associated with a hospital where patients have their blood drawn for testing at a commercial laboratory or it may be an area of the hospital where outpatients have their blood drawn. A phlebotomist usually carries blood-drawing equipment to the patient's room in a blood collection tray as shown in figure 6-2.

Figure 6-2
A blood collection tray.

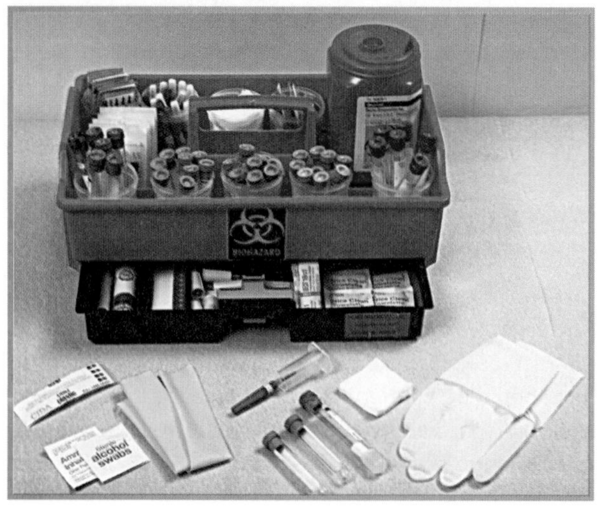

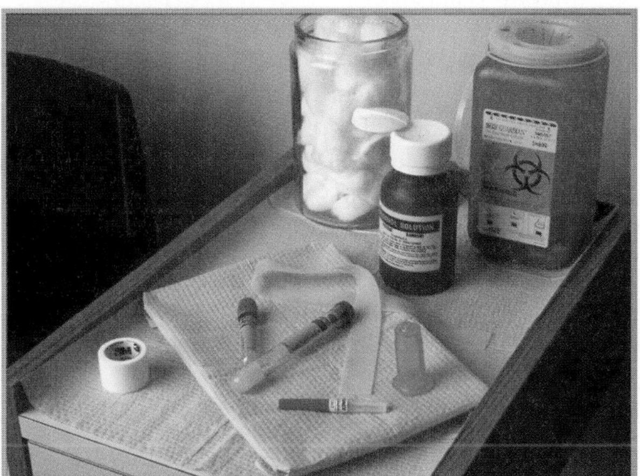

Figure 6-3
A typical blood-drawing station.

A blood collection tray is used to carry the venipuncture equipment from one patient room to the next. These trays are lightweight and should be made of a material that can be disinfected. The trays can also be divided into numerous compartments to help the phlebotomists organize their equipment. If blood collection is taking place in a blood-drawing center or an outpatient facility, supplies are usually kept on a countertop within easy reach of the venipuncture chair. Figure 6-3 depicts a typical blood-drawing station.

Evacuated Tube Method

The evacuated tube method is the most commonly used method of venipuncture. The equipment used in this method is depicted in figure 6-4. It consists of three main components:

- Needle
- Holder
- Vacuum tube with a rubber stopper

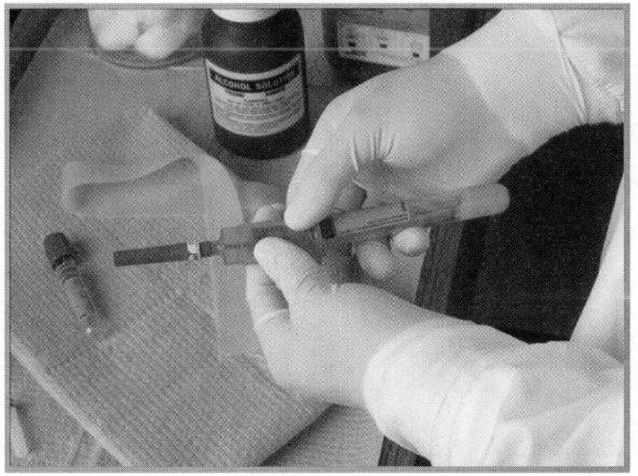

Figure 6-4
Equipment used in the evacuated tube method.

One of the main advantages of the evacuated system is that blood for many different tests can be collected with only one venipuncture. Many different manufacturers sell an evacuated tube system. To avoid problems, all components should be from the same manufacturer.

The evacuated tube system needle has sharp points at both ends and threads in the middle. The longer point enters the vein, and the shorter end punctures the rubber stopper on the evacuated tube. The threads permit the needle to screw securely into the needle holder. There are two types of evacuated tube system needles: single draw and multidraw. Single-draw needles are used when only one evacuated tube of blood is needed. Multidraw needles are used when multiple tubes of blood must be drawn at the same time. A multidraw needle has a plastic sleeve over the shorter end that punctures the evacuated tube. The plastic sleeve prevents blood from dripping into the holder as the tubes are being changed.

Needle Holders

Needle holders, sometimes called adapters, have a small threaded opening at one end for the needle and a large opening at the other end for the evacuated tube. Holders are made of plastic and do not have to be changed between patients as long as they are not contaminated with blood. If the holder becomes contaminated, it may be disinfected or discarded. The larger end of the holder has extensions on both sides that are used to steady the system when changing tubes. Holders come in two sizes: the small size is to hold pediatric-sized evacuated tubes, and the larger size accommodates adult-sized tubes. Manufacturers have begun to market disposable holders that will safely resheath needles, as shown in figure 6-5.

Evacuated collection tubes contain a vacuum. As the needle punctures the vein, the vacuum draws the blood from the vein into the tube. This creates a closed system and limits the phlebotomist's exposure to blood. The vacuum on the tube is guaranteed by the manufacturer until the expiration date, but occasionally the vacuum dissipates earlier. If the tube no longer contains a vacuum, blood will not flow into the tube even if the needle is in the vein. Thus phlebotomists always have extra evacuated tubes on the blood collection tray. Adult-sized evacuated tubes vary in the length of the tube so the total volume of blood drawn can range from 2 to 15 mL. Most evacuated tubes are sterile, and many are coated with silicon. The silicon coating prevents blood from sticking to the inner surface of the tube and helps prevent red blood cell **hemolysis,** or the destruction of red blood cells.

Figure 6-5
Disposable holders that will safely resheath needles. (Becton Dickinson VACUTAINER Systems)

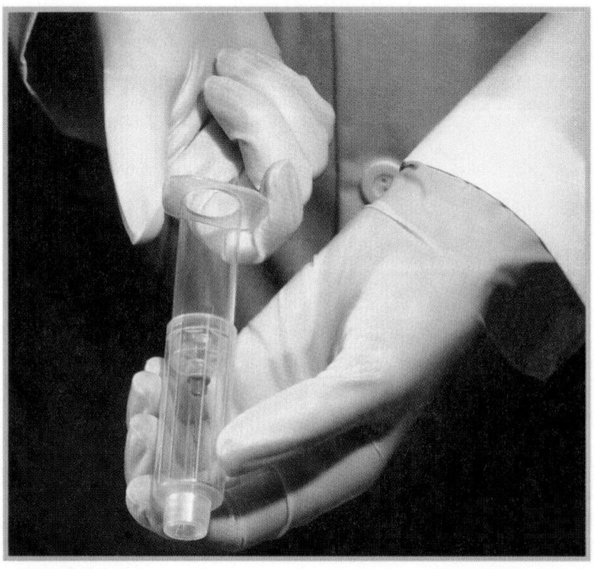

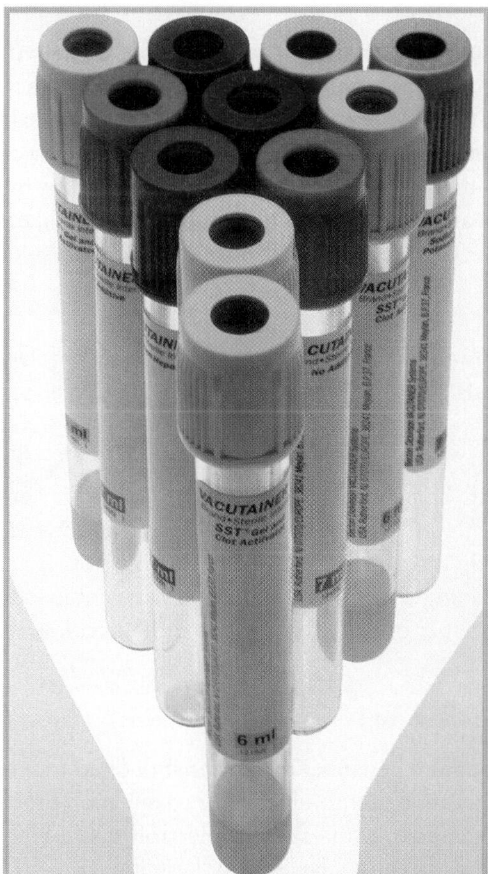

Figure 6-6
Examples of many of the different types of evacuated tubes. (Becton Dickinson VACUTAINER Systems.)

Evacuated Tubes

Examples of many of the different types of evacuated tubes are found in figure 6-6. Evacuated tubes can have two different types of stoppers. One type is a thick rubber stopper, and the other is a plastic cap that covers the stopper. The plastic cap helps prevent the specimen from splattering when the tube is opened. Both types of stoppers are color coded as to the type of additive found in the tube. The additives are usually either an anticoagulant or a preservative. Anticoagulants prevent blood from clotting and are used when blood plasma is required for testing. There are many different types of anticoagulants, and the choice of anticoagulants depends on the ordered laboratory test. Preservatives will slow the metabolic activity of blood cells and keep various blood constituents stable.

Lavender Tubes

Tubes with lavender-colored stoppers contain sodium or potassium ethylenediaminetetraacetic acid (EDTA). EDTA is an anticoagulant that prevents blood from clotting by binding calcium, and it also prevents platelet aggregation (clumping). Most hematology tests, such as a complete blood count (CBC), require an EDTA specimen because EDTA also preserves the shapes of blood cells.

Light Blue Tubes

Tubes with light blue stoppers are used for coagulation studies. These tubes contain the anticoagulant sodium citrate, which also prevents coagulation by binding calcium. EDTA cannot be used for coagulation studies because it affects coagulation factor V, one of the proteins involved in coagulation. It is always important to fill evacuated tubes completely, but it is even more important for coagulation studies. The ratio of sodium citrate to blood in the typical adult-sized tube should be 4.5 mL of blood to 0.5 mL of anticoagulant, or 9 parts blood to 1 part anticoagulant. If the tube does not fill completely, the ratio of blood to anticoagulant will be incorrect, which may affect coagulation test results.

Black Tubes

Tubes with black stoppers also contain sodium citrate, but the ratio of blood to anticoagulant is 4:1 instead of the 9:1 ratio found in blue stoppered tubes. This greater ratio is needed for the Westergren sedimentation rate.

Gray Tubes

Tubes with gray stoppers contain both an anticoagulant and a cell preservative. They may contain either potassium oxalate and sodium fluoride or lithium iodoacetate and heparin. The additives inhibit the glycolytic activity of cells, which helps maintain the glucose level for a minimum of 24 hours. Blood alcohol levels should be drawn in tubes containing sodium fluoride, which also inhibits bacterial growth. Some bacteria produce alcohol as a by-product of metabolism, and if the bacteria were permitted to grow, they would alter the alcohol test result.

Green Tubes

Tubes with green stoppers contain either sodium heparin, lithium heparin, or ammonium heparin. Heparin prevents coagulation by inhibiting the action of thrombin in the coagulation process. These tubes are used for various chemistry tests that require plasma such as electrolyte and blood urea nitrogen (BUN) assays. Specimens collected with heparin cannot be used for hematology slides because the heparin interferes with the hematology stain. Sodium heparin cannot be used for electrolyte evaluation, and lithium heparin should not be used to determine blood lithium levels.

Dark Blue Tubes

Tubes with dark blue stoppers are either anticoagulant free or contain the anticoagulant sodium heparin or disodium EDTA. These tubes and stoppers are chemically cleaned to avoid any stray traces of materials. Dark blue–topped tubes are used for toxicology studies, trace metal assays, and nutritional analysis.

Brown Tubes

Tubes with brown stoppers contain heparin and are chemically cleaned and certified to contain less than 0.1µg/mL lead. These tubes are used to determine lead levels in cases of suspected lead poisoning.

Yellow Tubes

Tubes with yellow stoppers are sterile tubes containing sodium polyanetholesulfonate (SPS). These evacuated tubes are used to draw blood for the microbiology laboratory, where the blood will be cultured for bacteria. SPS is an anticoagulant that also protects bacteria from the effects of the antibacterial properties of blood.

Red Tubes

A number of different colored stoppered tubes do not contain an anticoagulant and yield serum. Tubes with red tops do not contain any additives and are referred to as plain tubes. These tubes are used for

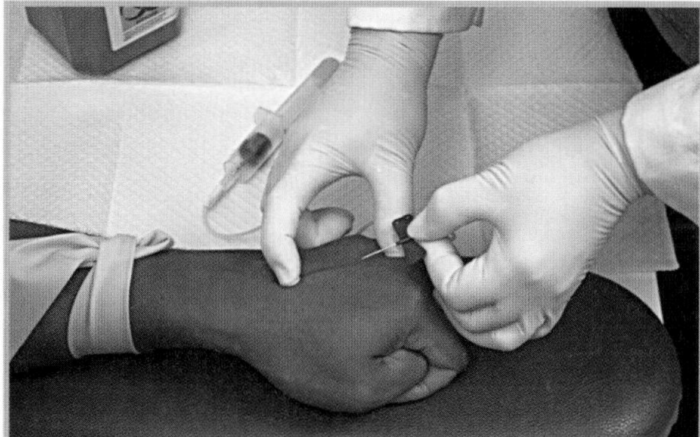

Figure 6-7
An example of a butterfly set.

serology tests, serum chemistry tests, and in the blood bank for blood typing when both cells and serum are needed. Many evacuated tubes contain clot activators that speed up the clotting process. Clot activators are substances that increase platelet activation and include silica, celite, and glass particles. Another additive that may be found in serum tubes is a gel-like substance that forms a barrier between the cells and serum on centrifugation. These tubes are referred to as serum separator tubes (SSTs). The colors of the stoppers for tubes with clot activators and serum separators may be red and gray (commonly referred to as speckled or tiger striped) or gold.

Winged Infusion [Butterfly] Method

A winged infusion set, commonly called a butterfly, is used to establish intravenous (IV) lines or to draw blood from small veins. An example of a butterfly set is shown in figure 6-7. The winged infusion set is composed of a needle with two plastic extensions (thus the name butterfly) attached to a long plastic tube. The typical butterfly needle is a 23-gauge needle and 1/2 to 3/4 inch long. The end of the plastic tubing is usually fitted with a **Luer adapter** (a device that connects the needle to the blood collection container) that can attach to either a syringe or an evacuated tube. The small needle and the extensions permit the lower angle of entry needed to puncture smaller veins. Some manufacturers are making a safer butterfly needle in which the needle is automatically covered on withdrawal from the vein. These safety needles will help reduce the incidence of needle stick injuries.

Syringe Method

Syringes are used to collect blood from small or weak veins that might collapse under the pressure exerted by an evacuated tube. The syringe method of venipuncture uses a single sample needle, syringe, and evacuated tubes (see figure 6-8). Syringe needles vary in length and gauge the same as evacuated tube needles. The difference is that these needles are not double pointed and are designed to attach to the tip of the syringe. Syringes used for venipuncture range in size from 2 to 20 mL and are packaged as single-use, disposable, sterile units. A syringe consists of the barrel and a plunger. An example of a syringe is found in figure 6-9. The needle screws into the threads on the tip of the barrel. When the vein is entered, the plunger is pulled back and a vacuum is created within the barrel. This vacuum pulls the blood from the vein into the barrel of the syringe. After the specimen is drawn, the blood is transferred to the appropriate evacuated tube by piercing the stopper with the syringe needle. The vacuum in the tube will pull the blood from the syringe into the tube.

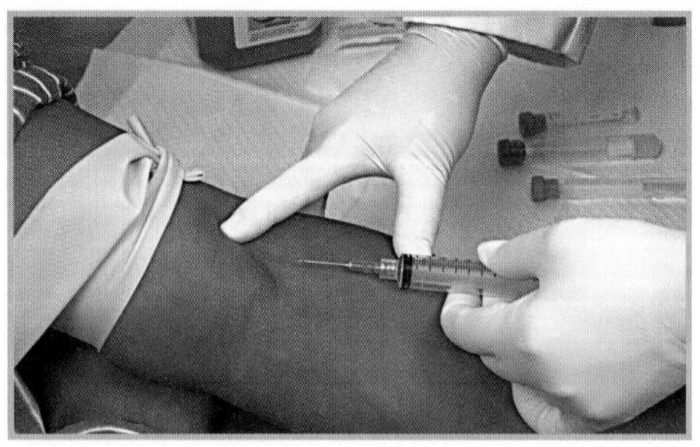

Figure 6-8
The syringe method of venipuncture uses a single sample needle, syringe, and evacuated tubes.

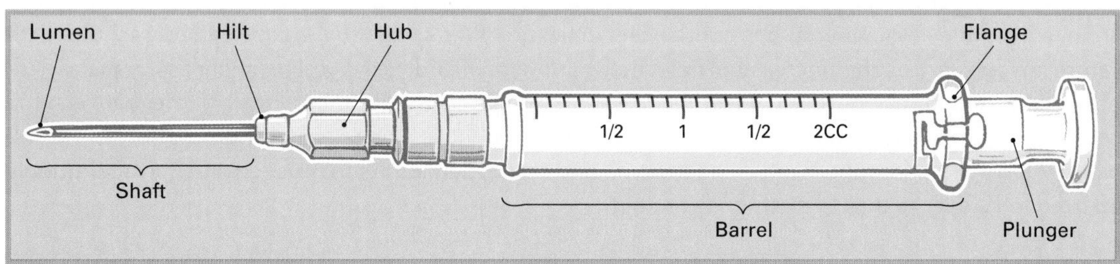

Figure 6-9
An example of a syringe.

Prepuncture Procedure

All venipunctures begin with a physician's requisition ordering that blood be drawn on a patient for specific laboratory tests. Once the requisition is received, it is the responsibility of the phlebotomist to ensure that all of the required equipment is either on the phlebotomy tray or within easy reach of the venipuncture chair. It is imperative that a phlebotomist not begin a venipuncture and then realize that equipment is missing. In fact, most phlebotomists have several of the same evacuated tubes close at hand. Sometimes the vacuum in the tube has dissipated and a fresh tube is necessary to collect the specimen. Requisitions are more fully discussed in chapter 5.

Patient Preparation for Venipuncture

Preparing the patient for the venipuncture is the next step in the process. The phlebotomist should greet the patient and identify himself or herself to the patient. The phlebotomist then must carefully check the patient's identification, as discussed in chapter 5. After the identification process is complete, the phlebotomist will then safely position the patient for the procedure. A hospitalized patient usually requires very little positioning other than to straighten the patient's arm. A towel or pillow may be placed under the arm to keep it from moving during the procedure. If it is necessary to lower a bed rail to have easier access to the patient, it is important to remember to return the bed rail to the original position after the procedure is completed.

Outpatients are usually either seated in a venipuncture chair or reclining on a lounge or examination table. Venipuncture chairs have armrests to support the patient's extended arm. There is also a strap or belt to hold the patient in the chair if he or she feels faint. In some models, the armrest is used to restrain the patient in the chair. Some patients may tell the phlebotomist that the sight of needles or blood makes them faint. These patients should be placed in a reclining position on their backs with the face upward (**supine**) for venipuncture to prevent injury from the side effect of **syncope** (fainting). Once the patient has been properly positioned, the phlebotomist should refer to the requisition and assemble all of the equipment needed for the procedure.

MED TIP

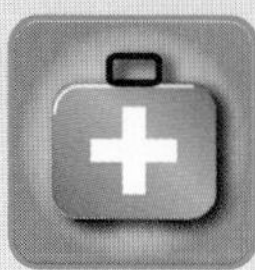

Never perform venipuncture on a patient who is standing or sitting on a stool due to the possible side effect of fainting (syncope).

Tourniquet Application

A tourniquet is a tightly applied band or strap that increases pressure in the veins of the arm, thereby making them more prominent for easier **palpation** (examine by touching). Tourniquets are placed 3 to 4 inches above the venipuncture site. For proper placement of the tourniquet see figure 6-10. A properly applied tourniquet should feel tight but not painful. Care should be taken not to pinch the patient's skin in the tourniquet or to place it over burns or sores. A tourniquet should be placed on the patient's arm so it can be released by the phlebotomist with one hand because the phlebotomist's other hand will hold the venipuncture equipment steady in the patient's arm.

Tourniquets should never be left on for more than 1 minute or **hemoconcentration** will occur. Hemoconcentration is a condition in which plasma enters the tissues, resulting in a higher than normal concentration of the cellular components of blood. To prevent hemoconcentration, the tourniquet is placed on the patient's arm while the phlebotomist palpates the arm and selects a vein. The tourniquet is then removed while the phlebotomist gloves and assembles the appropriate equipment. The issue of

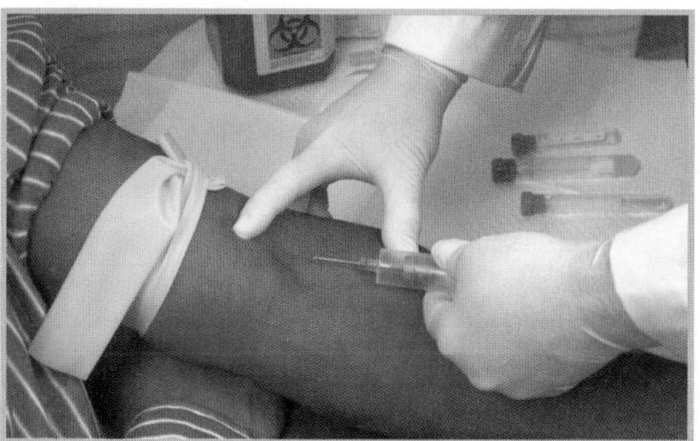

Figure 6-10
A tourniquet should be placed on the patient's arm so it can be released by the phlebotomist with one hand because the phlebotomist's other hand will hold the venipuncture equipment steady in the patient's arm.

when to put on gloves is controversial. Some phlebotomists glove before they apply the tourniquet. Others glove after they have selected the vein because they believe that gloves interfere with the sense of touch and make palpation more difficult. The tourniquet is then reapplied just prior to the phlebotomist beginning the actual venipuncture.

MED TIP

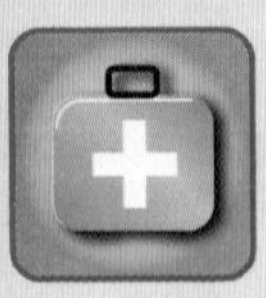

Regardless of when gloves are applied, never begin the actual venipuncture procedure without gloving.

SITE SELECTION

The most common site for a venipuncture is the antecubital fossa of the arm. At this site, three major veins—the cephalic, basilic, and median cubital—lie close to the surface of the skin. (See figure 6-11 for an illustration of the major veins of the arm).

The phlebotomist feels or palpates for the veins by using the index and middle finger and firmly pressing the area. The thumb should not be used for **palpation** because it has a pulse. Most phlebotomists find that applying a tourniquet and having patients clench their fists aids in selecting a vein. Patients should not continually clench and unclench their fists because doing so will cause hemoconcentration. Some experts recommend that patients' fists remain closed until the end of the procedure. Others believe that once blood flow has begun it is no longer necessary to have patients clench their fists. With experience, phlebotomists will decide which method works best for them. Veins should not be selected based on their appearance, but on how they feel on palpation. A good vein for venipuncture should feel firm yet spongy to the touch and should not roll or move when palpated. Once a vein is located, its path should be traced several times with the index finger, so the phlebotomist is familiar with the direction of the vein. Arteries are usually much deeper than veins and will pulsate. Tendons feel like hard, taut ropes. Veins that are hard or **sclerosed** (hard and gnarled) or have **hematomas** (bruises) from previous venipunctures should not be selected. If finding an appropriate site for venipuncture is difficult, applying a warm compress to the area for a few minutes may make the veins more prominent. Several commercial products are available for site warming, but a warm, damp washcloth provides the same effect.

MED TIP

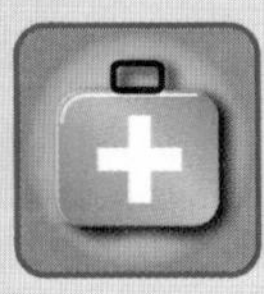

Remember that most patients have two arms. If the veins in the first arm do not appear to be satisfactory, try the patient's other arm.

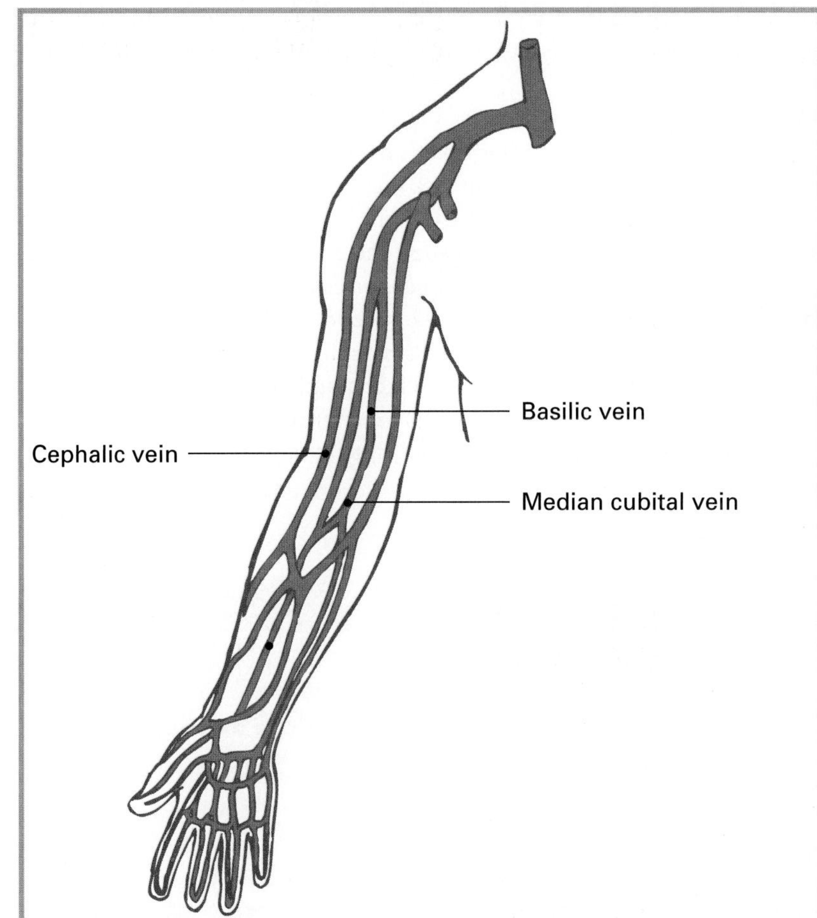

Figure 6-11
Illustration of the arm showing the veins that may be used for venipuncture.

If neither of the patient's arms appears suitable for venipuncture, the veins on the dorsal side of the wrist or hand may be used. These veins are much smaller and tend to roll, so a winged infusion set is the preferred method of drawing blood from the wrist. If the wrist is unsuitable for venipuncture, the veins of the ankle may be examined. Most hospitals require that the phlebotomist check with the patient's physician before using a vein in the foot for venipuncture.

There are other factors to consider in selecting a venipuncture site besides the characteristics of the vein. An area that has extensive scarring or burns should not be selected. If a patient has an IV in one arm, the other arm should be used for blood collection. If the patient has IVs in both arms, blood should be collected from below the IV site. Blood should never be collected from above the IV site because it may provide erroneous test results. If a patient has had a mastectomy, blood should not be drawn from that side because **lymphostasis** (obstruction of the normal flow of lymph), a result of the surgery, may harm the patient and make the specimen unsuitable for testing. Blood should not be drawn from an area that has a hematoma or **edema** (an accumulation of fluid in tissues). Sclerosed veins or those with hematomas are difficult to palpate, and erroneous test results may occur from samples drawn from those areas. If a patient has a **cannula, fistula,** or vascular graft in his or her arm, the phlebotomist must first consult with the patient's physician before drawing blood. A cannula is a temporary surgical connection between an artery and a vein, and a fistula is an artificial connection between an artery and vein. Both may be found in patients who require long-term dialysis or long-term IV medication.

Cleansing the Venipuncture Site

Once an appropriate vein has been selected, the site should be cleansed to reduce the microbial population on the skin. Proper cleansing of the area will reduce the risk that the blood specimen will be contaminated with bacteria. Most hospitals and drawing centers use a commercially prepared alcohol pad that comes in a sterile package. In addition, one may use a gauze pad saturated with 70 percent isopropyl alcohol or 0.5 percent chlorhexidine in alcohol. The site should be cleaned by using a circular motion starting at the center and moving outward with increasingly larger circles. The alcohol should be allowed to air dry because evaporation of the alcohol helps in the disinfecting process. The phlebotomist should not blow on the area to speed drying because doing so will recontaminate the site with bacteria. If the site is punctured while the alcohol is still wet, the patient will experience a burning sensation and the specimen may be hemolyzed. If the phlebotomist finds it necessary to repalpate the site after cleansing, it is important to clean the gloved finger first with alcohol.

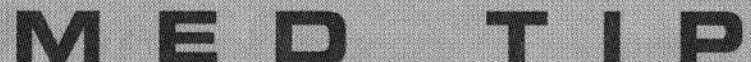

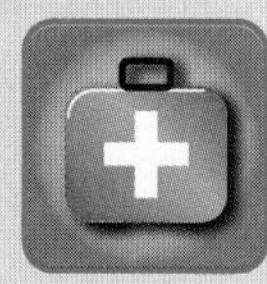

Never blow on the alcohol-prepared site because it will contaminate the area.

Procedures for Puncturing the Vein

Regardless of the method used to perform the venipuncture, all needles should be checked for irregularities before use. If a syringe is to be used, the plunger should move freely within the barrel. The thumb of the nondominant hand should be firmly placed on the selected vein approximately 2 inches below the intended venipuncture site to prevent the vein from rolling or moving during the procedure. It is imperative that the phlebotomist be gloved before beginning to puncture the vein. Some phlebotomists prefer to glove as soon as they enter the patient's room, whereas others glove after the vein has been selected.

Evacuated Tube Method

The phlebotomist breaks the sterility seal on the needle by holding each end in a hand and turning in opposite directions. Once the seal is broken, the shorter plastic sleeve is removed and the needle is threaded into the holder until it is secure. The evacuated tube is inserted into the holder and pushed onto the needle only up to the recessed guideline on the holder. If the tube is pushed past this point, the vacuum in the tube will be broken and blood will not flow into the tube. The phlebotomist should remove the long plastic sleeve and visually examine the bevel of the needle for any irregularities.

Now we will describe the most common method for holding venipuncture equipment, although there are many variations on this method. The tube, holder, and needle assembly are held using the dominant hand by placing the thumb on top, the third and fourth fingers on the bottom of the holder, and the index finger along the needle-holder connection to help guide it. The phlebotomist must make certain that

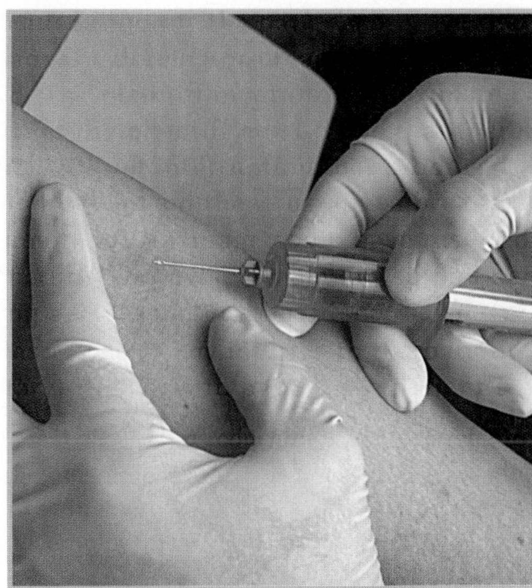

Figure 6-12
The proper angle of the needle insertion.

the bevel of the needle is facing upward and the needle is aligned in the same direction as the vein. At this point, the phlebotomist should warn the patient to expect a small pinch. Holding the needle assembly at a 15- to 30-degree angle directly above the vein, the vein is punctured in one smooth, swift movement. To view the proper angle of the needle insertion, see figure 6-12. The phlebotomist may feel a slight lessening of resistance against the needle once it enters the vein. The angle of insertion depends on the depth of the vein.

MED TIP

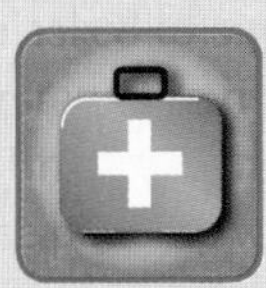

For a shallow vein, use a smaller angle of insertion. For a deeper vein, use a more severe angle of insertion.

The arm and needle assembly must always be held in a downward position so that blood will flow into the bottom of the tube first. This positioning prevents blood from the tube from flowing back into the vein (reflux). Once the phlebotomist believes the needle is in the vein, the nondominant hand may release the anchored vein and grasp the flange of the needle holder. Then the evacuated tube is pushed forward until the end of the needle punctures the stopper. This step requires some pressure, and it is important that the needle does not move deeper into the vein. To prevent deep penetration, the hand holding the needle assembly must hold it very firmly and prevent it from being pushed forward. If the needle has punctured the vein, blood will begin to flow into the evacuated tube. Once blood flow has been established, the patient may be instructed to open his or her fist and the tourniquet should be removed.

Evacuated tubes automatically stop filling when the proper amount of blood has entered the tube, even if the tube does not appear full. Physicians often order multiple tests on their patients, and consequently more than one tube of blood will be needed. Once the first tube is full, the phlebotomist securely holds the needle assembly with one hand and with the other hand removes the full tube using a slight twisting motion and backward pressure. Many phlebotomists find it helpful to push backward on the extension of the holder with their thumb while removing the full tube. If the tube contains an additive, the tube should be inverted gently several times for thorough mixing. The tube should not be shaken rapidly or the specimen may hemolyze. Note: Lavender-topped tubes, which contain EDTA, must be inverted eight to ten times. The next tube is placed in the holder and the process continues until all the required tubes have been filled. It is very important that the needle remain steady during the removal and insertion of the evacuated tubes. If the needle is moved in this process, it may either be pushed all the way through the vein or pulled out of the vein. After all of the tubes have been drawn, the last tube is gently disengaged from the needle before removing the needle from the patient's arm. Failure to do so may cause the patient to feel unnecessary discomfort. The evacuated tube method is described in procedure 6-1.

Winged Infusion (Butterfly) Method

The butterfly method or winged infusion set is used on smaller veins, especially in pediatric patients. The needles used with this method are shorter and have a smaller diameter. The needles range from 1/2 to 3/4 inch long and have a gauge between 21 and 25 versus 1 1/2 inch and 21 gauge for a standard needle used in the evacuated tube method. The shorter needle permits a smaller angle of insertion, making it easier to puncture small veins and less painful for the patient. The winged infusion or butterfly method is fully described in procedure 6-2.

The winged infusion set is removed from its sterile wrapper, and the needle is examined for irregularities. The two winged needle attachments are held together during insertion to guide the needle into the vein. Once the needle is in the vein, a small amount of blood will be seen in the plastic tubing. The opposite end of the tubing is fitted with a Luer adapter that permits the blood to flow into either evacuated tubes or a syringe. Once blood flow has been established, the winged attachments are lowered and flattened against the patient's skin. The attachments help prevent the needle from moving.

It is extremely important to use extra care when disposing of a winged infusion set. Because the needle may dangle from the long plastic tubing, it is strongly recommended that winged infusion sets with resheathing devices be used. These resheathing devices permit the phlebotomist to cover the needle with one hand immediately after it is withdrawn from the vein, thereby preventing a needle stick injury.

MED TIP

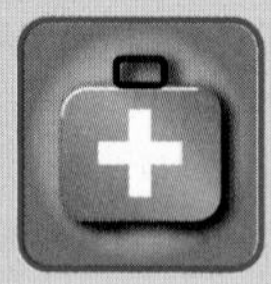

Winged infusion sets can be awkward to handle. Be extra careful in disposing of the set in the sharps container.

PROCEDURE 6•1

VENIPUNCTURE BY THE EVACUATED TUBE METHOD

Purpose:

To collect a venous blood sample that is needed to perform many diagnostic tests.

Terminal Performance Competency:

Perform a venipuncture correctly by using the evacuated tube method.

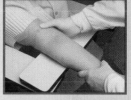

Position patient's arm.

Equipment:

Requisition, gloves, sharps container, alcohol wipes containing 70 percent isopropyl alcohol, sterile cotton balls or sterile gauze, tourniquet, evacuated tubes, needles and tube adapters, bandages, specimen labels, and pen.

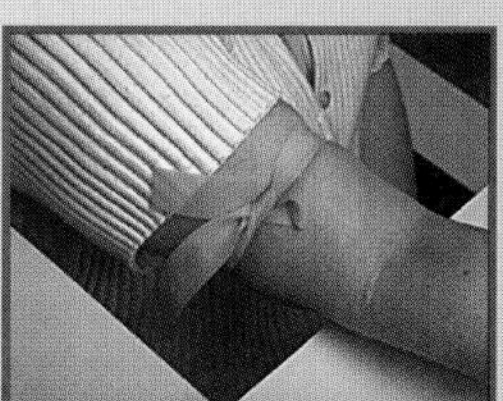

Tie tourniquet above antecubital fossa.

Procedure:

1. Obtain the patient requisition.
2. Greet and identify the patient.
3. Wash hands.
4. Assemble supplies for the ordered laboratory tests.
5. Position patient properly.
6. Apply tourniquet 2 inches above the antecubital fossa.
7. Palpate the veins and select the site for venipuncture.
8. Remove tourniquet. *Rationale: Tourniquet cannot be left on for more than 1 minute or hemoconcentration will occur.*
9. Cleanse site by using an alcohol wipe in a circular motion beginning at the insertion site.
10. Put on disposable gloves (if not done earlier). *Rationale: Protective equipment must be worn when handling blood or body fluids.*
11. Inspect needle and equipment. *Rationale: Always check needles for burrs or irregularities.*
12. Reapply tourniquet and, if the site must be repalpated, wipe your gloved finger with alcohol before retouching the site.

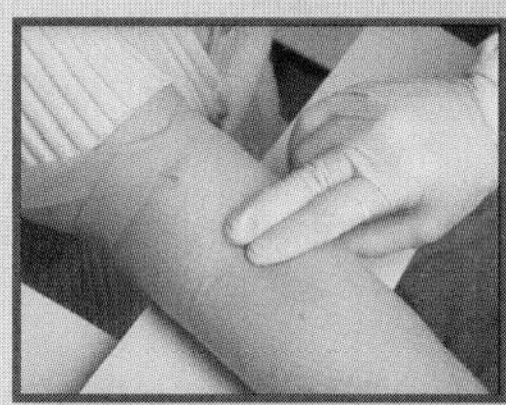

Palpate for vein.

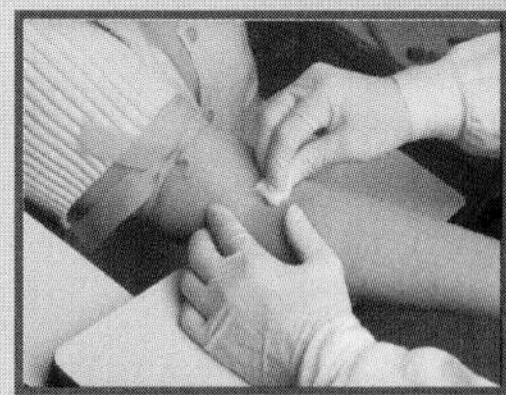

Cleanse the site with antiseptic.

(continued)

PROCEDURE 6•1 *(continued)*

13. Anchor the vein by placing the thumb of the nondominant hand 2 inches below the site and using the fingers of that hand to tightly hold the skin on the back of the arm. *Rationale: The skin is pulled taut to prevent the vein from moving, and the holding finger is placed below the site, not above, to prevent accidentally sticking the finger with the needle.*

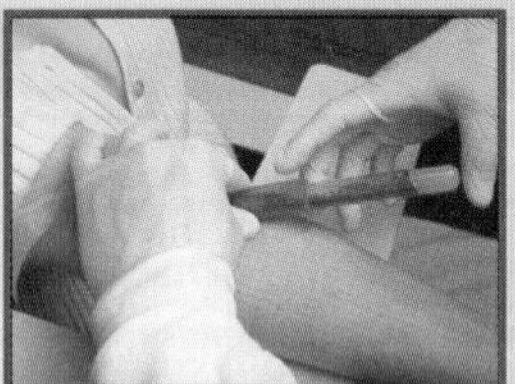

Hold adapter firmly while advancing tube.

14. Using the dominant hand, insert the needle with the bevel up at a 15- to 30-degree angle into the selected vein.
15. Holding the tube adapter firmly, advance the evacuated tube forward until the needle has punctured the rubber stopper.
16. Release the tourniquet as soon as blood flow is established.
17. Carefully remove the tubes when full. *Rationale: The tube will automatically stop filling when the vacuum is gone, leaving the tube approximately three-fourths full.*

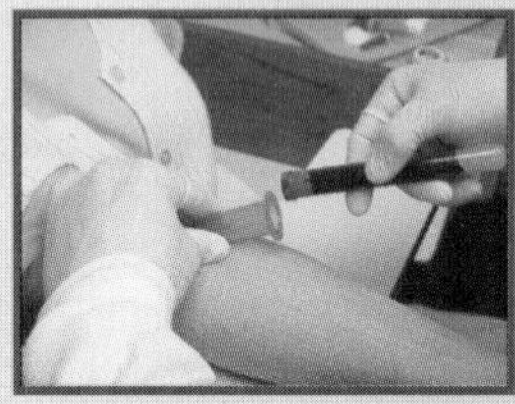

Gently remove the tube without disturbing the needle.

18. Carefully remove the tube without dislodging the needle.
19. Gently mix any tubes with additives as soon as they are removed. *Rationale: Forceful mixing of the tube contents may cause cell lysis.* Note: EDTA tubes must be inverted eight to ten times.
20. If more than one evacuated tube of blood is required, carefully advance the next tube into the adapter until the vacuum is broken by the needle.

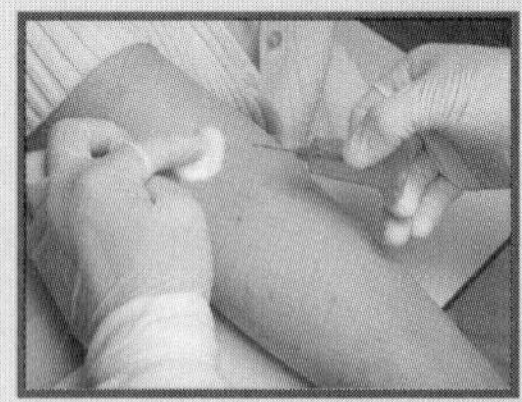

Withdraw the needle.

21. After the last evacuated tube is filled, place sterile gauze gently over the site.
22. Remove the needle.
23. Apply pressure to the site with the sterile gauze. *Rationale: Pressure on the puncture site will help prevent the formation of a hematoma.*

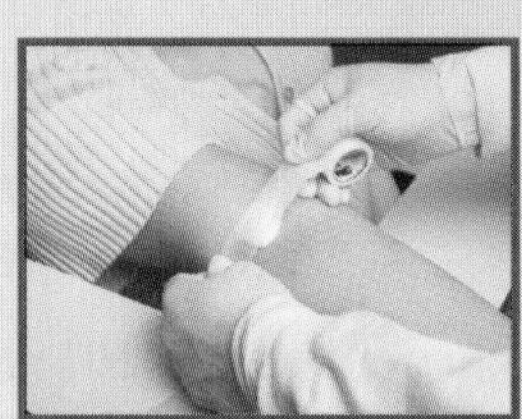

Apply bandage.

24. Carefully dispose of the needle in a sharps container.
25. Check to determine if the patient has stopped bleeding. If he or she has, apply a bandage. If the patient is still bleeding, apply continuous pressure to the site until bleeding has stopped.
26. Remove gloves.
27. Label the tubes with the patient's name and ID number, date, time of collection, and phlebotomist's identification.
28. Check if any of the evacuated tubes require special handling such as being kept cold or placed in the dark.
29. Properly dispose of all trash and contaminated materials in biohazard container.
30. Wash hands.
31. Thank the patient before leaving.

PROCEDURE 6 • 2

VENIPUNCTURE BY WINGED INFUSION (BUTTERFLY) METHOD

Terminal Performance Competency:

Perform a venipuncture correctly by using the butterfly method.

Equipment:

Requisition, gloves, sharps container, alcohol wipes containing 70 percent isopropyl alcohol, sterile cotton balls or sterile gauze, tourniquet, butterfly needle and attached tubing, Luer adapter, evacuated tubes, bandages, specimen labels, and pen.

Procedure:

1. Obtain the patient requisition.
2. Greet and identify the patient.
3. Wash hands.
4. Assemble supplies for the ordered laboratory tests.
5. Position patient properly.
6. Apply tourniquet 2 inches above the antecubital fossa.
7. Palpate the veins and select the site for venipuncture.
8. Remove tourniquet. *Rationale: Tourniquet cannot be left on for more than 1 minute or hemoconcentration will occur.*
9. Cleanse site by using an alcohol wipe in a circular motion beginning at the insertion site.
10. Put on disposable gloves (if not done earlier). *Rationale: Protective equipment must be worn when handling blood or body fluids.*
11. Inspect needle and equipment. *Rationale: Always check needles for burrs or irregularities.*
12. Reapply tourniquet and, if the site must be repalpated, wipe your gloved finger with alcohol before retouching the site.
13. Anchor the vein by placing the thumb of the nondominant hand 2 inches below the site and pulling the skin taut. *Rationale: The skin is pulled taut to prevent the vein from moving, and the holding finger is placed below the site, not above, to prevent accidentally sticking the finger with the needle.*

(continued)

PROCEDURE 6 • 2 *(continued)*

14. Using the dominant hand, hold the winged attachments and insert the needle with the bevel up at a 15- to 30-degree angle into the selected vein.

15. If the needle is in the vein, a small amount of blood will appear in the tubing.

16. Push the evacuated tube onto the Luer adapter, breaking the vacuum in the tube.

17. Flatten the winged attachments against the patient's skin.

18. Release the tourniquet once blood flow is firmly established.

19. Carefully remove the tubes when full. *Rationale: The tube will automatically stop filling when the vacuum is gone, leaving the tube approximately three-fourths full.*

20. Carefully remove the tube without dislodging the needle.

21. Gently mix tubes with additives as directed as soon as they are removed.

22. If more than one evacuated tube of blood is required, carefully push the next tube onto the Luer adapter until the vacuum is broken by the needle.

23. After the last evacuated tube is filled, place sterile gauze gently over the site.

24. Remove the needle.

25. Apply pressure to the site with the sterile gauze. *Rationale: Pressure on the puncture site will help prevent the formation of a hematoma.*

26. Carefully dispose of the needle in a sharps container.

27. Check to determine if the patient has stopped bleeding. If he or she has, apply a bandage. If the patient is still bleeding, apply continuous pressure to the site until bleeding has stopped.

28. Properly dispose of all trash and contaminated material.

29. Remove gloves.

30. Label the tubes with the patient's name and ID number, date, time of collection, and phlebotomist's identification.

31. Check if any of the evacuated tubes require special handling such as being kept cold or placed in the dark.

32. Wash hands.

33. Thank the patient before leaving.

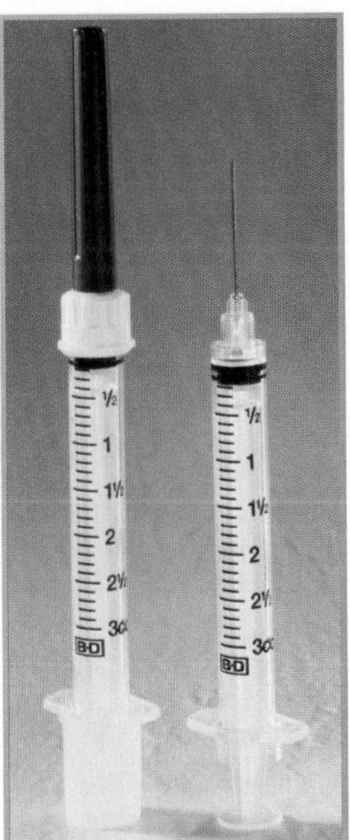

Figure 6-13
A syringe may be used to obtain a venous blood sample on a patient with weak veins. (Courtesy of Becton Dickinson and Company.)

Syringe Method

A syringe is the preferred method of venipuncture for individuals (usually the elderly or infants) with extremely weak veins that may collapse from the pressure of an evacuated tube. By using a syringe, the phlebotomist can control the pressure exerted on the vein, and weaker veins may be punctured without danger of collapse. The phlebotomist begins by removing the needle and syringe from their sterile wrappers and attaching them together. The needle should remain covered until immediately prior to use. The plunger should be drawn back and forth a few times within the barrel of the syringe to ensure that it moves freely and easily. The plunger is then pushed forward (toward the hub of the needle) as far as possible. A needle and syringe are illustrated in figure 6-13.

The phlebotomist anchors and enters the vein as in the evacuated tube method. Blood will appear in the hub of the needle if the vein has been punctured. Pulling back slowly on the plunger draws blood into the syringe. Care must be taken not to pull the plunger back too rapidly because the vein may collapse or the blood may hemolyze in the syringe. Once the appropriate amount of blood has been drawn, the needle and syringe can be withdrawn from the patient's arm.

The blood in the syringe is transferred to an evacuated tube by inserting the needle through the rubber stopper on the tube. The vacuum in the tube will force the blood to flow from the syringe into the tube. The plunger should not be used to push blood from the syringe into the tube because the extra pressure may cause the cells to hemolyze. To prevent needle stick injuries, the evacuated tube should be placed on a rack rather than held while transferring blood from the syringe.

Occasionally more than one syringe of blood must be drawn to fill all of the ordered tests. In this situation, the phlebotomist will need an assistant. After the first syringe is filled, sterile gauze is placed on the patient's arm under the hub of the needle. The syringe is carefully unscrewed and handed to the assistant. A fresh syringe is then screwed onto the needle that has been held steady to prevent movement within the vein. While the second syringe is being filled, the assistant screws a new sterile needle onto the first syringe and fills the appropriate evacuated tubes. This is a difficult procedure and, if possible, should be avoided by using a larger syringe. The syringe method of collection is described in procedure 6-3.

Postpuncture Procedure

After the required amount of blood has been drawn, a gauze square or cotton ball is carefully placed over the venipuncture site and the needle is gently withdrawn from the patient's arm. The phlebotomist immediately applies pressure to the gauze square or cotton ball for 3 to 5 minutes. Pressure should be continually applied to the site until all bleeding has stopped. If the patient is taking anticoagulation medication, it may take longer for the bleeding to stop. If bleeding persists longer than 10 minutes, the nursing staff should be notified. If the patient is able to help, he or she may apply pressure to the site while the phlebotomist completes the procedure. The patient should not bend his or her arm at the elbow because bleeding may recur when the arm is straightened.

To prevent a needle stick injury, all needles should be disposed of promptly into a puncture-resistant container (sharps container). Phlebotomists usually have a sharps container in their phlebotomy tray; however, some hospital rooms have sharps containers attached to the wall. If a syringe was used to draw blood, the entire device (needle and syringe) is disposed of in the sharps container. If a needle does not fall to the bottom of the container but is stuck on the rim, the phlebotomist should use the needle holder rather than his or her hand to knock the needle into the container. If a needle must be resheathed, a one-handed technique should be used.

MED TIP

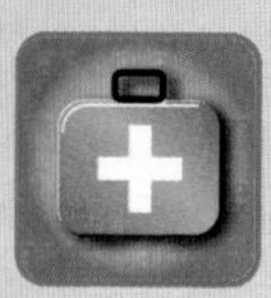

Never bend, cut, or break needles and never remove them from the disposal container.

The newly drawn evacuated tubes should be well mixed and labeled before leaving the patient's bedside or before the patient leaves the outpatient drawing area. Labels may be either computer generated or handwritten. They should contain the patient's name and hospital identification number, date, time of collection, and phlebotomist identification. (See chapter 5 for more information about specimen labels.) The phlebotomist should check to see if any of the evacuated tubes require special handling (i.e., cold or dark).

PROCEDURE 6 • 3

VENIPUNCTURE BY SYRINGE METHOD

Terminal Performance Competency:

Perform a venipuncture correctly by using the syringe method.

Equipment:

Requisition, gloves, sharps container, alcohol wipes containing 70 percent isopropyl alcohol, sterile cotton balls or sterile gauze, tourniquet, syringe, syringe needles, bandages, specimen labels, and pen.

Procedure:

1. Obtain the patient requisition.
2. Greet and identify the patient.
3. Wash hands.
4. Assemble supplies for the ordered laboratory tests.
5. Position patient properly.
6. Apply tourniquet 2 inches above the antecubital fossa.
7. Palpate the veins and select the site for venipuncture.
8. Remove tourniquet. *Rationale: Tourniquet cannot be left on for more than 1 minute or hemoconcentration will occur.*
9. Cleanse site by using an alcohol wipe in a circular motion beginning at the insertion site.
10. Put on disposable gloves (if not done earlier). *Rationale: Protective equipment must be worn when handling blood or body fluids.*
11. Inspect needle. *Rationale: Always check needles for burrs or irregularities.*
12. Assemble needle and syringe and check the syringe by moving the plunger back and forth a few times. Push the plunger forward as far as possible.
13. Reapply tourniquet and, if the site must be repalpated, wipe your gloved finger with alcohol before retouching the site.

(continued)

PROCEDURE 6 • 3 *(continued)*

14. Anchor the vein by placing the thumb of the nondominant hand 2 inches below the site; use the fingers of that hand to tightly hold the skin on the back of the arm and pull the skin taut. *Rationale: The skin is pulled taut to prevent the vein from moving, and the holding finger is placed below the site, not above, to prevent accidentally sticking the finger with the needle.*

15. Using the dominant hand, insert the needle with the bevel up at a 15- to 30-degree angle into the selected vein. Blood will appear in the hub of the needle if the vein has been punctured.

16. Slowly pull back on the plunger to draw the blood into the syringe.

17. Release the tourniquet as soon as blood flow is firmly established.

18. When the syringe is full, place sterile gauze gently over the site.

19. Remove the needle and syringe.

20. Apply pressure to the site with the sterile gauze. *Rationale: Pressure on the puncture site will help prevent the formation of a hematoma.*

21. Transfer the blood in the syringe to the appropriate evacuated tube by inserting the needle through the rubber stopper on the evacuated tube. *Rationale: The vacuum in the tube will force the blood from the syringe into the tube.*

22. Gently mix all evacuated tubes that contain an additive.

23. Carefully dispose of the needle and syringe in a sharps container.

24. Check to determine if the patient has stopped bleeding. If he or she has, apply a bandage. If the patient is still bleeding, apply continuous pressure to the site until bleeding has stopped.

25. Remove gloves.

26. Label the tubes with the patient's name and ID number, date, time, and phlebotomist's identification.

27. Check if any of the evacuated tubes require special handling such as being kept cold or placed in the dark.

28. Properly dispose of all trash and contaminated materials.

29. Wash hands.

30. Thank the patient before leaving.

Before leaving the patient's side, the phlebotomist checks the phlebotomy site and, when the bleeding has stopped, applies tape or an adhesive bandage over the pressure pad. Children under the age of 2 should not get a bandage because they may swallow it. Patients are instructed to leave the bandage on for a minimum of 15 minutes. The phlebotomist must make certain that all materials are properly disposed of and nothing is left on the patient's bed, tray, or nightstand. Contaminated material is placed in a biohazard container; uncontaminated paper and plastic may be placed in the regular trash. If a patient asks for water or has another request, the phlebotomist should tell him or her that the request will be passed on to the nurse. The patient may have restrictions that the phlebotomist is unaware of and complying may inadvertently interfere with the patient's treatment. Before leaving the patient's room, the phlebotomist should thank the patient for his or her cooperation.

Multiple Sample Collection

Many times, blood for multiple tests is drawn at the same time, thereby subjecting the patient to only one venipuncture. The order in which the evacuated tubes are collected is very important. It is possible for additives in one tube to be transferred to the next tube by the end of the needle that punctures the stopper on the evacuated tube. This cross-contamination between additives may cause erroneous test results in the blood specimen. Sterile specimens such as blood cultures are always drawn first, regardless of whether the evacuated tube method or the syringe method is used.

Evacuated Tube Method

The recommended order of draw for the evacuated tube method is as follows:

1. Sterile specimens such as blood culture tubes
2. Nonadditive tubes or serum tubes (red stopper, gel separator)
3. Coagulation tubes or those with citrate (light blue stopper)
4. Heparin tubes (green stopper)
5. Ethylenediaminetetraacetic acid (EDTA) tubes (lavender stopper)
6. Oxalate or fluoride tubes (gray stopper)

Note: If only a tube for coagulation studies (light blue stopper) is needed, a serum tube must be drawn first and then discarded. This technique prevents thromboplastin, a coagulation factor, released during the initial vein puncture from contaminating the needle and interfering with the coagulation tests. The order for a multiple sample draw for blood collected by the winged infusion method is the same because the blood sample is still collected in evacuated tubes.

Syringe Method

When collecting blood with a syringe the order of filling the evacuated tubes differs from that used when collecting blood with the evacuated tube method. Blood may begin to clot as soon as it enters the syringe; therefore, it is important to quickly fill tubes with anticoagulants before serum tubes.

The recommended order of filling the evacuated tubes with blood collected using the syringe method is as follows:

1. Sterile specimens such as blood cultures
2. Coagulation tubes or those with citrate (blue stopper)
3. EDTA tubes (lavender stopper)
4. Heparin tubes (green stopper)
5. Oxalate or fluoride tubes (gray stopper)
6. Serum tubes (red or red and gray stopper)

When filling evacuated tubes with blood drawn in a syringe, no pressure on the plunger is needed. The vacuum in the evacuated tube will cause the blood to flow from the syringe into the tube. Tubes with additives should be gently mixed as soon as they are filled to prevent the specimen from clotting.

CHAPTER REVIEW

Summary

There are currently three methods in use to collect a venous blood sample. The most common method is the evacuated tube method. The winged infusion method is commonly used on children and those with weak or fragile veins. The third method of collection is the syringe method. Phlebotomists must be familiar with the equipment and the procedures for all three methods.

Competency Review

1. Define hemoconcentration and discuss how it can be prevented.
2. Describe five commonly used evacuated tubes and tell when they are used.
3. Describe the order of draw for the evacuated tube method and the syringe method.
4. Explain the difference between the evacuated tube and syringe methods.
5. Explain the reasons for using the butterfly method and syringe method of blood collection.

Examination Review Questions

1. **The primary methods of performing a venipuncture include**
   (A) syringe method
   (B) butterfly method
   (C) evacuated tube method
   (D) finger stick method
   (E) a, b, and c

2. **The preferred method used for cleaning the venipuncture site is with**
   (A) soap and water
   (B) 10 percent isopropyl alcohol
   (C) 70 percent isopropyl alcohol
   (D) zephrin chloride
   (E) betadine

3. **If a venipuncture patient has a cannula already in the vein, the phlebotomist must**
   (A) proceed into the cannula with caution
   (B) ask the patient if other phlebotomists have used the cannula when drawing blood
   (C) go ahead and use the other arm for venipuncture
   (D) consult with the patient's physician before drawing blood
   (E) none of the above

4. **The evacuated tube method for venipuncture is based on the principle that**
   (A) a vacuum is created when the needle is pushed beyond the recessed guideline on the holder
   (B) a vacuum exists in the tube that allows for blood to flow from the patient into the tube
   (C) a syringe must be used to actually enter the vein
   (D) the color of the tube indicates if a vacuum exists within the tube
   (E) the phlebotomist will feel increased resistance against the needle once it enters the vein

5. **If the phlebotomist repalpates the venipuncture site after the initial cleansing**
   (A) the gloved finger must be recleaned with alcohol
   (B) no recleaning is necessary if the alcohol is still wet on the site
   (C) the patient's arm must be recleaned
   (D) it is not necessary to reclean the site since alcohol will last on the skin for 30 minutes
   (E) none of the above is correct

6. **The maximum amount of time a tourniquet can be left on without causing hemoconcentration is**
   (A) 30 seconds
   (B) 1 minute
   (C) 2 minutes
   (D) 5 minutes
   (E) 10 minutes

7. **Syringes are usually used to draw blood in all of the following cases except**
   (A) elderly patients
   (B) children
   (C) adults in their twenties
   (D) those with weak veins
   (E) those with veins that tend to collapse

8. **A winged infusion set with a Luer adapter can be used to fill**
   (A) evacuated tubes
   (B) syringes
   (C) a and b
   (D) sterile test tubes
   (E) none of the above

9. **The proper method of locating a vein for venipuncture is**
   (A) palpation
   (B) applying cold water to the site
   (C) applying hot water to the site
   (D) using a blood pressure cuff
   (E) all of the above

10. **The evacuated tube that is used for coagulation studies is the**
    (A) red stoppered tube
    (B) lavender stoppered tube
    (C) green stoppered tube
    (D) yellow stoppered tube
    (E) light blue stoppered tube

Getting Connected

Multimedia Extension Activities

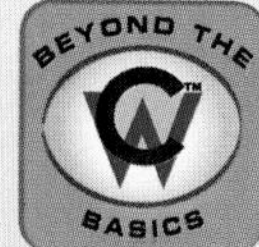

www.prenhall.com/fremgen

Use the address above to access the free, interactive Companion Website created specifically for this textbook. Enhance your studying by answering practice quiz questions, with hints and instant feedback related to chapter 6. If you would like to gain a deeper understanding of selected topics within this chapter, be sure to click on the **Beyond the Basics** feature, which provides more details for further learning. If you do not have a web connection, you may use the CD-ROM enclosed in the back of this book to take advantage of the same features off-line.

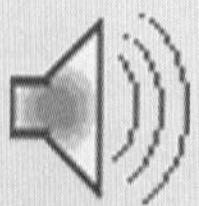

Audio Glossary

Use the CD-ROM enclosed with your textbook to hear the pronunciation of the key terms in the chapter. You may also access this material on the Companion Website www.prenhall.com/fremgen.

Bibliography

Bishop, M., J. Duben-Englekirk, and E. Fody. *Clinical Chemistry: Principles, Procedures, Correlations*, 3rd ed. Philadelphia: Lippincott-Raven, 1996.

Henry, J. B. *Clinical Diagnosis and Management by Laboratory Methods*, 19th ed. Philadelphia: W. B. Saunders, 1996.

Lehmann, C. A. *Saunders Manual of Clinical Laboratory Science*. Philadelphia: W. B. Saunders, 1998.

National Committee for Clinical Laboratory Standards. *Procedures for the Collection of Diagnostic Blood Specimens by Venipuncture*, 3rd ed. (document H3-A3). Villanova, Pa.: National Committee for Clinical Laboratory Standards, July 1991.

Stienne-Martin, E. A., C. A. Lotspeich-Steininger, and J. A. Koepke. *Clinical Hematology Principles, Procedures, and Correlations*, 2nd ed. Philadelphia: Lippincott-Raven, 1998.

CHAPTER 7

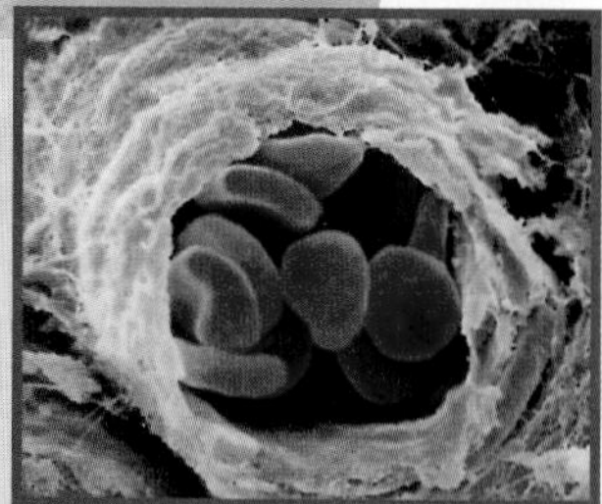

Dermal (Capillary) Puncture

Chapter Outline

- Introduction
- Composition of a Capillary Specimen
- Reasons for Dermal Punctures
- Equipment
- Site Selection
- Finger Puncture Procedure
- Heel Puncture Procedure
- Cleansing the Site
- Puncturing the Skin
- Collecting the Sample
- Postpuncture Procedure
- Order of Draw
- Summary
- Competency Review
- Examination Review Questions
- Bibliography

Learning Objectives

After completing this chapter, you should be able to

1. Define and spell the glossary terms listed in this chapter.
2. Describe the reasons for dermal punctures.
3. List the supplies needed for a dermal puncture.
4. Identify the most common dermal puncture sites.
5. Describe the dermal puncture procedure for both a finger puncture and a heel puncture.
6. Describe the order of draw in a dermal puncture.

GLOSSARY

ARTERIOLES the smallest arteries.

ARTERIOSPASM involuntary contraction of an artery.

CALCANEUS heel bone.

GERIATRIC pertaining to the elderly.

INTERSTITIAL space between cells or tissue.

OSTEOMYELITIS infection of bone.

PALMAR palm side of the hand.

PLANTAR sole side of the foot.

VENULES the smallest veins.

INTRODUCTION

In the previous chapter we discussed the protocol for performing a venipuncture by the evacuated tube method, the butterfly method, and the syringe method. In this chapter we introduce the reader to the procedure for obtaining a blood specimen by the capillary or dermal puncture method.

Composition of a Capillary Specimen

A specimen obtained from a dermal puncture is composed of **interstitial** fluid, which is a is found between cells and tissues, and small amounts of blood from capillaries, **venules** smallest veins and arteries). In fact, arterial blood makes up the majority of the dermal more arterial blood than venous blood is found in capillaries. If the puncture site has been warmed prior to the incision, the percentage of arterial blood in a capillary specimen will be even higher. Because of the mixture of bloods and fluid, some test results will be different if performed on a capillary specimen or a venous specimen. The amount of glucose will be higher in a capillary specimen than in a venous specimen, whereas total protein (TP), calcium (Ca^{2+}) and potassium (K^{+}) will be lower in the capillary specimen.

Reasons for Dermal Punctures

A dermal puncture is the method of choice for obtaining blood from infants and children under the age of 2 years. Children under 2 years have extremely small veins, and venipuncture is very difficult even when using a small-gauge needle and the butterfly method. In some cases, venipuncture in children under 2 years can cause serious complications such as cardiac arrest, hemorrhage, reflex **arteriospasm** (involuntary contraction of an artery), and infection. Young children have a small total blood volume, but fortunately most laboratory tests can be done using microcollection techniques found in dermal punctures. Traditional venipuncture with evacuated tubes may require more blood than small children can safely lose and can lead to anemia. Even filling two 5-mL evacuated tubes may use 5 to 10 percent of a premature infant's total blood volume.

MED TIP

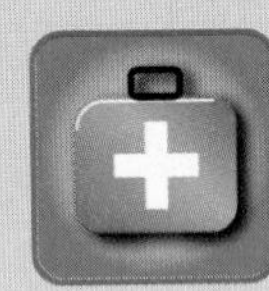

Dermal punctures should be the method of choice to collect blood specimens on children under the age of 2 years.

Dermal punctures are occasionally performed on adults when a suitable vein for venipuncture cannot be located or for patients whose veins must be reserved for intravenous (IV) therapy such as chemotherapy. Dermal punctures are also performed on adults with extremely weak or fragile veins, commonly found in **geriatric** (elderly) patients. These veins may collapse under the vacuum produced by an evacuated tube or a syringe.

Testing methodologies have become increasingly more sophisticated, and most tests can easily be done on the small amount of blood obtained from a dermal puncture. Some laboratory tests, including coagulation studies, erythrocyte sedimentation rate (ESR), and blood cultures, cannot be performed on a specimen from a dermal puncture. The dermal puncture procedure is described in procedure 7-1.

Equipment

Much of the equipment used in a dermal puncture is the same as that used in a venipuncture—disposable loves, alcohol wipes, sterile gauze pad or cotton balls, adhesive bandages, and a sharps container. This ment is illustrated in figure 7-1. Equipment unique to the capillary puncture includes skin puncture and microspecimen collection containers.

PROCEDURE 7•1

DERMAL PUNCTURE

Purpose:

In patients in whom venipuncture is difficult or ill advised (i.e., the elderly and the very young) the method of choice to obtain a blood specimen for diagnostic testing is by dermal (capillary) puncture.

Terminal Performance Competency:

Use aseptic technique while performing a capillary puncture and obtain an appropriate specimen.

Equipment:

Requisition, disposable gloves, sharps container, lancet, capillary tubes or microspecimen tubes, alcohol wipes containing 70 percent isopropyl alcohol, sterile cotton balls or gauze pads, bandages, specimen labels, and pen.

Procedure:

1. Obtain the patient requisition.
2. Greet and identify the patient.
3. Wash hands.
4. Explain the procedure to the patient.
5. Assemble the supplies needed for the ordered tests.
6. Select the site for capillary puncture.
7. Warm the puncture site (if necessary for specimen collection).
8. Clean site with alcohol.
9. Put on disposable gloves (if not done earlier). *Rationale: Protective equipment must be worn when handling blood or body fluids.*
10. Using a disposable lancet, make the incision.
11. Dispose of the lancet in the sharps container.
12. Wipe away the first drop of blood with sterile gauze or cotton. *Rationale: The first drop of blood cannot be used for testing because it is contaminated with tissue fluid.*
13. Collect specimen in capillary tubes or microcollection containers, avoiding air bubbles by keeping the capillary tube opening in the blood and not exposed to the air.
14. Elevate the site and apply pressure until bleeding stops.
15. Label specimens with patient name and ID number, date, time of collection, type of specimen, and phlebotomist's identification.
16. Check if a specimen requires special handling.
17. Bandage site if patient is over 2 years old.
18. Properly dispose of trash and contaminated materials.
19. Wash hands.
20. Thank the patient before leaving.

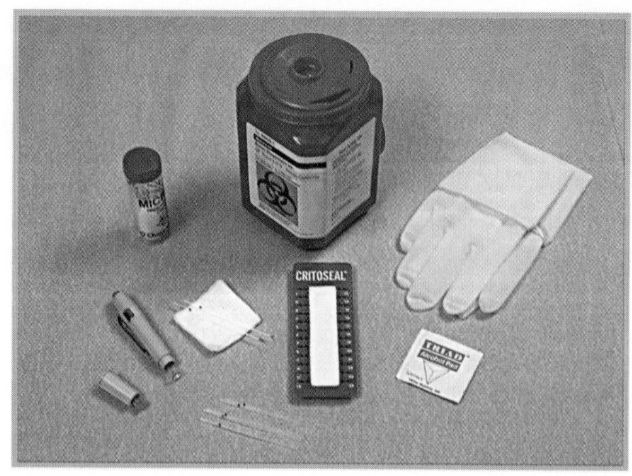

Figure 7-1
Equipment used in a dermal puncture.

Skin Puncture Devices

Many different types of disposable skin puncture devices are on the market today. These devices range from a simple manual lancet to an automatic spring-loaded retracting device. One common feature that the spring-loaded devices share is that the depth of the incision is controlled. Dermal puncture devices can make incisions ranging from 0.85 mm for premature babies to 3.0 mm for deeper incisions on adults. The most common incision depth is 2.4 mm. It is important when performing a dermal puncture to control the depth of the incision so as not to puncture a bone. Besides being extremely painful, puncturing the bone may cause a very serious bone infection, called **osteomyelitis**.

A lancet is the simplest of the skin-puncturing devices. It is a single-use, sterile, disposable metal blade that comes individually wrapped. Some lancets are all metal and come in individual foil pouches. Others are plastic and the sterile metal blade is exposed by twisting off a plastic cover. The puncture depth of a lancet is controlled by the length of the blade. There are also spring-loaded skin-puncturing devices in which the blade is automatically released by the phlebotomist activating the trigger once the device is held firmly against the patient's skin. Figure 7-2 shows a series of spring loaded lancets. The different colors identify the depth of the puncture made by the blade. In most of the spring-loaded devices, the blade automatically retracts into the device after the incision is made. Another type of spring-activated device allows the phlebotomist to set the depth of the incision by selecting the platform that is positioned over the site. The platform and the lancet can then be ejected into a sharps container after using by pressing a button on the device.

Microcollection Tubes

Many types of microspecimen collection containers, including microcollection tubes, microhematocrit tubes, capillary tubes, and micropipettes with an attached dilution system, are available for use. These small specimen containers can be used for a variety of hematology and chemistry tests. See figure 7-3 for an illustration of microcollection containers with a centrifuge.

Microcollection tubes are disposable plastic tubes that contain many of the same additives as evacuated tubes. The caps of these microcollection tubes are color coded in the same manner as evacuated

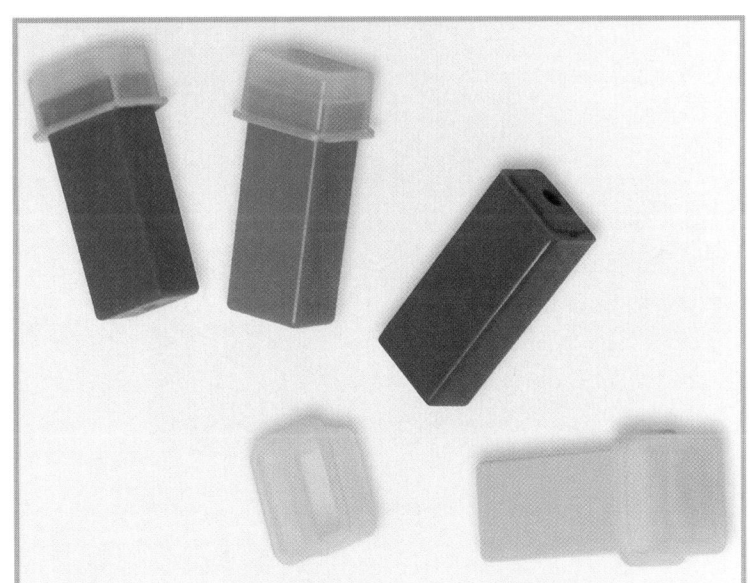

Figure 7-2
Spring loaded lancets.

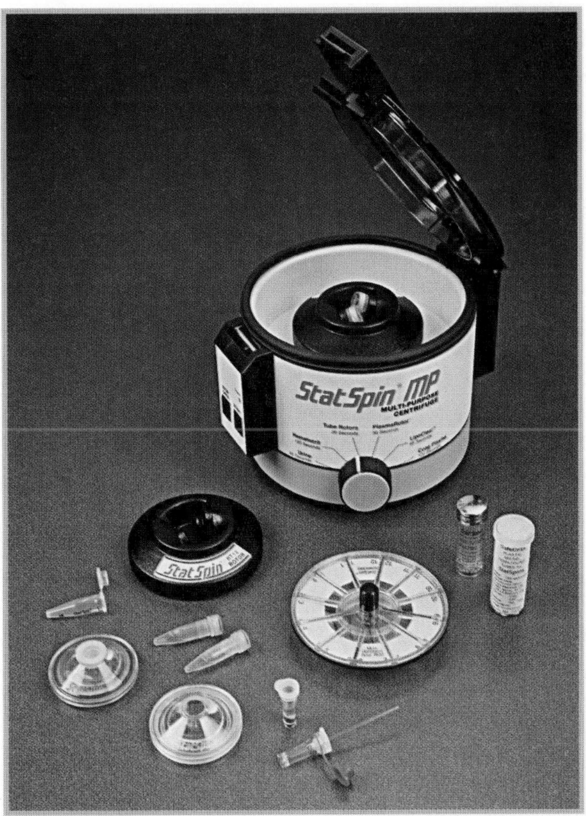

Figure 7-3
Microcollection containers with a centrifuge. (Photos of StatSpin products provided by StatSpin, Inc., a wholly owned subsidiary of IRIS, Chatsworth, CA.)

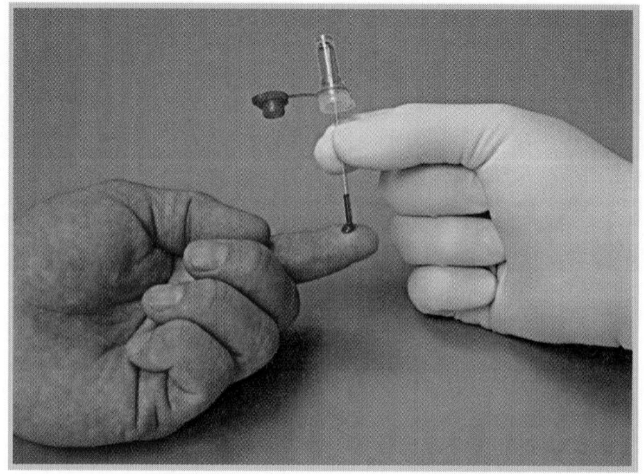

Figure 7-4
Microcollection tube filling by capillary action. (Photos by StatSpin products provided by StatSpin, Inc., a wholly owned subsidiary of IRIS, Chatsworth, CA.)

tubes. For example, a red-topped microspecimen tube is used to collect a serum sample. There are currently two main methods used to fill these small tubes. Some tubes are topped with little scoops that are used to pick up the blood drop from the skin surface. After the tube is full, the scoop is replaced with a color-coded plastic cap. Other tubes have a built-in collection tip that fills the tube by capillary action. After the tube is full, it is placed within a larger tube for transporting to the laboratory.

Capillary tubes are small, disposable glass or plastic tubes that fill by capillary action. Figure 7.4 illustrates a microcollection tube being filled by capillary action. These tubes are frequently referred to as microhematocrit tubes because they are centrifuged to determine the patient's hematocrit or packed cell volume. These tubes can also be used to collect blood for other tests. Some tests require plasma, so a capillary tube with heparin would be used. Heparinized tubes have a red band. Other tests require serum, so a plain or blue-banded capillary tube would be required.

When testing requires a larger blood sample than can be supplied by a microhematocrit tube, a Caraway or Natelson tube may be used to collect the specimen. These tubes are much larger than microhematocrit tubes and are tapered at one end to fill by capillary action. Natelson tubes are longer than Caraway tubes and have a greater capacity. Both tubes have a yellow band, indicating the anticoagulant lithium heparin; a red band, indicating ammonium heparin; or a blue band, indicating no anticoagulant.

A micropipette with a dilution system is a two-part system that collects the sample and stores it in a vial of diluting fluid for future testing. The system consists of a calibrated capillary pipette and a vial of diluting fluid. The size of the capillary pipette and the amount and type of diluting fluid differ for each laboratory test. This system is frequently used for hematology tests on small blood samples.

Site Selection

The area selected for capillary puncture should be free of scars, bruises, or rashes. An area that is swollen or edematous is not appropriate for dermal puncture because that blood sample will be too diluted with interstitial fluid. If possible, a site that is warm and pink rather than cold and blue should be selected. Skin-warming devices may be used to increase arterial blood flow to the site. Two main sites that are most frequently used for capillary puncture are the third or fourth fingertip and the heel in those under 1 year. Occasionally the **plantar** (sole-side) surface of the big toe or the earlobe is used as a dermal puncture site.

MED TIP

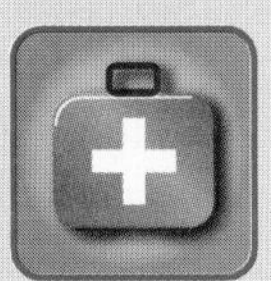

Warming the skin increases blood flow to the area and makes sample collection easier. Use warm, moist towels. You may also place the extremity in warm water.

Finger Puncture Procedure

Finger punctures may be performed on those over 1 year of age. The distal end of the third or fourth finger is the most commonly used site. The very tip of the finger should not be punctured because there is a greater chance of puncturing bone because the bone is close to the skin surface. The little finger is not used for the same reason. The index finger is not usually selected because it may be calloused and because the finger is used so frequently that the puncture may cause the patient discomfort. The fleshy pad on the end of the finger, slightly off center, should be punctured. The incision should be perpendicular to the lines of the fingerprint to help the blood flow into the collection container rather than under the fingernail. Different dermal puncture sites are pictured in figure 7-5.

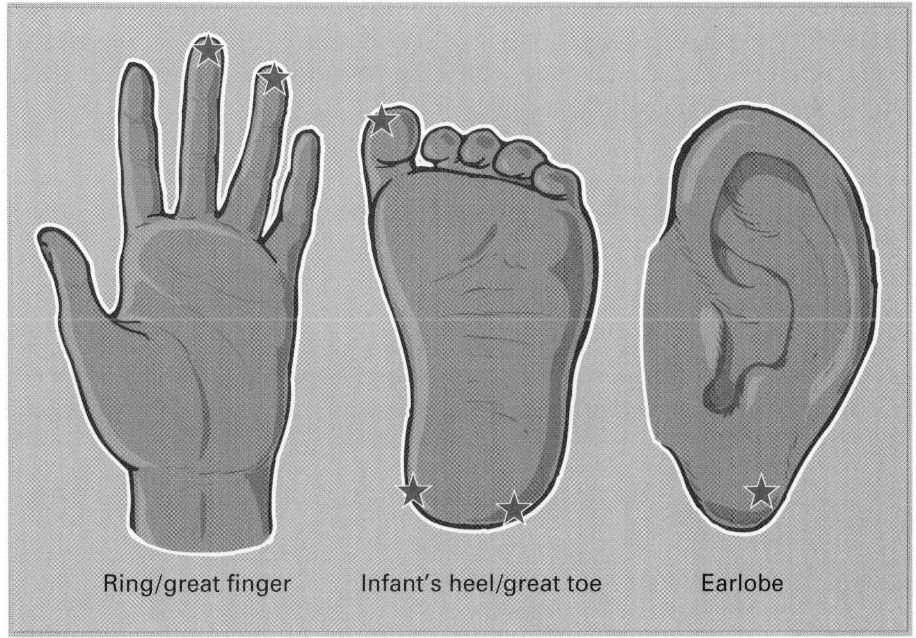

Figure 7-5
Different dermal puncture sites.

Heel Puncture Procedure

Heel punctures are performed on infants under 1 year of age. The puncture site must be carefully selected to avoid puncturing the **calcaneus** (heel bone). No puncture should be deeper than 2.4 mm (shallower in premature infants) to prevent puncturing the calcaneus. The arch of the foot should be avoided to prevent damaging nerves and tendons. The back of the heel should also be avoided because the calcaneus is very close to the surface of the skin. Punctures should be performed on the most medial or most lateral portion of the plantar surface of the foot. Sometimes infants may need more than one heel stick during their hospital stay. The phlebotomist should not puncture a previous unhealed site because infection may result.

If the selected site, either finger or foot, appears cold, warming the skin will increase the blood flow to the area and make sample collection much easier. Commercial skin warmers are available, or a warm, damp towel may be placed on the site for at least 3 minutes. It is recommended that a longer warming period be used for specimens for pH or blood gas analysis.

Cleansing the Site

Cleansing the site for a capillary puncture follows the same procedure as for a venipuncture. The site is cleaned using a prepared sterile alcohol (70 percent isopropanol) pad in a circular motion. It is important to make certain that the site is thoroughly dry before beginning the puncture. Residual alcohol will hemolyze the blood sample and cause a burning sensation at the puncture site. Also, if the alcohol contaminates the blood sample, it will cause an error in glucose testing.

Puncturing the Skin

Dermal punctures can be extremely messy because blood is allowed to collect on the surface of the skin and then flow into the microspecimen container. Although it has been strongly recommended that phlebotomists always wear gloves when collecting any type of blood specimen, it is extremely important that gloves always be worn when performing a dermal puncture.

Finger Puncture

For a finger puncture, the patient's arm is extended with the **palmar** (palm) surface up. The phlebotomist firmly supports the arm and grasps the patient's finger between the thumb and index finger. The finger is gently massaged first to increase blood flow, and the incision is made perpendicular to the fingerprint swirls. The procedure for a finger puncture is illustrated in figures 7-6 through 7-8. If a manual lancet is used, the incision is made with one smooth, swift motion. If an automatic lancet is used, the device is placed in firm contact with the skin before the incision is made. As soon as the incision is made, the lancet is discarded in the sharps container. If another incision is required, a fresh lancet must be used.

MED TIP

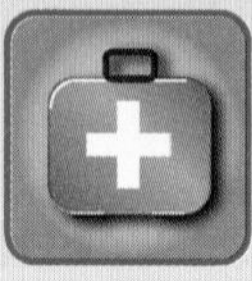

Carefully select a lancet that makes an incision at the appropriate depth for the patient.

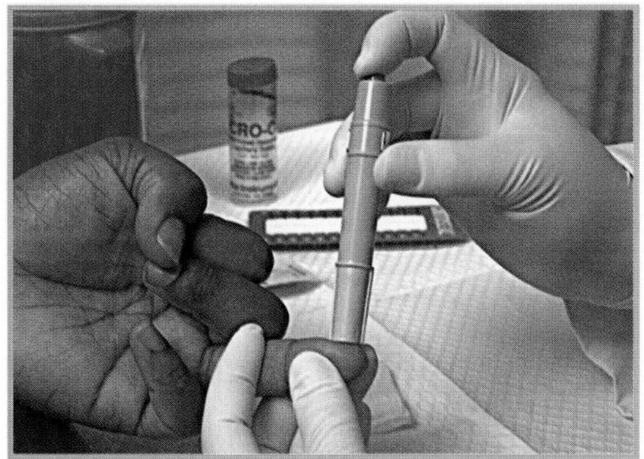

Figure 7-6
Grasp the patient's finger between the thumb and index finger.

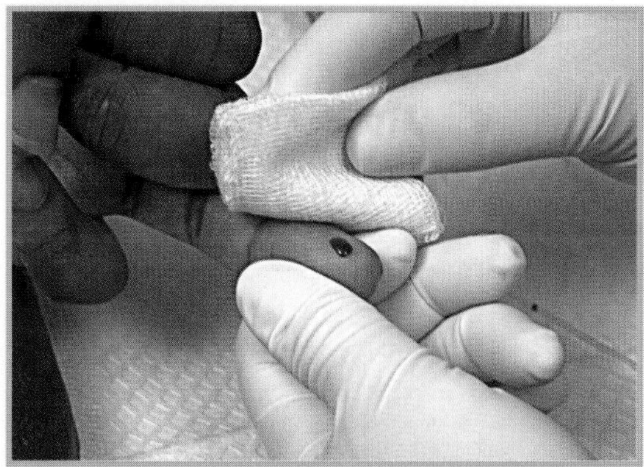

Figure 7-7
The first drop of blood is not used because it is too dilute for testing.

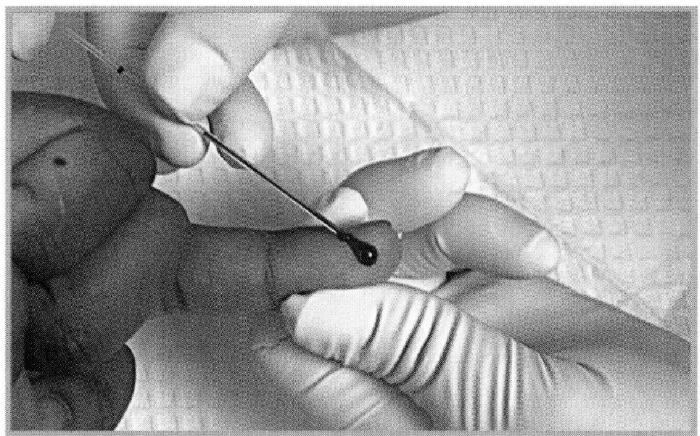

Figure 7-8
The collection tube fills by capillary action.

Heel Puncture

For a heel puncture, the infant's heel is held firmly in the nondominant hand with the thumb below the heel and the index finger over the arch. The heel is held firmly but not too tightly or blood flow to the foot may be stopped. The dominant hand places the puncture device firmly against the skin perpendicular to the heel. Pediatric lancets are usually spring loaded and make an incision no deeper than 2.4 mm. A shallower device is suggested for a premature infant. The lancet should be properly disposed of in a sharps container as soon as the incision is made. A lancet should never be used more than once. An illustration of a heel puncture is shown in figure 7-9.

Collecting the Sample

The first drop of blood that appears is wiped away using sterile gauze or cotton. This drop is heavily contaminated with tissue fluid and makes the blood sample too diluted for testing. The finger or heel may be gently squeezed and then released to ensure adequate blood flow, but it is important

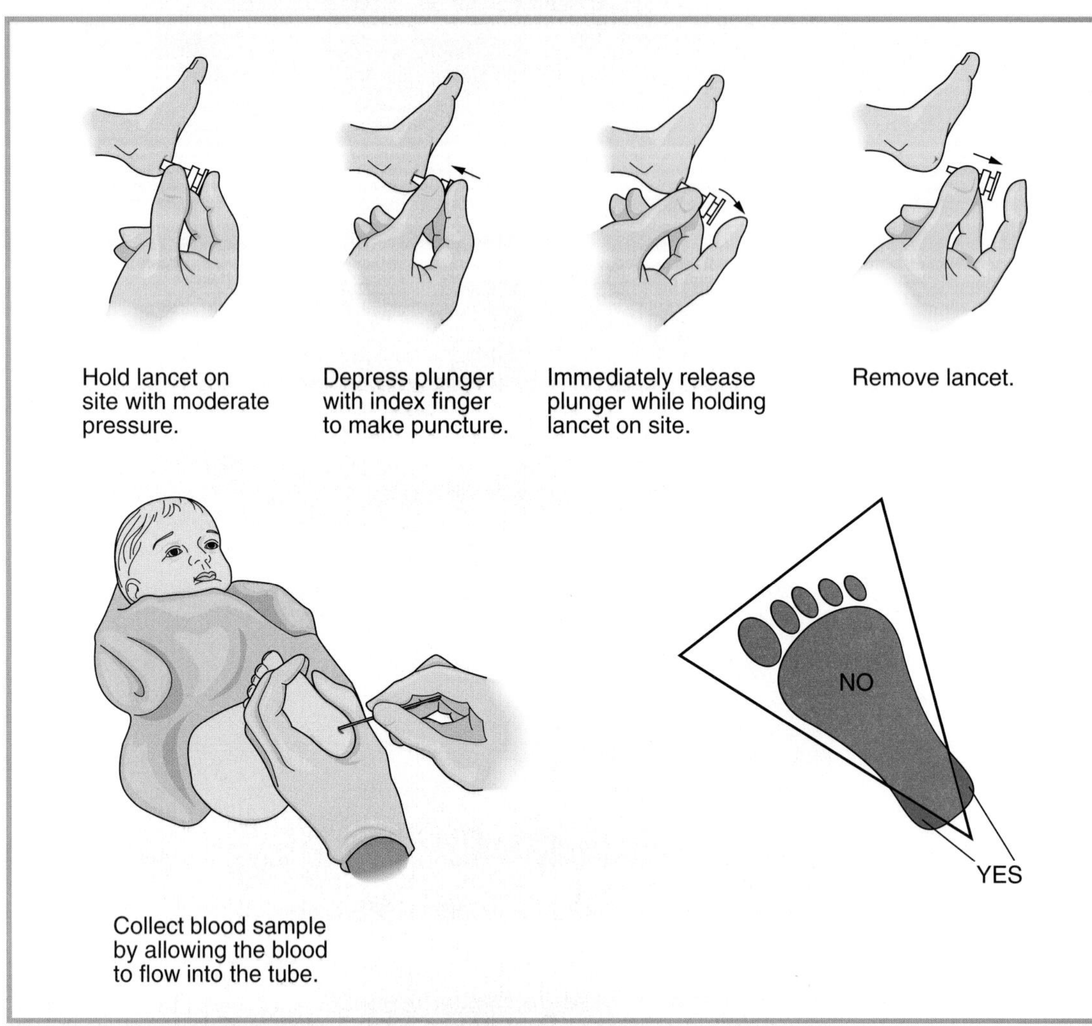

Hold lancet on site with moderate pressure.
Depress plunger with index finger to make puncture.
Immediately release plunger while holding lancet on site.
Remove lancet.
NO
YES
Collect blood sample by allowing the blood to flow into the tube.

Figure 7-9
An illustration of a heel puncture.

not to "milk" the site. Milking the site may cause the sample to hemolyze or become diluted with excess interstitial fluid.

Most microspecimen collection containers fill by capillary action. The opening of the container is held below the puncture site and touched to the drop of blood. The blood should flow into the collection container. If the microspecimen container has a scoop or capillary tube attached to the collection tube, the skin should not be touched because doing so will contaminate the specimen. As the drop of blood touches the scoop, it should roll down the side of the tube.

MED TIP

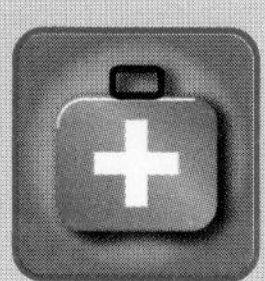

If the blood drop does not fall to the bottom of the microspecimen container, gently tap the bottom of the tube until the drop rolls to the bottom.

Postpuncture Procedure

After the sample has been collected, the phlebotomist elevates the finger or heel and applies pressure with sterile gauze or cotton. He or she continues to apply pressure until bleeding has stopped and then applies an adhesive bandage to the site if the patient is over age 2. The phlebotomist should check with nursery personnel before applying a bandage on a neonate because an infant's skin is so fragile that it might be damaged by the adhesive bandage.

The microspecimen collection containers should be labeled before the phlebotomist leaves the patient's side. The label must contain the same information as a label for a venipuncture. Labels may be wrapped entirely around the microtubes. If capillary tubes are collected, they are usually placed in a larger labeled tube for easier transportation to the testing laboratory. Before leaving the patient's room, the phlebotomist must make certain that all trash has been disposed of in the appropriate container, wash his or her hands, and thank the patient and the patient's parents (if appropriate) for their cooperation.

Order of Draw

Platelets will quickly begin to accumulate around the dermal puncture site. Therefore, any specimen that evaluates platelets should be collected first. If a blood smear is required, the smear is the first specimen collected (see chapter 8). The blood smear is followed by specimens collected in diluting chambers or specimens with ethylenediaminetetraacetic acid (EDTA) and then others. Coagulation studies cannot be performed on capillary specimens due to the interstitial fluid in the sample.

CHAPTER REVIEW

Summary

Dermal (capillary) punctures are the method of choice for obtaining a blood sample on infants, children under 2 years of age, or those in whom venipuncture is exceedingly difficult. As equipment and testing methodologies in laboratory science become more sophisticated, smaller quantities of blood can be used for clinical testing. In this chapter we discussed the specialized equipment required for dermal puncture and provided a step-by-step procedure for performing a finger puncture.

Competency Review

1. Describe the contents of capillary blood.
2. List the tests that cannot be performed on capillary blood.
3. List three types of microspecimen containers.
4. Explain why a dermal puncture site should not be milked.
5. List four reasons for rejecting a site for dermal puncture.

Examination Review Questions

1. The average depth of incision in a dermal puncture is

(A) 0.85 mm
(B) 1.5 mm
(C) 2.4 mm
(D) 3.4 mm
(E) 4.0 mm

2. The preferred finger selection when performing a dermal puncture is the

(A) index finger
(B) thumb
(C) little finger
(D) third or fourth finger
(E) all of the above are acceptable sites

3. The preferred site for dermal puncture on an infant under the age of 1 year is

(A) the ear
(B) the lateral portion of the heel
(C) the scalp
(D) the finger
(E) the back of the heel

4. At the dermal puncture site, the alcohol needs to dry before beginning the test because

(A) residual alcohol may cause a burning sensation on puncture
(B) residual alcohol will hemolyze the blood sample
(C) residual alcohol may cause an error in glucose testing
(D) a and b
(E) a, b, and c

5. Milking the dermal puncture site

(A) forces a better supply of blood into the tip of the finger
(B) may cause the blood sample to hemolyze
(C) is to be avoided
(D) may cause dilution with tissue fluid
(E) b, c, and d

6. Some laboratory tests cannot be performed on blood obtained from capillary puncture because

(A) more red blood cells are needed
(B) the pH of capillary blood is too high
(C) the pH of capillary blood is too low
(D) more blood is needed for the test than can be obtained by capillary puncture
(E) more platelets are needed

7. **When performing a heel puncture, care should be used to avoid puncturing the calcaneus because doing so might cause**
   (A) too small of a sample
   (B) osteomyelitis
   (C) a low glucose reading
   (D) too few platelets in the sample
   (E) the sample to clot too quickly

8. **One way to increase the blood flow to a dermal puncture site is to**
   (A) warm the site
   (B) cool the site
   (C) rub the site
   (D) select sites farther away from the center of the body
   (E) perform the procedure shortly after the patient awakes

9. **The first drop of blood that appears after a dermal puncture is not used because**
   (A) it contains too many cells
   (B) alcohol may be present
   (C) the glucose level will be too high
   (D) it contains too much oxygen because the child was crying
   (E) it is diluted with interstitial fluid

10. **To stop the bleeding after a finger puncture, the phlebotomist should**
   (A) immediately place a bandage on the site
   (B) elevate the finger
   (C) place the finger in warm water
   (D) place the finger in cool water
   (E) wipe the finger with alcohol

Getting Connected

Multimedia Extension Activities

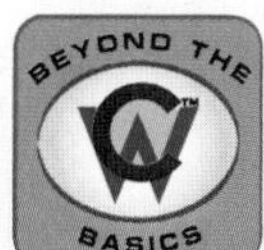

www.prenhall.com/fremgen

Use the address above to access the free, interactive Companion Website created specifically for this textbook. Enhance your studying by answering practice quiz questions, with hints and instant feedback related to chapter 7. If you would like to gain a deeper understanding of selected topics within this chapter, be sure to click on the **Beyond the Basics** feature, which provides more details for further learning. If you do not have a web connection, you may use the CD-ROM enclosed in the back of this book to take advantage of the same features off-line.

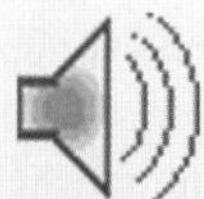

Audio Glossary

Use the CD-ROM enclosed with your textbook to hear the pronunciation of the key terms in the chapter. You may also access this material on the Companion Website www.prenhall.com/fremgen.

Bibliography

Bishop, M., J. Duben-Engelkirk, and E. Fody. *Clinical Chemistry: Principles, Procedures, Correlations,* 3rd ed. Philadelphia: Lippincott-Raven, 1996.

Henry, J. B. *Clinical Diagnosis and Management by Laboratory Methods,* 19th ed. Philadelphia: W. B. Saunders, 1996.

Lehman, C. A. *Saunders Manual of Clinical Laboratory Science.* Philadelphia: W. B. Saunders, 1998.

National Committee for Clinical Laboratory Standards. *Procedures for the Collection of Diagnostic Blood Specimens by Skin Puncture,* 3rd ed. (document H4-A3). Villanova, Pa.: National Committee for Clinical Laboratory Standards, July 1991.

Stienne-Martin, E. A., C. A. Lotspeich-Steninger, and J. A. Koepke. *Clinical Hematology Principles, Procedures, and Correlations,* 2nd ed. Philadelphia: Lippincott-Raven, 1998.

CHAPTER 8

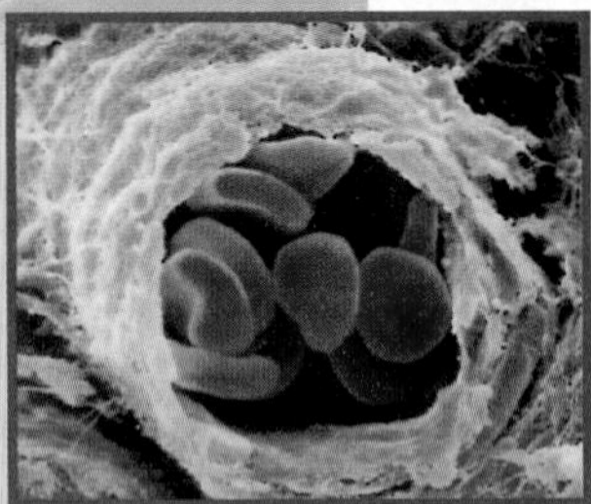

Special Blood Collection Procedures

Chapter Outline

- Introduction
- Timed Specimens
- Therapeutic Drug Monitoring
- Blood Cultures
- Bleeding Time Test
- Blood Donor Collection
- Blood Smears
- Neonatal Screening
- Arterial Blood Gas
- Specimens in Legal Cases
- Point of Care Testing
- Summary
- Competency Review
- Examination Review Questions
- Bibliography

Learning Objectives

After completing this chapter, you should be able to

1. Define and spell the glossary terms listed in this chapter.
2. Discuss the importance of timed specimens.
3. Explain the principles of therapeutic drug monitoring.
4. Explain the reason for drawing blood cultures and describe the procedure.
5. Explain the reason for performing a glucose tolerance test and describe the procedure.
6. Describe the procedure for the bleeding time test.
7. Explain the reasons for careful blood donor selection.
8. Describe the procedure for making a blood smear.
9. Explain the reasons for drawing blood for arterial blood gases and describe the procedure.
10. Discuss the importance of neonatal screening for phenylketonuria.
11. Explain when the chain-of-custody protocol is required.
12. Describe point of care testing and list the commonly performed tests.

GLOSSARY

ABGs arterial blood gases.

Allen test test used to determine if an artery is safe to use for an arterial blood gas test.

Autologous donation donating blood for one's own use.

CBC complete blood count.

Chain of custody a specific protocol for legal specimens that documents the specimen from collection to the final test result.

Collateral circulation more than one artery supplies blood to the same area.

Diabetes mellitus a condition in which there is impaired carbohydrate metabolism due to lack of insulin.

Differential test in which blood is stained on a microscope slide and the white blood cells, red blood cells, and platelets are observed.

FUO fever of an undetermined origin.

Glycolysis process of breaking down glucose.

Hemostasis process by which one stops bleeding.

Hypoglycemia condition in which the amount of sugar in the blood is too low.

Hypothyroidism condition in which the function of the thyroid gland is impaired.

Keloid thick, raised scar.

Myeloproliferative disease chronic malignant disorder due to an abnormal proliferation of a cell line.

Phenylketonuria hereditary metabolic disease due to lack of the enzyme phenylalanine hydroxylase that can cause severe mental retardation if not detected soon after birth.

Point of care testing laboratory testing performed at the patient's bedside rather than in the laboratory.

Postprandial after eating.

Septicemia bacterial infection of the bloodstream.

Sphygmomanometer instrument for determining blood pressure.

STAT derived from the Latin word meaning immediately.

TAT an acronym for *turnaround time.*

TDM therapeutic drug monitoring.

Therapeutic phlebotomy drawing blood for the purpose of treating a medical condition.

Introduction

Venipunctures and dermal (capillary) punctures are the two most common procedures a phlebotomist will perform; however, a competent phlebotomist must also be familiar with other procedures and special tests that are part of the scope of a phlebotomist's practice.

Timed Specimens

Frequently, a laboratory requisition will state that a blood specimen be drawn at a particular time. The phlebotomist must be aware of the drawing time and prioritize the work accordingly. He or she must record the time the specimen is drawn on the requisition. Requisitions for timed specimens range from determining the blood level of a medication to measuring the body's ability to metabolize a carbohydrate.

Stat Specimens

The word ***stat*** comes from the Latin word meaning immediately. A stat specimen is one in which the results must be known as soon as possible in order to treat a critically ill patient. When a stat laboratory requisition is received, the phlebotomist must draw the blood immediately and quickly deliver the specimen to the laboratory. Some hospitals have a separate stat laboratory in which the **turnaround time (TAT)** for test results is much faster than normal. If the hospital does not have a stat laboratory, a stat specimen is processed as soon as it arrives in the main laboratory. Although stat specimens must be drawn and processed quickly, the proper procedures must always be followed. A phlebotomist must not sacrifice proper procedure in the rush to quickly get the specimen to the laboratory because serious errors can occur.

MED TIP

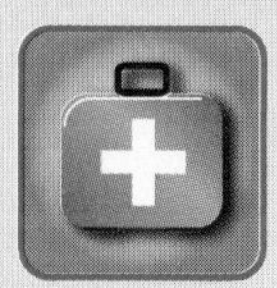

A stat specimen takes precedent over all other work.

Fasting Specimens

A fasting specimen requires that patients eat or drink nothing other than water for a certain period of time (usually 8 to 12 hours) prior to having their blood drawn. The most common tests performed on fasting specimens are cholesterol, triglycerides, and glucose determinations. It is the phlebotomist's responsibility to ask patients if they have followed the test protocol and fasted. If they have not fasted, the phlebotomist should check with a supervisor to see if the blood should still be drawn. If the blood specimen is drawn, a note on the requisition must state that the specimen was nonfasting.

Two-Hour Postprandial Glucose Test

The 2-hour **postprandial** glucose test is a screening test for diabetes. A 2-hour postprandial test would take place 2 hours after eating. A patient with normal glucose metabolism will have a normal blood glucose level 2 hours after eating. In the 2-hour postprandial test, the patient is instructed to eat a high-carbohydrate diet for 2 to 3 days prior to the test. The morning of the test, the patient is given instructions to eat a breakfast that contains approximately 100 g glucose. Two hours later, that patient's blood is drawn for a glucose determination. If the glucose level is abnormally high, a more specific test, the glucose tolerance test, should be performed. Besides drawing the blood specimen, the phlebotomist has the additional task of determining whether the patient has followed the test instructions and if it has been 2 hours since the patient has eaten breakfast. If the specimen is drawn before the 2 hours have passed, the results will be inaccurate.

Glucose Tolerance Test

The glucose tolerance test is the primary test used to diagnose carbohydrate metabolism disorders such as **diabetes mellitus** and **hypoglycemia.** Diabetes mellitus is a condition due to lack of insulin in which there is impaired carbohydrate metabolism. It is related to hypoglycemia, a condition in which the amount of sugar in the blood is too low. In this test, a fasting patient is given a standard amount of glucose. Blood and urine samples are then taken at periodic intervals to determine how long it takes the patient to metabolize the glucose. The length of the test may vary from 3 to 6 hours. The phlebotomist is usually responsible for giving the patient test instructions as well as collecting the specimens at the appropriate times. For a sample schedule of a glucose tolerance test see table 8-1.

The test protocol calls for the patient to eat well-balanced meals for 2 or 3 days prior to the test. The patient is then required to fast for the 12 hours preceding the test. The patient may not smoke or chew gum during the fasting period because these activities may stimulate digestion and interfere with the test results. However, the patient is encouraged to drink water for the duration of the test. The test begins with the collection of a fasting blood specimen and a urine sample. The patient is given a standard dose of glucose (typically 75 g for adults and 1.0 g/kg of body weight for children) to drink within 5 minutes. Commercially prepared glucose beverages are available, and they are more palatable if very cold. Some patients

TABLE 8-1 Sample Schedule of a Glucose Tolerance Test

Fasting blood specimen and urine specimen	8:00 A.M.
Began drinking glucose	8:10 A.M.
Finished glucose	8:15 A.M.
Half-hour blood specimen and urine specimen	8:45 A.M.
One-hour blood specimen and urine specimen	9:15 A.M.
Two-hour blood specimen and urine specimen	10:15 A.M.
Three-hour blood specimen and urine specimen	11:15 A.M.
Four-hour blood specimen and urine specimen	12:15 P.M.
Five-hour blood specimen and urine specimen	1:15 P.M.

have a difficult time swallowing the glucose beverage and may vomit. If that happens, the phlebotomist should notify the physician and ask whether to continue the test. Timing for collecting the specimens begins as soon as the glucose solution is consumed. A blood specimen and a urine specimen are collected at 30 minutes and then at hourly intervals for the remainder of the test.

All specimens should be labeled as to the time they were drawn and their order in the test (e.g., 11:15 A.M., 3 hours). It is also important to collect the same type of specimen each time. That means if the fasting specimen was from a capillary puncture, all of the other specimens should be from capillary punctures. If capillary blood and venous blood results are used in the same tolerance test, the results will be misleading. The specimen is usually collected in a gray-topped tube containing sodium fluoride which inhibits **glycolysis,** the process of breaking down sugar. The glucose test result will be more accurate than if collected in a red-topped tube. If a red-topped tube is used it should be centrifuged immediately after clotting, and the serum should be removed and refrigerated until laboratory testing. This will slow down the glycolytic action of the red blood cells.

The results of a glucose tolerance test are usually put in graph form as shown in figure 8-1. In a patient with normal glucose metabolism, the glucose level will peak between 30 minutes and 1 hour after ingest-

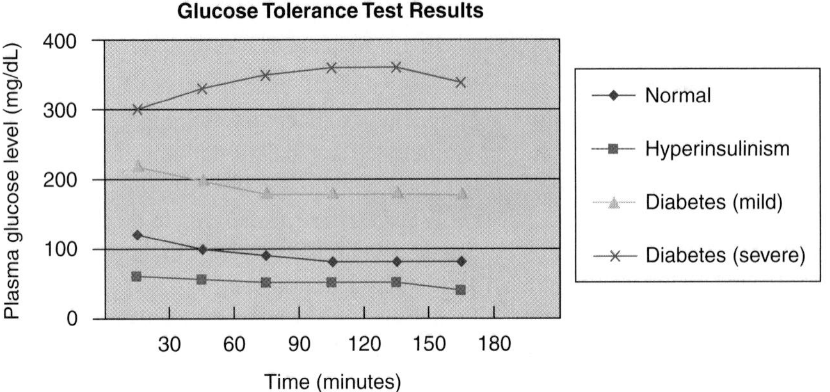

Figure 8-1 Results of a glucose tolerance rest.

ing the glucose solution. The glucose level should drop to the fasting level within 2 hours, and glucose should never be found in any of the urine specimens. If the patient has diabetes, the peak glucose level will be much higher due to the lack of insulin and will take much longer to return to the fasting level. In a patient with hypoglycemia, the glucose level will remain fairly close to the fasting level for the entire test.

Lactose Tolerance Test

A lactose tolerance test is used to diagnose lactose intolerance (a condition in which individuals cannot digest lactose [milk sugar]). The day prior to the lactose tolerance test, the patient has a 3-hour glucose tolerance test to determine if he or she has normal glucose metabolism. The lactose tolerance test follows the same 3-hour protocol as the previous day's glucose tolerance test. The patient ingests a set amount of lactose, and blood samples are drawn at periodic intervals. If the patient has normal lactose metabolism, the lactose curve will be similar to the curve in the glucose tolerance test. If the patient cannot metabolize lactose, the curve will appear flattened and there will be no more than a 20-mg/dL rise from the fasting level. If the patient has lactose intolerance, he or she may experience severe gastrointestinal discomfort during the test. False-positive results may occur in this test with patients who have slow gastric emptying.

Epinephrine Tolerance Test

The epinephrine tolerance test is used to determine the amount of glycogen stored in the liver. When the body needs glucose, the stored glycogen is broken down into glucose with the help of the hormone epinephrine. The patient must fast for 12 hours, and then a specimen is drawn for a fasting blood glucose test. The venipuncture is followed by an intravascular injection of epinephrine hydrochloride. Thirty minutes later another specimen to determine blood glucose level is drawn. If the patient has normal glycogen stores, the second blood sample should indicate a minimum increase of 30 mg/dL of glucose over the first sample. No increase in the second glucose level or a slight increase may be indicative of a glycogen storage disease or liver disease.

Glucagon Tolerance Test

The glucagon tolerance test also is used to test liver glycogen stores. The test is similar to the epinephrine tolerance test except that glucagon is injected instead of epinephrine. Test results are interpreted in the same manner as for the epinephrine tolerance test.

MED TIP

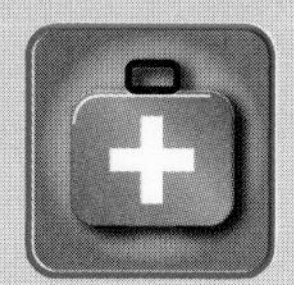

It is your responsibility to ask the patient if he or she has followed the pretesting instructions.

Therapeutic Drug Monitoring

Therapeutic drug monitoring (TDM) is a test that measures the amount of a particular medication in the patient's bloodstream. People metabolize medicine at different rates depending on their age, metabolic rate, kidney function, general state of health, and other factors. Physicians use TDM to determine the optimal dose of a medication for a patient. Physicians want to ensure that the medication in the patient's blood has reached the most effective level for treatment without being toxic to the patient. Normally two blood samples are needed to determine the proper dose of the medication for the patient. These two samples are known as the trough and peak levels. The trough level is the least amount of the medication found in the blood; it is determined from the specimen drawn just prior to administration of the next dose of medication. The peak level occurs when the largest amount of the medication is found in the bloodstream. The drawing time of the peak level varies with the type of medication, the route of administration (intravenous, intramuscular, or oral), and the half-life of the medication. Drugs that require monitoring include certain antibiotics such as gentamycin, tobramycin, and vancomycin and medications such as digoxin and theophylline.

Most TDM is performed on serum drawn in plain red-topped evacuated tubes. Tubes with gel serum separators should be avoided because it appears that the serum separators falsely lower the results for some tests. The stoppers on the evacuated tubes may also interfere with some testing; therefore, to minimize this effect, the tubes must be kept upright after the sample has been drawn. The phlebotomist has the added responsibility of recording the time the specimen was drawn and the time and method of administration of the last dose of the medication on both the requisition and the specimen label.

MED TIP

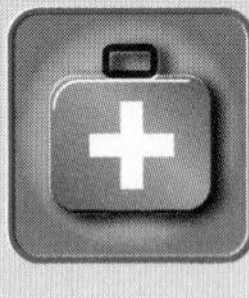

To ensure that therapeutic drug monitoring is done correctly, the process requires additional communication between the pharmacy, nursing staff, and phlebotomist.

Blood Cultures

A physician may order a blood specimen for microbiological culture (blood culture) to aid in diagnosing **septicemia** (bacterial infection of the blood) or the patient may have the presumptive diagnosis of a **fever of undetermined origin (FUO).** A patient's fever often spikes (increases) at certain times during the day. The optimal time to draw blood to increase the chance of identifying bacteria is during a fever spike. When the patient's temperature is high, more bacteria are in the bloodstream than when the patient's temperature is low. Many times a blood culture is ordered just prior to a fever spike and then half an hour to an hour later. If the requisition calls for two sets of blood cultures to be drawn at the same time, they should be drawn from different sites. Typically two blood samples are drawn at the same time. After being received in the microbiology laboratory, one blood sample will be incubated in an aerobic environment and the other in an anaerobic environment. Blood cultures require a strict skin-disinfecting procedure to prevent the blood specimen from becoming contaminated with the normal bacteria that reside on the skin. Procedure 8-1 describes the skin-disinfecting procedure.

PROCEDURE 8 • 1

DISINFECTING SKIN FOR BLOOD CULTURES

Purpose:

To properly cleanse the skin prior to collecting a blood specimen for blood culture.

Terminal Performance Competency:

Collect a specimen for a blood culture by correctly using the appropriate equipment.

Equipment:

Requisition, gloves, sharps container, alcohol wipes containing 70 percent isopropyl alcohol, povidone-iodine solution, sterile cotton balls or sterile gauze, tourniquet, evacuated tubes, needles and tube adapters, bandages, specimen labels, and pen.

Procedure:

1. Obtain the patient requisition.
2. Greet and identify the patient.
3. Wash hands.
4. Assemble the supplies for the ordered laboratory tests.
5. Position the patient properly.
6. Apply the tourniquet 2 inches above the antecubital fossa.
7. Palpate the site and select the site for venipuncture.
8. Remove the tourniquet. *Rationale: A tourniquet cannot be left on for more than 1 minute or hemoconcentration will occur.*
9. Cleanse site by using an alcohol wipe in a circular motion beginning at the insertion site. *Rationale: The alcohol removes dirt and skin oils from the skin.*
10. Next apply the povidone-iodine solution to the site in concentric circles.
11. Allow the solution to dry for at least 30 seconds.
12. Perform a third disinfection with alcohol if required by your institution.
13. Put on disposable gloves (if not done earlier). *Rationale: Protective equipment must be worn when handling blood or body fluids.*
14. Wipe the tops of the evacuated tubes with a povidone-iodine solution and then alcohol prior to use.
15. If you must touch the site again prior to venipuncture, clean your gloved finger with the alcohol solution.
16. Proceed with the normal procedure for venipuncture.

MED TIP

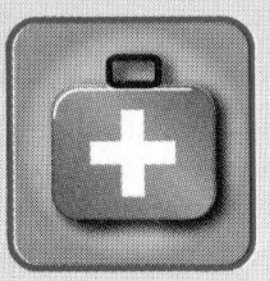

The most important step in drawing a blood culture is to carefully follow the skin-disinfecting procedure.

The remainder of the blood culture procedure is the same as for a routine venipuncture with the exception of the specimen containers. Some health care institutions draw blood for microbial cultures into yellow-topped evacuated tubes that contain sodium polyanetholsulfonate (SPS). SPS acts as an anticoagulant and does not inhibit bacterial growth like some other anticoagulants. The SPS tubes are sent to the laboratory, where the blood is transferred to the appropriate microbiological media to grow bacteria. Other health care institutions draw the blood specimen directly into the microbiological media or else inoculate the media at the patient's bedside. Some blood culture media are in flat-bottomed bottles with a long neck that fits into the evacuated tube holder and the blood specimen is drawn directly into the bottle. Winged infusion sets and syringes can also be used to draw specimens for blood culture. When the blood culture medium is inoculated at the patient's bedside, the anaerobic culture is always done first to limit the blood's exposure to air.

Bleeding Time Test

The bleeding time test is a screening test that assesses the status of the patient's **hemostasis,** the process by which one stops bleeding. The bleeding time test procedure is detailed in procedure 8-2. The bleeding time test is part of a standard presurgical workup and is used to diagnose coagulation disorders. In the template bleeding time test, a standardized incision is made in the patient's arm, and the phlebotomist records the time it takes to stop bleeding. A normal bleeding time is between 2 and 9 minutes. Patients should be warned that a small scar might result from this test, especially in those who are prone to form **keloids.** Keloids are thick, raised scars. Patients should avoid aspirin or aspirin-containing products for 1 week before the test because aspirin will affect platelet function and interfere with the test results.

Bleeding time tests have been performed since the early part of the twentieth century. Early methods used the earlobe as the puncture site, and an incision was made with a scalpel. These tests were unreliable because the depth of the incision could not be controlled and would vary from patient to patient.

Note: If bleeding does not stop in 15 minutes, discontinue the test and apply pressure to the site. Report the result as greater than 15 minutes.

MED TIP

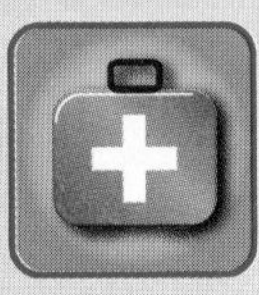

The use of a butterfly bandage helps to prevent scarring at the site of a bleeding time test.

PROCEDURE 8 • 2

TEMPLATE BLEEDING TIME TEST

Purpose:

To determine how long it takes a patient to stop bleeding from a standard-sized incision.

Terminal Performance Competency:

Perform a bleeding time test on a patient following the standard protocol.

Equipment:

Disposable gloves, alcohol wipes, blood pressure cuff (**sphygmomanometer**), stopwatch, filter paper discs, disposable trigger lancet that makes an incision 5 mm long by 1 mm deep, butterfly bandage, sharps container, and pen.

Procedure:

1. Obtain the requisition.
2. Greet and identify the patient.
3. Assemble the needed supplies.
4. Wash hands.
5. Put on disposable gloves.
6. Position the patient's arm on a steady support with the volar surface facing up. The preferred site is in the middle of the arm approximately 5 cm below the antecubital crest. Avoid areas that are burned, scarred, or have hematomas. If the area is hairy, shave the site because hair will interfere with the test.
7. Place the sphygmomanometer on the upper arm and inflate it to 40 mm Hg. The cuff should remain at this pressure for the entire test.
8. Clean the area with the alcohol wipe and allow it to dry.
9. While the alcohol is evaporating, remove the bleeding time device from its sterile wrapper and remove the safety clip. Be careful not to touch the blade end of the device because it will become contaminated with bacteria. Rest the device horizontally on the patient's arm and place it in firm contact with the patient's skin.
10. Press the trigger of the device and start the stopwatch simultaneously.
11. Discard the bleeding time device in the sharps container.
12. At 30-second intervals, touch the drop of blood that forms at the incision site to the filter paper. The filter paper will wick the blood away from the incision. Be careful not to touch the filter paper to the incision because doing so may disturb the forming platelet plug and delay clotting.
13. Continue until the filter paper is no longer stained with blood. Record the bleeding time to the nearest 30-second interval.
14. Remove the blood pressure cuff.
15. Clean the area with alcohol, being careful not to disturb the incision.
16. Cover the site with the butterfly bandage and instruct the patient to leave it on for 24 hours to prevent scarring.

Blood Donor Collection

Phlebotomists may be employed in blood donor stations such as the Red Cross or by hospitals that also draw blood to be used for transfusions. Any site that draws blood for donation must follow guidelines established by the American Association of Blood Banks (AABB) and the U.S. Food and Drug Administration (FDA). Blood drawn for donation is collected in a special sterile bag and called a unit. A unit of blood is approximately 450 mL of blood and 63 mL of the anticoagulant–cell preservative mixture found in the sterile bag.

The blood donation process begins with donor selection. Proper donor selection should protect both the recipient and the donor of the blood. The donor should not experience any ill effects from donating blood, and the recipient's condition should not worsen from receiving the donated blood.

Donor selection begins with a medical history including information about current medications and a series of questions about intravenous drug use and sexual practices. The latter information is used to protect recipients from blood that may be contaminated with bloodborne pathogens. The person interviewing the prospective donors should impress on them the importance of answering truthfully. Donors also have the opportunity of privately indicating that their blood should not be used for transfusion. The second part of the donor selection process is a minor physical examination that includes a record of age (17–65), weight (>110 pounds), blood pressure (≤180/100 mm Hg), temperature (<99.5°F or <37.5°C), and hemoglobin (≥12.5 g/dL) or hematocrit (≥38 percent). The prospective donor's arm is also checked for skin lesions, rashes, and needle marks. After the unit of blood is collected, it is tested for all bloodborne pathogens for which testing is available.

Blood for donation is collected into one large sterile plastic bag called a unit to which multiple smaller bags are attached. The smaller bags are used to make various products from whole blood without exposing it to air. This system is called a closed system, and it helps to keep the blood sterile. Typically, a unit of blood will be processed into packed cells, plasma, plasma products, and platelets. The patient is placed in a supine position, and the collecting bags are hung below the patient and fill by gravity. The bags are usually placed on a device similar to a scale that will stop blood flow when the bag reaches its filled weight. If the blood flow stops before the bag is filled, another venipuncture cannot be performed to fill the remainder of the bag. That blood collection would end with a partially filled bag. A unit or full bag of blood contains approximately 450 mL of blood.

Venipuncture for blood donation is similar to venipuncture for diagnostic purposes; the preparation of the puncture site is a two-step process similar to that used in blood culture collection. The antecubital fossa is first scrubbed for 30 seconds with a 0.7 percent aqueous scrub solution of an iodophor compound. The excess foam is removed with sterile gauze. Then the area is wiped with a stronger iodine complex and allowed to dry for a minimum of 30 seconds. If the venipuncture is not going to take place immediately, the site must be covered with sterile gauze.

After the site has been prepared, the tourniquet is replaced and a 15- to 17-gauge needle is used. Special 17-gauge thin-walled needles are preferred for blood donation. These needles have the external diameter of a 17-gauge needle but the internal diameter of a 15-gauge needle. With this needle, blood flow is rapid but there is less discomfort to the patient because the external diameter of the needle is smaller. After blood flow begins, the needle is taped to the patient's arm and covered with sterile gauze. The patient should be encouraged to slowly open and close his or her fist during the process because this action encourages blood flow. It normally takes about 7 minutes to draw a unit of blood. The phlebotomist should never leave the patient alone during the drawing process and should closely watch the patient for dizziness for 10 to 15 minutes after the draw is completed. Patients should also be advised to drink more fluids than usual for the next few days to replace the fluid volume that was lost.

Autologous Donation

A patient who is undergoing elective surgery may wish to donate blood prior to surgery for his or her own use. This process is called **autologous donation.** Autologous donation has become more popular recently with the increasing fear of transmitting bloodborne pathogens through a blood transfusion. Autologous donation may take place several weeks to 72 hours before surgery. For an autologous transfusion, the patient requires his or her doctor's permission and a minimum hemoglobin level of 11 g/dL. If the patient does not use the blood and has met all of the donor requirements, the blood may be added to the general blood supply in the blood bank.

Therapeutic Phlebotomy

Therapeutic phlebotomy is drawing blood from a patient for the purpose of treating a medical condition. Therapeutic phlebotomy is used in the management of patients with **myeloproliferative** diseases such as polycythemia vera. A myeloproliferative disease is a chronic malignant disorder due to an abnormal proliferation of a cell line. This blood should not be used for transfusion but discarded. The procedure for a therapeutic phlebotomy is the same as that for blood donation. The patient, however, may not be in good health and should be closely watched for signs of any adverse reactions.

Blood Smears

A blood smear is a glass microscope slide that has a drop of blood spread on its surface. Blood smears are part of a **complete blood count (CBC).** The blood smear is read under the microscope, and the white blood cells are classified by type and counted. Red blood cell morphology is examined, and the number of platelets is estimated. These results are collectively known as a **differential.** Blood smears may be made at the patient's side from capillary blood or in the hematology laboratory from venous blood collected in an ethylenediaminetetraacetic acid (EDTA) evacuated tube. If the blood smear is being prepared from an EDTA evacuated tube, the smear should be made within an hour of drawing the sample or the blood cells will be distorted. See procedure 8-3 for the step-by-step procedure for making a blood smear and illustrations of the process.

A properly made blood smear begins approximately 1 inch from the edge of the slide and covers about one-half the slide. It ends in a feathered edge where the cells are one layer thick and there are no holes or lines running through the surface of the smear. The smear should be made on a clean, dust-free glass slide. Learning to make a proper blood smear requires considerable practice and patience.

Neonatal Screening

Most states require that all newborns be tested for **phenylketonuria (PKU)** and congenital **hypothyroidism.** Both of these conditions, if left untreated, can lead to mental retardation. Phenylketonuria is a hereditary metabolic disease caused by lack of the enzyme phenylalanine hydroxylase and can result in severe mental retardation if not detected soon after birth. If a special diet that is low in phenylketones is begun early, mental retardation can be prevented. Congenital hypothyroidism is a condition in which the thyroid gland is impaired due to production of defective enzymes. Newborns should be tested for these diseases between the ages of 24 and 72 hours.

Hospital nurseries have special filter paper specimen collection cards that have three to five circles on them. Blood obtained from a heel stick is touched to one of the circles on the card. The blood drop should be large enough to entirely fill the circle and soak through to the other side of the paper. If the

PROCEDURE 8•3

MAKING A BLOOD SMEAR

Purpose:

To place blood on a glass slide so it can be stained and viewed under a microscope.

Terminal Performance Competency:

Prepare a blood slide using correct aseptic technique without error.

Equipment:

Clean glass slides, whole blood (EDTA evacuated tube), disposable gloves, biohazard container, laboratory coat, pen or marker, and dropper or two wooden applicator sticks.

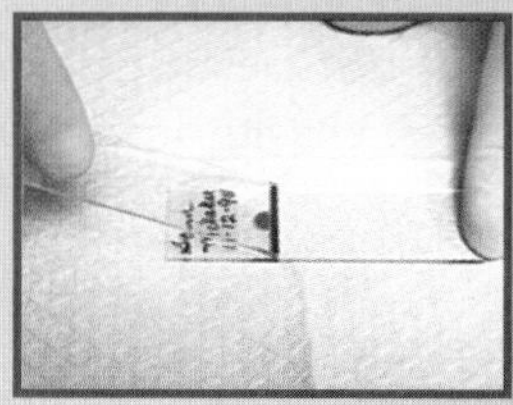

Place spreader in front of first blood drop.

Performance:

1. Place a drop of blood approximately 1 to 2 mm in diameter in the center of the slide approximately 1 inch from the end or 1/4 inch from the frosted band. If capillary blood is used, wipe away the first drop and hold the finger upside down and touch the blood drop to the slide.
2. Place a second clean slide (spreader) in front of the first drop and pull back until it touches the blood drop. Allow the blood to spread along the entire width of the spreader slide.
3. Hold the spreader slide at a 30- to 45-degree angle and with virtually no pressure glide the spreader quickly and evenly along the length of the smear slide.
4. Allow the slide to air dry and label it. Never blow on the slide to dry it. *Remember to wear gloves for the entire process because the blood on the slide is infectious until it is stained.*

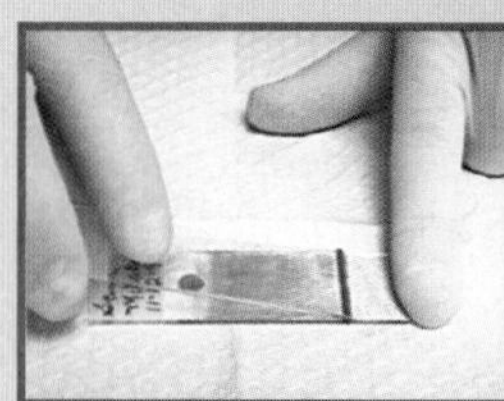

Glide the spreader quickly.

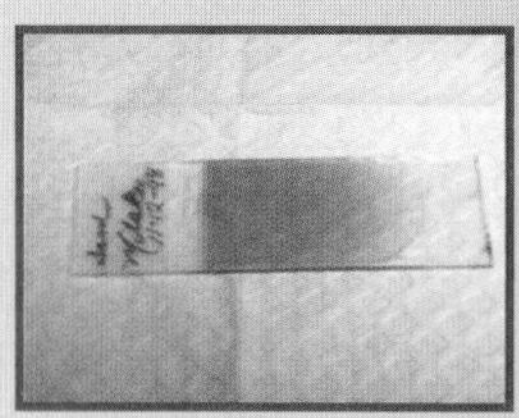

Allow the slide to air dry and label it.

circle does not fill completely, more blood should not be added. The phlebotomist can try filling another circle with a larger drop of blood. Blood may also be collected in a heparinized capillary tube and transferred to the filter paper. Care must be taken not to scratch the surface of the filter paper with the end of the capillary tube when transferring the blood.

Arterial Blood Gas

Arterial blood gas (ABG) tests are used to monitor the patient's respiration status. The results obtained from this testing are the P_{O_2} (partial pressure of oxygen), the P_{CO_2} (partial pressure of carbon dioxide), and the pH of blood. This information is used to analyze the patient's degree of oxygenation and the acid-base balance of the blood. Arterial blood is used for these determinations because the composition of arterial blood is constant throughout the body, whereas the composition of venous blood varies with its location.

The blood used for ABGs is obtained by an arterial puncture. Special training is required to perform arterial punctures, and phlebotomists do not usually perform them. Arterial punctures are usually performed by physicians, nurses, and respiratory therapists. In some specialized settings, however, phlebotomists with additional training may perform arterial punctures.

Not all arteries can be used for arterial punctures. The three most common sites are the radial artery on the thumb side of the wrist, the brachial artery on the median aspect of the antecubital fossa, and the femoral artery located in the groin. The criteria for an artery to be used for puncture include large enough for a 23-gauge needle, located near the surface of the skin, and an area where there is **collateral circulation.** Collateral circulation occurs when more than one artery supplies blood to the same area. The artery selected for the arterial puncture may be damaged during the procedure, and collateral circulation is critical to keep the area supplied with blood.

Before performing an arterial puncture on the radial artery, the **Allen test** must be performed. The Allen test is used to determine if an artery is safe to use for an ABG. It determines if there is collateral circulation to the selected area and checks that both the ulnar artery and the radial artery are supplying blood to the area. The procedure for the Allen test is as follows:

1. Support the patient's wrist and, with the palmar surface up, have them make a fist.
2. Using the second and third fingers of both hands (not the thumb, because it has a pulse) occlude both the ulnar and radial arteries.
3. Have the patient slowly open and close his or her fist several times until the palm pales.
4. Release the pressure on the ulnar artery while keeping the radial artery occluded.
5. If the ulnar artery is functioning, color should return to the palm within 5 to 15 seconds. If the ulnar artery is not functioning, an arterial puncture should not be performed on the radial artery.

Once the site is selected, it is carefully cleansed to prevent infection. First the area is wiped with alcohol and then with povidone-iodine. If the site is touched after cleansing, the gloved fingers should be treated in the same manner. Sometimes a local antiseptic such as lidocaine is injected under the skin.

The arterial sample is collected using a 1- to 5-mL syringe with a 21- to 23-gauge needle. The syringe is precoated with liquid lithium heparin to prevent the sample from clotting. The skin over the site is then pulled taut and the syringe is held like a dart with the bevel of the needle facing up. The artery is pierced at a 45-degree angle for the radial artery and at a 90-degree angle for the femoral artery. Blood will flow into the tip of the syringe if the artery has been pierced. The force of the blood flow in the artery will push the blood into the syringe. There is no need to pull back on the plunger of the syringe.

After the sample has been collected, the needle is removed and pressure is immediately applied to the site with sterile gauze. Pressure should be applied for 5 minutes, and a longer period may be required if the patient is taking anticoagulation medication. With the free hand, the excess air is expelled from the syringe and the needle is safely recapped or covered. The specimen is gently mixed with the heparin and placed in ice. When both hands are available, the needle is safely removed and properly disposed of in a sharps container. The syringe is capped with a Luer adapter, labeled, and replaced in the ice. The patient is checked for bruising or swelling at the site. The povidone-iodine is removed with alcohol and a pressure bandage is applied. The phlebotomist should check for a pulse below the site of the puncture; if it is absent, he or she must notify the nurse at once. The specimen should be kept on ice and taken to the laboratory for testing as soon as possible, preferably within 10 minutes.

Specimens in Legal Cases

Usually laboratory tests are ordered by physicians for medical reasons, but sometimes laboratory test results are required for legal reasons. Specimens that are collected for evidence in legal proceedings are called forensic specimens. The most commonly ordered forensic specimens are alcohol levels, drug screenings, and blood for DNA analysis. Phlebotomists who collect laboratory specimens that are tested for legal purposes must follow a specific protocol that documents the location of the specimen at all times and who has access to it from collection to the final test result. This process is called **chain of custody.** The chain of custody requires that a record be kept of the specimen from the time it is collected until after the laboratory test is performed. The chain of custody documents the travels of the specimen and who had access to it. Usually a law enforcement officer must be present when the specimen is obtained. Special seals close the specimen container and special forms accompany the specimen.

Blood that is to be tested for an alcohol level should be collected using an evacuated tube that contains sodium fluoride (gray top). Alcohol wipes should never be used to cleanse the skin because residual alcohol may contaminate the sample and cause erroneous results. Soap and water are usually the substitute used for alcohol.

Once a specimen for drug screening was only considered for legal purposes, but now many companies and athletic associations require a drug screen for employment or to participate in athletic competition. The National Institute on Drug Abuse (NIDA) has established guidelines for specimen collection, processing, and testing. These guidelines include tamper-proof containers, proper labeling of the specimen, and following the chain-of-custody protocol. Drugs that are tested for in a drug screening include alcohol, amphetamines, barbiturates, benzodiazepines, cocaine, cannabinoids, methadone, and opiates.

Point of Care Testing

Point of care testing is a new development in health care in which the clinical testing is done at the patient's side rather than in the clinical laboratory. Other names for this new trend include ancillary or bedside testing and alternate site testing. Small, portable clinical instruments have made bedside testing possible. Point of care testing may be performed by nurses, nursing aides, medical assistants, phlebotomists, or laboratory personnel. Special training in instrumentation, preventive maintenance, and quality control procedures is required for the personnel who perform point of care testing. Point of care testing falls under the auspices of the Clinical Laboratory Improvement Act of 1988 (CLIA 1988). For more information on CLIA 1988 see chapter 3. Figure 8-2 is an example of a common instrument used for point of care glucose testing.

Point of care testing can occur in many situations besides the patient's bedside. Emergency rooms, critical care units, clinics, and nursing homes are providing point of care testing for some basic laboratory procedures. The most frequently performed point of care test is a glucose level. Diabetic patients have been monitoring their glucose levels at home for years. There are many different types of small, portable glucose instruments that require a single drop of capillary blood. Other laboratory tests that have been adapted for point of care testing include blood gas analysis, coagulation tests such as pro-

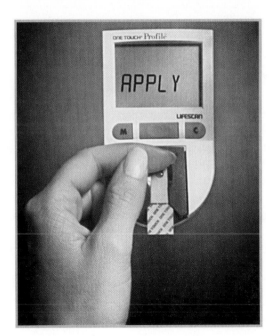

Figure 8-2
An example of a common instrument used for point of care glucose testing. (ONE TOUCH Profile Diabetes Tracking System, courtesy LifeScan, Inc.)

times (PT) and activated partial thromboplastin times (APTT), and common chemistry tests such as for electrolytes and cardiac enzymes.

Point of care testing has reduced the turnaround time for test results, which has facilitated better medical care for patients by reducing hospital stays and providing information faster in a medical crisis. Properly trained personnel are necessary for quality laboratory results. A training program that includes proper specimen collection, instrument operation and calibration, and a strictly enforced quality control program is essential for laboratory results that are reliable, reproducible, and accurate.

CHAPTER REVIEW

Summary

The phlebotomist's scope of practice is much larger than the collection of blood by either the venipuncture or dermal puncture method. The phlebotomist is also responsible for performing many tests directly at the patient's side. In addition, the phlebotomist is responsible for many laboratory tests that require special attention to timing or the collection procedures.

Competency Review

1. Explain the importance of the cleansing procedures for drawing blood cultures and blood for donation.
2. Explain why the 2-hour postprandial glucose test is a screening test and the glucose tolerance test is a more definitive test.
3. Explain the importance of the disposable trigger lancets used in the bleeding time test.
4. Describe the Allen test and explain its significance.
5. Describe the information that can be obtained from a properly made blood smear.

Examination Review Questions

1. Fasting for 12 hours prior to blood collection is a necessary requirement for

(A) the bleeding time test
(B) blood donation
(C) the glucose tolerance test
(D) autologous blood donation
(E) therapeutic phlebotomy

2. Therapeutic drug monitoring (TDM) requires that a ________ be drawn.

(A) fasting specimen
(B) specimen in an SPS evacuated tube
(C) peak and trough specimen
(D) capillary specimen
(E) 2-hour postprandial specimen

3. The bleeding time test is used to assess the patient's

(A) ability to stop bleeding
(B) ability to bleed
(C) oxygen level of blood
(D) arterial blood gas level
(E) red blood cell count

4. In a glucose tolerance test

(A) the amount of glucose ingested is important
(B) the amount of glucose is not important
(C) the length of fast is unimportant as long as it is at least 6 hours
(D) an infant may drink from a bottle
(E) lactose may be substituted for glucose

5. The most frequently performed point of care test is a

(A) chemistry electrolyte test
(B) coagulation test
(C) glucose test
(D) arterial blood gas analysis
(E) CBC

6. The Allen test is used to determine if

(A) a therapeutic phlebotomy is needed
(B) the patient has phenylketonuria
(C) the patient has low oxygen levels
(D) the patient requires a CBC
(E) there is collateral circulation in the wrist and hand area.

7. **The turnaround time (TAT) is significant**
   (A) only for stat specimens
   (B) only for PKU testing
   (C) for all laboratory specimens
   (D) in the bleeding time test
   (E) when the patient is elderly

8. **The CBC includes all of the following except**
   (A) red blood cell count
   (B) white blood cell count
   (C) platelet count
   (D) differential
   (E) arterial blood gas analysis

9. **Chain of custody is always an important consideration in**
   (A) infant specimens
   (B) geriatric specimens
   (C) therapeutic phlebotomy
   (D) legal cases
   (E) point of care testing

10. **Blood that is being drawn for donation is collected in**
   (A) red-topped tubes
   (B) lavender-topped tubes
   (C) microspecimen containers
   (D) 50-mL syringes
   (E) sterile bags that contain an anticoagulant and preservative

Getting Connected

Multimedia Extension Activities

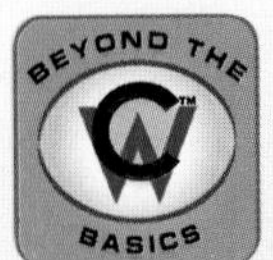

www.prenhall.com/fremgen

Use the address above to access the free, interactive Companion Website created specifically for this textbook. Enhance your studying by answering practice quiz questions, with hints and instant feedback related to chapter 8. If you would like to gain a deeper understanding of selected topics within this chapter, be sure to click on the **Beyond the Basics** feature, which provides more details for further learning. If you do not have a web connection, you may use the CD-ROM enclosed in the back of this book to take advantage of the same features off-line.

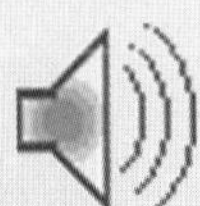

Audio Glossary

Use the CD-ROM enclosed with your textbook to hear the pronunciation of the key terms in the chapter. You may also access this material on the Companion Website www.prenhall.com/fremgen.

Bibliography

Baron, E. J., L. R. Peterson, and S. M. Finegold. *Bailey and Scott's Diagnostic Microbiology*, 9th ed. St. Louis: Mosby, 1994.

Bishop, M. L., J. L. Duben-Englekirk, and E. P. Fody. *Clinical Chemistry: Principles, Procedures, Correlations*, 3rd ed. Philadelphia: J. B. Lippincott, 1996.

Harmening, D. M., *Clinical Hematology and Fundamentals of Hemostasis*, 13th ed. Philadelphia: F. A. Davis, 1997.

Henry, J. B. *Clinical Diagnosis and Management by Laboratory Methods*, 19th ed. Philadelphia: W. B. Saunders, 1996.

National Committee for Clinical Laboratory Standards. *Percutaneous Collection of Arterial Blood for Laboratory Analysis* (document H11-1). Villanova, Pa.: National Committee for Clinical Laboratory Standards, 1985.

National Committee for Clinical Laboratory Standards. *Devices for Collection of Diagnostic Blood Specimens by Skin Puncture*, 3rd ed. (document H4-A3). Villanova, Pa.: National Committee for Clinical Laboratory Standards, 1991.

National Committee for Clinical Laboratory Standards. *Percutaneous Collection of Arterial Blood for Laboratory Analysis* (document H11-A2). Villanova, Pa.: National Committee for Clinical Laboratory Standards, 1992.

National Committee for Clinical Laboratory Standards. *Blood Gas Preanalytical Considerations: Specimen Collection, Calibration, and Controls* (document C27A). Villanova, Pa.: National Committee for Clinical Laboratory Standards, 1993.

National Committee for Clinical Laboratory Standards. *Ancillary (Bedside) Blood Glucose Testing in Acute and Chronic Care Facilities* (document C30–A). Villanova, Pa.: National Committee for Clinical Laboratory Standards, 1994.

National Committee for Clinical Laboratory Standards. *Performance of the Bleeding Time Test: Proposed Guidelines* (document H45–P). Villanova, Pa.: National Committee for Clinical Laboratory Standards, 1995.

Quinley, E. D. *Immunohematology: Principles and Practice*. Philadelphia: J. B. Lippincott, 1993.

Walker, R. H., ed. *American Association of Blood Banks Technical Manual*, 11th ed. Arlington, Va.: American Association of Blood Banks, 1993.

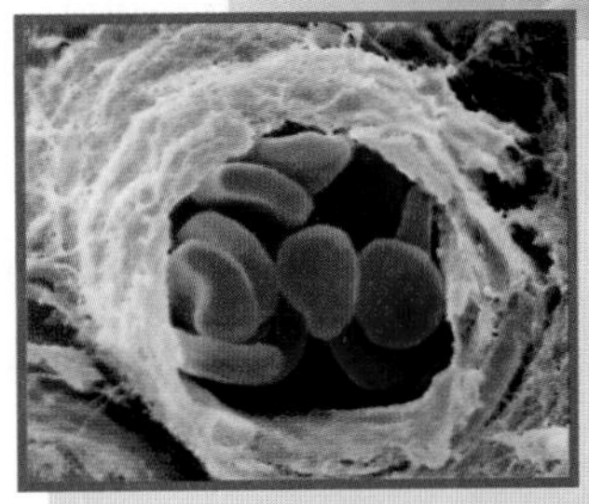

Special Patient Populations

Chapter Outline

Learning Objectives

After completing this chapter, you should be able to

1. Define and spell the glossary terms listed in this chapter.
2. Describe when a venipuncture, heel puncture, and finger puncture are used for pediatric patients.
3. Discuss the techniques available to immobilize a pediatric patient.
4. Discuss the special precautions that should be used during venipuncture on a geriatric patient.
5. Explain why infection control is extremely important in a nursery.
6. Describe some of the different methods of communicating with a hearing impaired patient.
7. List five guidelines for working with a visually impaired patient.
8. Describe how to communicate with a non-English-speaking patient.
9. Discuss the best way to diffuse a tense situation with an angry patient.
10. List the extra equipment needed by a traveling phlebotomist.
11. Explain why there is a need for traveling phlebotomists.

GLOSSARY

CANNULA a temporary device implanted in a vein for attachment to dialysis equipment.

FISTULA permanent surgical fusion of a vein and artery.

GERIATRIC pertaining to the elderly.

IATROGENIC physician induced.

ISOLETTE individual clear plastic basket used in nurseries for newborns.

PHENYLKETONURIA (PKU) hereditary metabolic disorder.

SCLEROSED scarred.

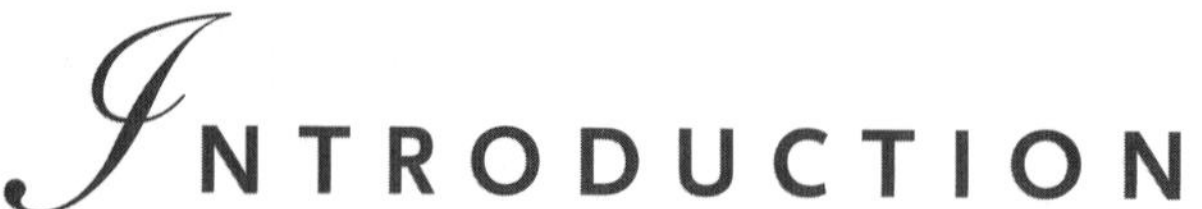

Health care in the United States is undergoing dramatic changes. Due to advances in medicine, the number of laboratory tests for the pediatric population is growing, and, consequently, the number of pediatric phlebotomies is increasing. Although the number of pediatric patients is increasing, the population of the United States is aging. Currently, 15 percent of the population in the United States is over 65 years of age, and the U.S. Census Bureau predicts that by 2023, 20 percent of the population will be over 65 years. In addition, more patients are recovering from surgery or illness at home, thereby creating a need for home health care. A competent phlebotomist must be able to successfully obtain a blood specimen from all patient populations and in many different settings, some of which may be nontraditional.

The Pediatric Patient

As it becomes possible for more and more laboratory tests to be performed on small quantities of blood, more children are being seen for venipuncture at sites other than pediatric hospitals. These sites include doctors' offices, blood-drawing centers, and local hospital outpatient laboratories. Although pediatric venipuncture has its own unique challenges, all phlebotomists should become experienced in pediatric phlebotomy. Figure 9-1 illustrates a pediatric patient who will experience venipuncture as part of her treatment. Developing the necessary skills for pediatric phlebotomy takes time. It requires excellent interpersonal communication and patience. Most phlebotomists gain experience with older children before attempting to collect blood from toddlers. The protocol for venipuncture and dermal puncture is the same for adults and children and was discussed in detail in chapters 6 and 7. A pediatric phlebotomist must become experienced in calming both young children and parents while working under possibly stressful conditions.

One characteristic unique to pediatric phlebotomy is that the phlebotomist must communicate with both the patient and the patient's parent or guardian. The phlebotomist must explain the procedure to both and gain the trust of both the child and the adult in an attempt to limit their anxiety. Trust is gained by greeting the patient and accompanying adult in a warm, pleasant manner and matter-of-factly explaining the procedure. Usually, parents or guardians are quite helpful in calming their children and relieving their fears; however, if the phlebotomist feels that the adult is making the child more anxious, he or she can politely ask the adult to wait outside until the procedure is finished.

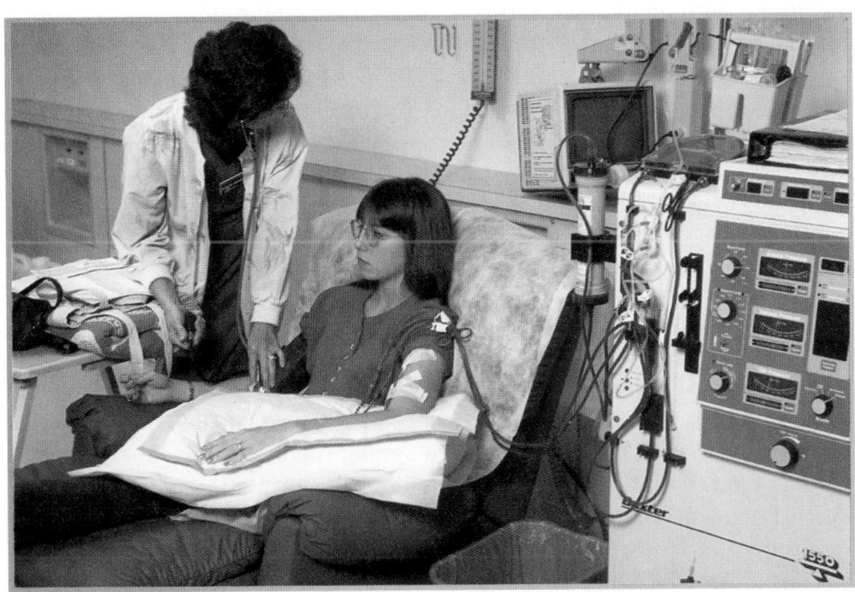

Figure 9-1
Proficiency in pediatric phlebotomy is becoming increasingly important.

Many children have never had their blood drawn before and associate needles with an injection. The phlebotomist may find it helpful to demonstrate the procedure to the child using a stuffed animal or doll. It is very important to explain the procedure in words that the child will understand and at the same time not be condescending to the child. The phlebotomist should give the child the opportunity to ask questions about the procedure and provide honest answers. If asked if the needle will hurt, a truthful response is, "yes, but only for a moment." It may help reduce the child's anxiety if he or she is able to participate in the procedure. By asking the child to hold the bandage or cotton, the phlebotomist is hoping to distract the child from focusing solely on the needle.

The most common method of blood collection from a child under 2 years of age is a dermal (capillary) puncture. The usual guidelines are heel punctures on children under 1 year or 20 pounds and finger punctures from 1 to 2 years of age. Each blood-drawing center has its own guidelines for heel versus finger puncture collections. Children over 2 years may have a venipuncture using either the antecubital fossa or the dorsal veins of the hand. If a venipuncture is required for children under the age of 2 years, superficial veins are used and the procedure is usually performed by specially trained personnel.

Most experienced pediatric phlebotomists use a 23- to 25-gauge butterfly needle with pediatric-sized evacuated tubes. Many different types of evacuated tubes are available in adult and pediatric sizes. Some children may not sit quietly throughout the venipuncture procedure, and the long plastic tubing of the butterfly system permits some degree of movement without disrupting the procedure.

Some children are so terrified of the procedure that they are unable to cooperate with the phlebotomist. For those situations, in 1993, the U.S. Food and Drug Administration (FDA) approved the use of a topical anesthetic, EMLA. EMLA is a mixture of lidocaine and prilocaine, two previously approved anesthetics. EMLA is placed on intact skin and covered with a dressing. Optimal effectiveness is reached in 1 hour and lasts for 2 to 3 hours. EMLA may be used on children older than 1 month and with no known drug sensitivities. Disadvantages to using EMLA are that the exact area of venipuncture must be known and the child must wait for 1 hour for the EMLA to numb the skin.

Most young children must be immobilized to perform a safe and successful venipuncture. It is usually helpful to have the parent or another adult the child knows assist in the procedure. Immobilization can occur in two ways. The most common method is to have the child sit on the adult's lap. The adult can comfort the child while holding the arm that is not being used. In some cases, it may be necessary for the adult to restrain the child's legs by placing one of his or her own legs over the child's. The phlebotomist can steady the arm that is being used in the procedure. The other method of restraining a child requires the child to lie down on a bed. The adult, on the opposite side of the bed from the phlebotomist, leans over the child and restrains both arms. The phlebotomist then has both hands free to perform the venipuncture.

The Nursery Patient

Nurseries, which house the youngest patients in a hospital, vary in size and can hold anywhere from four to a dozen or more newborns. Each newborn is kept in an individual clear plastic basket called an **isolette** that is identified with the baby's name in a similar manner to the label on a bed in a patient's room. All states require that newborns be tested for **phenylketonuria (PKU)** (hereditary metabolic disorder), and many newborns are continually monitored for bilirubin levels or require other laboratory tests. Most newborns require very few blood tests, but when needed, blood

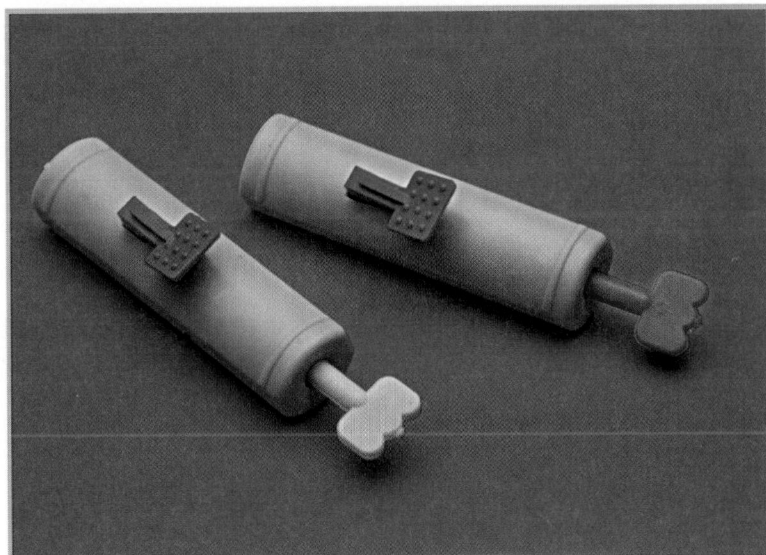

Figure 9-2
An illustration of a typical lancet used for a heel stick.

is usually obtained by a heel stick (see chapter 7). See figure 9-2 for an illustration of a typical lancet used for a heel stick. Unfortunately, some newborns require many laboratory tests; if so, a larger specimen is usually obtained by a venipuncture using a surface vein such as a dorsal hand vein or the cephalic vein. These specimens are usually drawn by specially trained nursery personnel. Depending on the policy of the nursery, heel sticks may be performed by nursery personnel or phlebotomists.

Although infection control is an important aspect of patient care, it is most important in a nursery. Newborns are extremely susceptible to infections, and multiple patients are kept in the same room. If an infection develops in one newborn, it can easily spread to others. To prevent an infection in the nursery, specialized infection control procedures have been developed to protect the infants. Those entering a nursery must wash their hands and cover their clothing with a disposable gown. Some nurseries also require head and shoe coverings. The phlebotomy tray must be left outside the nursery door, and only necessary supplies may be brought into the nursery. Some nurseries stock their own phlebotomy supplies to prevent any extraneous material from coming into the nursery.

MED TIP

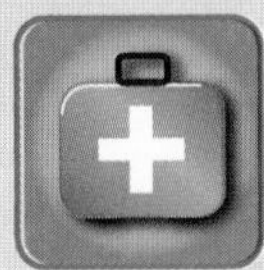

Although it is always important for you to change gloves and wash hands between patients, it is even more important when working in a nursery.

Infants are usually kept on their backs bundled in a receiving blanket in an isolette, as illustrated in figure 9-3. A cloth diaper or rolled blanket may be placed along side the newborn to help keep him or her from rolling over. It will be necessary to remove the blanket and perhaps roll the infant over onto his or her back to perform a heel stick. Upon completing the procedure, the infant is rewrapped in the receiving blanket and placed in the same position as he or she was originally found. All supplies and trash should be removed from the isolette.

MED TIP

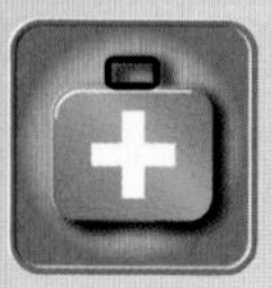

Do not use bandages on children under the age of 2 years because they may swallow them.

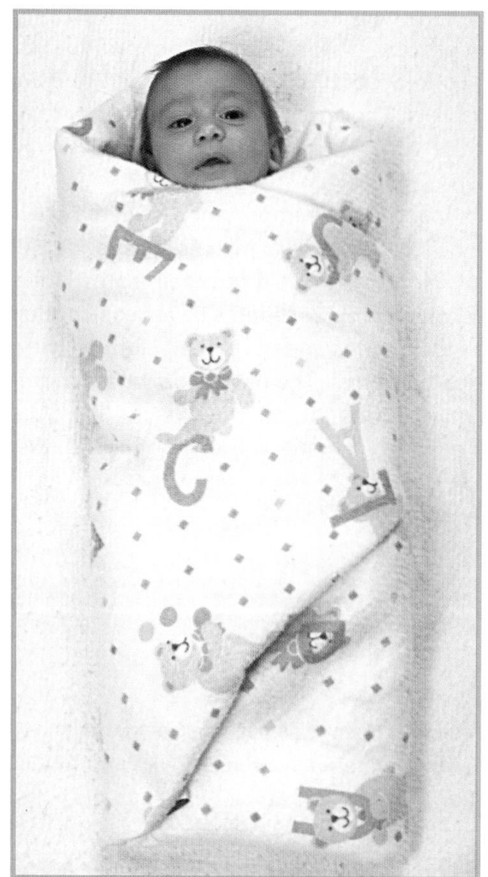

Figure 9-3
Infants are usually kept on their backs bundled in a receiving blanket in an isolette.

The Geriatric Patient

Just as in the pediatric patient, drawing blood from the **geriatric,** or elderly, patient may present a phlebotomist with special challenges that can easily be overcome with a little extra time and patience. The special problems that may be encountered with a geriatric patient are usually associated with the normal physiological aging process. See table 9-1 for a summary of critical points for geriatric venipuncture.

Communication may be more difficult with older patients. Hearing acuity may diminish with age; therefore, the phlebotomist must speak slowly and clearly. A stroke or Parkinson's disease may make a patient's speech difficult to understand. Difficulty in communication can be frustrating for both the patient and the phlebotomist. Patience and understanding on the part of the phlebotomist will help alleviate the difficulties. It is imperative that older adult patients understand the blood collection process and, if able, give informed consent to the procedure. It is extremely important that they not feel that they are being ignored; if possible, they should be made to feel that they are active participants in their health care.

Physiological changes that take place in the skin and musculature can make venipuncture more technically difficult in the geriatric patient. As one ages, skin cells are not replaced as rapidly as previously, and the skin becomes less elastic. Blood vessels also lose elasticity and may become more fragile. These changes, combined with the loss of collagen and muscle tissue, produce veins with a tendency to roll. Veins must be well anchored when performing a venipuncture, but care must be used not to bruise fragile skin. It is usually helpful to pull the skin taut on both sides of the vein rather than applying pressure above or below the venipuncture site.

MED TIP

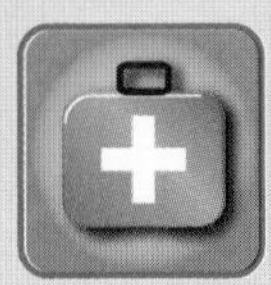

If the skin in the antecubital fossa has a hematoma, use another site for blood collection.

TABLE 9-1 Key Points for Venipuncture in the Geriatric Population

1. Assess the patient and determine if it is necessary to speak more slowly and carefully than usual.
2. Correctly identify the patient.
3. Use a tourniquet that fastens, not ties, and apply over clothing.
4. To aid in blood flow, gently massage the arm and apply heat.
5. Use the appropriate size of needle and evacuated tube.
6. Avoid probing for the vein with the needle.
7. If necessary, apply pressure for extra time to stop bleeding.
8. Use discretion in applying adhesive bandages.

Veins in the elderly may be **sclerosed** (scarred) and have poor blood flow. Butterfly needles or pediatric-sized evacuated tubes are usually helpful when obtaining blood from weak or sclerosed veins. Older adult patients may be unable to extend their arms, unclench their fists, or prevent their limbs from trembling due to stroke, arthritis, Parkinson's disease, or other neurological conditions. Acceptable drawing sites may also be limited in geriatric patients because of bruises, difficulty in locating a vein, or skin irritation, all of which are common in this patient population. Probing is not advised due to the discomfort and bruising it may cause. The phlebotomist may have to be creative in seeking a venipuncture site or have a coworker assist with the procedure.

Some techniques can be helpful in locating an appropriate site for venipuncture in the geriatric patient. Applying heat to the site will increase blood flow and make the veins more prominent, but tapping the patient's arm to dilate veins may cause bruising. Having the patient make a fist will help make locating a suitable vein easier. Painting the area with iodine also makes veins easier to visualize. This technique can only be used if the patient is not allergic to iodine and iodine will not interfere with any of the ordered laboratory tests.

Another normal aging process is a weakening of the immune system, which leaves a patient more susceptible to an infection and slower to recover from one. Hand washing and following sterile technique are always important, but they are even more critical with a geriatric patient. If the scheduled phlebotomist has a respiratory infection or any other infectious illness, he or she should avoid the geriatric patient and summon a coworker.

The coagulation time may be increased in the elderly patient. Delayed coagulation makes it especially important to apply pressure to the puncture site until all bleeding has stopped. If the patient has fragile skin, adhesive bandages or tape can damage the skin. In extreme cases, cloth tape can also damage the skin. If a geriatric patient has very delicate skin, an elastic bandage can be used to hold gauze in place without damaging the skin.

Geriatric patients may also suffer from emotional problems that may be exhibited as inappropriate behavior. The phlebotomist should be aware of these behavioral changes and speak to the patient in a calm, gentle tone. If the patient is not cooperative, a coworker should be called for assistance before beginning the procedure.

Another problem that may be encountered with the elderly is the difficulty in establishing patient identification. Geriatric outpatients may not have identification if they do not have a driver's license. Patients in nursing facilities may not have identification wrist bands. Inpatients may become confused and wander into the wrong room. It is imperative that the established protocol be followed to confirm the patient's identity. Immeasurable harm can occur if a patient is incorrectly identified and the specimen is mislabeled.

A common complication of frequent venipuncture in the elderly is anemia. **Iatrogenic** (physician-induced) anemia leads to the need for transfusion in 10 percent of the patients in intensive care units. This complication can be avoided by simply reducing the number of ordered laboratory tests and by using pediatric-sized evacuated tubes. The laboratory has the responsibility of monitoring the number of tests ordered on a patient and should consult with the physician if the number of tests appears to be excessive.

The Hearing Impaired Patient

Due to the high noise level in many cities and the amplification of music today, there is a large hearing impaired population, as pictured in figure 9-4. For guidelines on working with the hearing impaired patient refer to table 9-2. Hearing impaired patients may be unaware of their impairment or may be em-

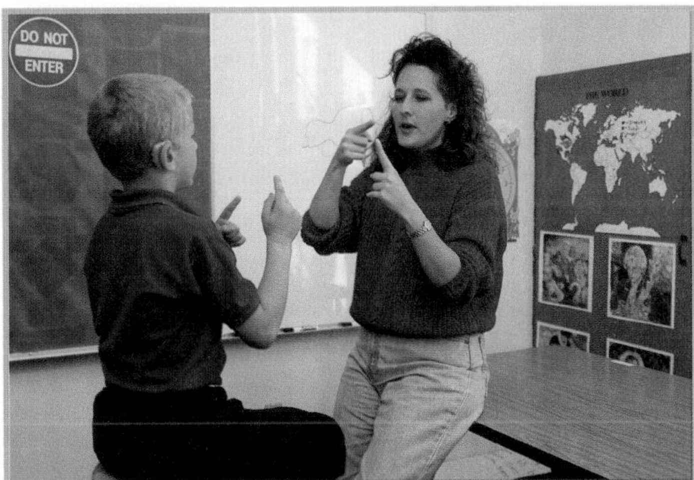

Figure 9-4
The number of hearing impaired patients is increasing.

TABLE 9-2	Guidelines for Helping the Hearing Impaired Patient
1.	Never shout; speak slowly and clearly.
2.	If the patient does not understand you the first time, rephrase the statement. The patient may not understand again if you use the same phrases and sounds.
3.	Explain everything carefully before beginning any procedure.
4.	Face the patient when you are speaking. Many hearing impaired persons have learned some lipreading.
5.	Have paper and pencil nearby so that you and the patient can communicate in writing.

barrassed by it. There are many compassionate methods for working with affected patients. The phlebotomist must remember to ask open-ended questions such as, "Please tell me your name" rather than "Is your name Mr. Jones?" He or she should always have paper and pencil available and try to communicate in writing with the hearing impaired patient. The phlebotomist should be aware that patients with impaired hearing are often very sensitive to nonverbal communication such as a frown. Other guidelines for working with the hearing impaired or deaf patient can be found in table 9-2.

The Visually Impaired Patient

Blindness may be present at birth or develop as a result of a disease such as diabetes mellitus. Patients who are blind can remain independent. Table 9-3 presents several guidelines for working with the visually impaired patient.

TABLE 9-3	Guidelines for Working with the Visually Impaired Patient

1. Always speak to announce your presence when you are near a blind person. The visually impaired patient may become startled if you touch him or her without announcing your presence.
2. Guide the patient into the laboratory or phlebotomy chair by offering your arm. A blind patient will prefer to hold onto your arm rather than having you grab his or her arm.
3. Try to face the patient and speak clearly. He or she is unable to read your lips as a sighted person can do.
4. Describe the patient's surroundings to him or her.
5. Try not to leave the patient alone for any length of time.
6. Explain everything carefully before beginning any procedure.

The Non-English-Speaking Patient

It is still possible to safely perform a laboratory procedure if the patient and the phlebotomist do not speak the same language. However, the phlebotomist must take extra time and patience to be sure the patient understands what is going to happen. Every effort must be made to use nonverbal language and sign language indicating that blood is going to be drawn for a test. The phlebotomist should have available a list of interpreters within the facility who may help in communicating with the patient. If available, an interpreter should be present. Every patient deserves compassionate care. The patient who does not understand English is often very fearful of medical procedures.

MED TIP

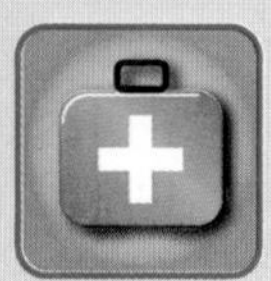

Remember that drawing blood from a patient without the patient's consent (implied or otherwise) can be considered assault and battery. Therefore, you must be able to communicate with every patient.

Ideally every institution has cards available with key phrases in various languages such as "Good Morning," "Good Afternoon," "What is your name?" "I work in the laboratory," "Have you had your breakfast?" and "I need a blood [urine] sample." (See appendix C for basic Spanish phrases.)

The Difficult Patient

One of the most difficult communication problems involves the angry patient. It can be a difficult task for the phlebotomist to refrain from taking the patient's comments personally. People have different styles and coping behaviors when they are frightened or angry. Many people who come in for a laboratory test are fearful of the diagnosis they will hear as a result of the test. Some patients are frightened of the equipment used for obtaining laboratory specimens or have an unwarranted fear of pain.

The phlebotomist's job is to remain calm and to use professional techniques to positively direct the patient's anger and/or fear. For example, many patients gain control over their anger when the phlebotomist offers a comment such as, "I'm really sorry you feel this way. Let's see if we can solve the problem."

The angry patient may have to be moved into a private area if he or she cannot be calmed immediately. Disruptive patients can upset other patients waiting to have laboratory work done. Although it is not necessary to give in to the unreasonable demands of a patient, the phlebotomist must realize that an upset patient is often expressing a need for the phlebotomist to listen carefully, without judgment, and to assist in solving the problem. Whenever possible, the patient's comments should be directed to the solution of the problem without arguing with the patient.

The Dialysis Patient

In an effort to monitor their health, dialysis patients (as pictured in figure 9-5) have frequent laboratory tests. Dialysis is a treatment that removes waste products from the blood of patients with end-stage kidney disease. The frequency of blood tests and the dialysis procedure severely limits the available venipuncture sites. Dialysis patients may have either a **cannula** or a **fistula** implanted to aid in the dialysis procedure. A cannula is a temporary device implanted in a vein for easy access during dialysis. Although a blood sample for laboratory testing can be obtained from a cannula, this procedure should only be performed by specially trained personnel. A fistula is a permanent surgical fusing of an artery and a vein. Blood should not be drawn from a fistula for laboratory testing because the specimen would contain a mixture of arterial and venous blood.

MED TIP

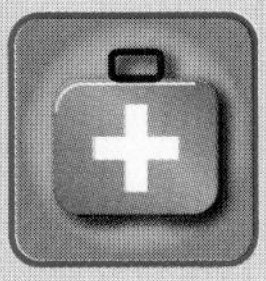

If one arm has a fistula or cannula and the other arm an intravenous (IV) tube, the specimen may be drawn on the arm with the IV, dorsal to the IV site.

Figure 9-5
In an effort to monitor their health, dialysis patients have frequent laboratory tests.

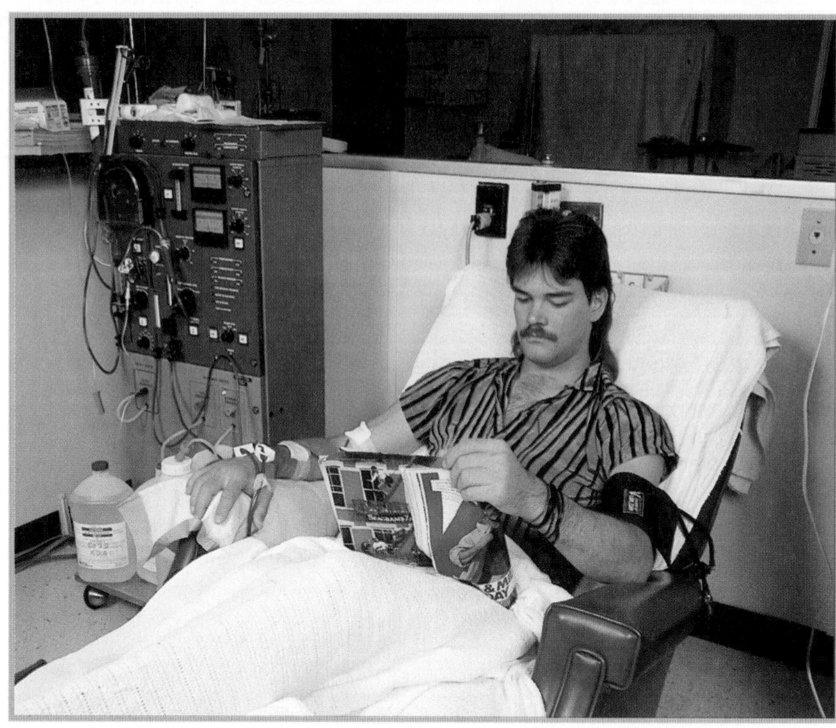

The Homebound Patient

Recent changes in heath care practices have drastically shortened the length of time patients spend in the hospital. Patients are being discharged from hospitals earlier than ever before. Many patients still require nursing care or laboratory services once they have been discharged from the hospital and sent home. An illustration of the homebound patient is found in figure 9-6. In an effort to serve these patients, nurses and other health care professionals visit patients at home to provide care that was once provided in the hospital setting. Many patients' conditions must be monitored with laboratory tests after they have been discharged, but they may be unable to return to the hospital's outpatient laboratory. To serve this population, some hospitals, private laboratories, and home health care agencies are hiring phlebotomists who travel to a patient's home to obtain a blood specimen and then return that specimen to the laboratory.

The traveling phlebotomist must be comfortable working in different situations throughout the day and apart from other health care professionals. Characteristics of a traveling phlebotomist include the ability to work independently, the ability to adapt to new situations, excellent organizational skills, and an attention to detail. The traveling phlebotomist must make certain that he or she has all the necessary supplies before going to a patient's house. The supplies the phlebotomist must carry include not only the actual venipuncture supplies but also the proper disposal equipment for sharps and contaminated waste, and specialized handling equipment to transport the specimen safely to the laboratory.

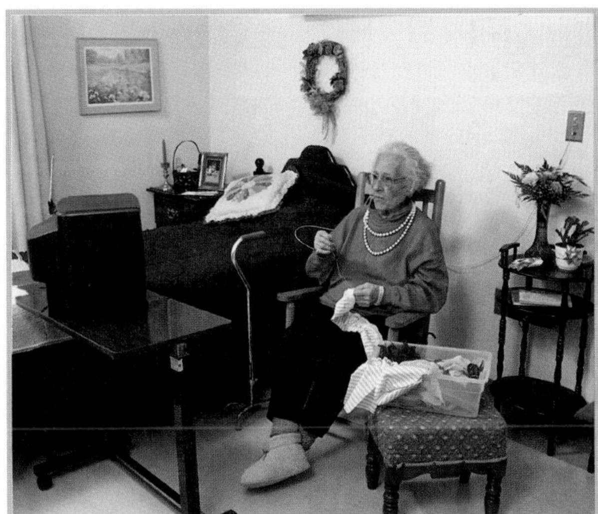

Figure 9-6
Homebound patient.

The traveling phlebotomist must be comfortable going into different households and performing technical duties under a wide range of conditions. Sometimes the patient may be in bed, and other times the phlebotomist may draw the patient's blood at a kitchen table. The house may be quiet or there may be a number of children eager to watch the procedure. The phlebotomist must firmly yet politely restrict family members or move to a different area of the house if it is in the best interests of the patient and the phlebotomist. After the blood sample has been collected, the phlebotomist must carefully dispose of any needles or lancets in an approved sharps container and remove all contaminated supplies in a biohazard container. The phlebotomist must also be aware of special handling conditions for the specimen (e.g., exposure to cold, protection from exposure to light) and transport the specimen to the laboratory under the proper conditions.

CHAPTER REVIEW

Summary

In today's changing health care environment, phlebotomists no longer care for only traditional adult inpatients or outpatients. Patients may be visited in their homes, large outpatient facilities, short-procedures units, or just about anywhere for blood collection. In addition, the age range of patients is expanding, with laboratory tests being ordered on hour-old newborns to patients in their nineties. Phlebotomists are expected to obtain a properly collected blood specimen from a wide range of patients in a variety of circumstances.

Competency Review

1. Discuss the equipment usually used in pediatric venipuncture.
2. Describe the special precautions that must be followed to enter a nursery.
3. Why may it be difficult to establish the identity of a geriatric patient?
4. How can the incidence of iatrogenic anemia be reduced in the elderly?
5. Describe the characteristics of a traveling phlebotomist.

Examination Review Questions

1. **All of the following are unique to pediatric phlebotomy except**
   (A) children are usually less cooperative than adults
   (B) the phlebotomist must deal with both the patient and an adult
   (C) the veins in children tend to roll
   (D) pediatric-sized evacuated tubes are difficult to work with
   (E) only a dermal puncture can be used on a pediatric patient

2. **Veins in a geriatric patient may have a tendency to roll because with age**
   (A) veins become less elastic
   (B) collagen is lost
   (C) skin becomes less elastic
   (D) muscle is lost
   (E) all of the above

3. **When dealing with a very angry patient, which of the following statements would best diffuse the situation?**
   (A) "Please come back some other time when you are less angry."
   (B) "I'm sorry you are upset about the length of time you have had to wait. Let me see if I can do this test quickly for you."
   (C) "I think you are angry because without a medical background like mine, you simply do not understand the situation."
   (D) "We are very busy, and you will just have to wait your turn."
   (E) It is best not to respond to an angry patient but to ignore the patient until his or her anger is spent.

4. In a dialysis patient blood can be drawn from all of the following except the

(A) fistula
(B) cannula
(C) dorsal side of the wrist
(D) antecubital fossa
(E) none of the above

5. When a phlebotomist performs a venipuncture at a patient's home

(A) the phlebotomist must always perform the procedure in a relatively sterile area like a bedroom
(B) the phlebotomist must carry equipment to safely dispose of sharps and contaminated trash
(C) the phlebotomist must always be willing to perform a venipuncture in front of family members
(D) the patient is usually too sick to be in a hospital
(E) phlebotomists only work in hospitals

6. When performing a venipuncture on a geriatric patient, all of the following are concerns except

(A) hematoma
(B) iatrogenic anemia
(C) sclerosed veins
(D) removing contaminated waste from the isolette
(E) easy bruising of the skin

7. The traveling phlebotomist carries extra supplies, including

(A) puncture-proof containers
(B) disposal equipment for contaminated trash
(C) specimen transportation containers
(D) extra evacuated tubes
(E) all of the above

8. The protocol for performing a dermal puncture on a pediatric patient

(A) differs from the adult procedure
(B) is the same as the adult procedure
(C) requires pediatric-sized evacuated tubes
(D) differs in the use of larger lancets
(E) does not require the use of an antiseptic

9. When performing a venipuncture on a child, the phlebotomist

(A) must never tell the child that the procedure will hurt
(B) must never wear gloves because that will frighten the child
(C) must answer all questions truthfully
(D) must ask the child's parent to leave the room because the presence of a parent will make the child more nervous
(E) all of the above

10. All of the following will help in locating a vein for venipuncture in an elderly patient except

(A) applying heat to the area
(B) gently tapping the area
(C) painting the area with iodine
(D) having the patient make a fist
(E) looking carefully at both arms

Getting Connected

Multimedia Extension Activities

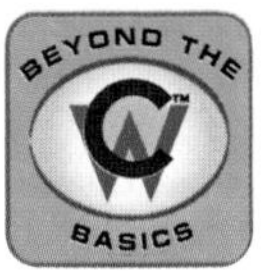

www.prenhall.com/fremgen

Use the address above to access the free, interactive Companion Website created specifically for this textbook. Enhance your studying by answering practice quiz questions, with hints and instant feedback related to chapter 9. If you would like to gain a deeper understanding of selected topics within this chapter, be sure to click on the **Beyond the Basics** feature, which provides more details for further learning. If you do not have a web connection, you may use the CD-ROM enclosed in the back of this book to take advantage of the same features off-line.

Audio Glossary

Use the CD-ROM enclosed with your textbook to hear the pronunciation of the key terms in the chapter. You may also access this material on the Companion Website www.prenhall.com/fremgen.

Bibliography

Farber, V. "Mastering Pediatric Phlebotomy." *Advance for Medical Laboratory Professionals*, January 27, 1997, 5–7.

Foulke, G. E., and D. J. Harlow. "Effective Measures for Reducing Blood Loss from Diagnostic Laboratory Tests in Intensive Care Unit Patients." *Critical Care Medicine* 17 (1989): 1143–1145.

Harden, L."Pediatric Phlebotomy: Great Expectations." *Advance for Medical Laboratory Professionals*, November 3, 1997, 12–13.

"Homelab Draws Blood in the Privacy of Home." *Detroit News*, March 20, 1996.

Klosinski, D. "Collecting Specimens from the Elderly Patient." *Laboratory Medicine* 28, no. 8 (1997): 518–522.

Miller, S. "Successful Aging in America." *Medical Laboratory Observer*, March 1997, 23.

Olds, S., M. London, and P. Ladewig. *Maternal-Newborn Nursing: A Family-Centered Approach*, 5th ed. Redwood City, Calif.: Addison-Wesley, 1996.

CHAPTER 10

The Care and Handling of Specimens

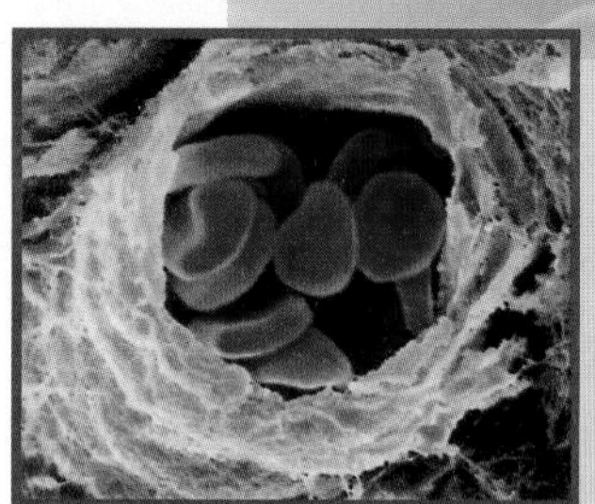

Chapter Outline

Learning Objectives

After completing this chapter, you should be able to

1. Define and spell the glossary terms used in this chapter.
2. Discuss the physiological factors that affect laboratory results.
3. Discuss the proper procedure for transporting a specimen within a health care facility.
4. Describe the procedure for shipping a diagnostic specimen.
5. Describe the role of the central processing area of the laboratory.
6. List conditions under which a specimen would be rejected by the laboratory.

GLOSSARY

AEROSOL a fine mist.

ALIQUOT a portion of a patient specimen used for testing.

ANALYTE term for a substance being tested.

BASAL STATE a resting metabolic state early in the morning and a minimum of 12 hours after eating.

CENTRIFUGATION the process of separating substances of different weights by spinning at high speeds.

DIURNAL daily.

NEONATE a newborn infant.

NORMAL VALUE the amount of a substance that is normally present.

QNS quantity not sufficient.

INTRODUCTION

The quality of the clinical laboratory's work depends on the quality of the specimen received. The phlebotomist is responsible for ensuring that the laboratory receives a high-quality specimen that has been properly handled. If a specimen is collected or handled incorrectly, the results of laboratory testing on that specimen may be erroneous and may lead to the patient receiving incorrect treatment.

Physiological Factors Affecting Laboratory Results

Test results on patient specimens are affected by a number of variables such as age, gender, diet, exercise, **diurnal** (daily) rhythms, medications, and even geographic factors such as altitude. Each clinical laboratory determines its own set of **normal values** for its patient population and the instrumentation used in testing. The normal value is the amount of a substance that is normally present. The normal values for laboratory tests are based on specimens that are drawn when the patients are in a **basal** state. The basal state is a resting metabolic state early in the morning before rising and at least 12 hours after eating. Most health care facilities attempt to draw inpatients' blood samples early in the morning when the patients are in a basal state. Unfortunately, it is usually not possible to draw outpatients' blood samples when the patients are in a basal state.

Many studies have been published about the effects of age and gender on laboratory test results. Laboratories have different sets of normal values for children versus adults and men versus women for tests that are affected by age and gender. For example, the normal red blood cell count is $4.6–6.2 \times 10^{12}/L$ for men, $4.2–5.4 \times 10^{12}/L$ for women, and $3.8–5.5 \times 10^{12}/L$ for children under 12 years of age. Diet has a significant impact on many laboratory results. In an effort to overcome the effects of this variable, many tests require a fasting specimen. A fasting specimen is one that is drawn after the patient has had nothing to eat or drink (except water) for 12 hours. Laboratory tests that can be significantly affected by diet are glucose, iron, alkaline phosphatase, triglyceride, and potassium levels. A protein-rich meal can affect the results of serum urea nitrogen and phosphorus tests for up to 12 hours. Moderate amounts of caffeine can increase plasma cortisol and lipid levels.

MED TIP

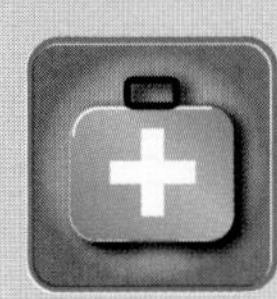

If the patient was to have fasted for a test and did not, make sure the requisition slip is marked nonfasting.

Moderate exercise can affect the levels of lactic acid, creatinine, protein, and some fatty acids for up to 1 hour. The levels of some enzymes, such as creatine phosphokinase (CPK), aspartate aminotransferase (AST), and lactate dehydrogenase (LD), can remain elevated for 24 hours after exercising. Even a change from lying in bed to sitting or standing (supine to erect) immediately prior to venipuncture can cause an increase in various analytes (e.g., albumin, calcium, cholesterol, lipids, potassium, and total protein).

Emotional stress can also affect a patient's laboratory values. Phlebotomists should do their best to reduce anxiety in their patients not only to make the procedure less stressful but also to prevent inaccurate test results. Patient stress has been shown to cause a short-term increase in white blood cell counts and adrenal hormone levels and a short-term decrease in the serum iron level. Crying can cause elevations in the white blood cell count of a **neonate,** a newborn infant. If at all possible, blood should not be drawn on a neonate for a white blood cell count until he or she has stopped crying for 1 hour.

Many blood **analyte** (substance being tested) levels fluctuate throughout the day. Levels of hormones such as testosterone, cortisol, and adrenocorticotropic hormone (ACTH) are highest in the morning, whereas the white blood cell count, eosinophil count, and serum iron levels are highest in the afternoon. If possible, the diurnal variation of specific analytes should be considered when drawing blood specimens, and the time of collection should correspond to the highest level of the analyte.

Many medications, both prescription and over-the-counter drugs, can alter the levels of various blood components. For example, the antibiotic penicillin, if given as an intramuscular injection, may cause an increase in lactate dehydrogenase (LD), and some diuretics may cause an elevation in calcium and glucose levels. Physicians should be aware of how various medications affect laboratory values. If possible, the patient may be told to stop taking the medication for 4 to 24 hours prior to blood collection or 48 to 72 hours prior to collection of a urine specimen. If it would be detrimental to the patient's health to stop the medication, the name of the medication should be noted on the requisition slip.

The phlebotomist is not able to control for many of the mentioned physiological factors that can affect laboratory levels. However, he or she can control for some of the conditions under which the specimen is obtained. In chapter 6, we discussed the complication of hemoconcentration. Hemoconcentration is an increase in blood components in an area caused by plasma moving from the circulatory system into tissues because of prolonged use of a tourniquet. Hemoconcentration may cause an increase in the levels of cholesterol, iron, lipids, and total protein and a decrease in the level of potassium. The phlebotomist alone controls the length of time a tourniquet remains on the patient's arm.

Handling of Specimens

Specimens are collected into a primary container (e.g., evacuated tube). The primary container must have a stopper to prevent spillage and to protect the specimen from evaporation and contamination. The primary container is then placed in a leak-proof plastic bag, and the requisition slip is attached to the outside of the plastic bag. The plastic bag protects the requisition slip and health care workers from contamination if the primary container breaks or leaks. Evacuated tubes should always be kept in an upright position. The upright position also aids in specimen clotting and prevents the stopper from contaminating the specimen. Keeping the evacuated tube in a vertical position also helps prevent hemolysis. Many facilities use a transportation block that holds blood specimens upright and protects them from rough handling.

The National Committee for Clinical Laboratory Standards (NCCLS) has established guidelines that all accredited laboratories must follow. These guidelines have set a limit of 2 hours from the time the specimen is drawn until the cells are separated from the serum or plasma. Blood cells are still metabolically active after the specimen is drawn, and certain test results (glucose, calcitonin, aldosterone, phospherus, and enzymes) may be inaccurate if the cells remain in contact with the serum or plasma for an extended time. Most laboratories strive for a 45-minute delivery period to the laboratory and a total time of 1 hour from collection until centrifugation. If a specimen is collected off-site and transportation to the laboratory will take longer than 2 hours, the specimen should be centrifuged at the collection site and the cells and serum or plasma separated before being transported to the clinical laboratory.

Specimen Transportation

Proper specimen transportation is just as important as proper specimen collection. The specimen must be kept under the appropriate environmental conditions for the ordered laboratory test(s), and it is essential that safety precautions be followed to prevent contamination of the specimen and to protect the person who transports the specimen.

On-Site

Each health care facility has its own procedures for the transportation of specimens to the laboratory. In some facilities the phlebotomist is responsible for transporting specimens to the laboratory; the phlebotomist will see all of the patients for whom he or she has requisitions and then transport all of the collected specimens to the laboratory. In other facilities, a transportation team or the laboratory has that responsibility. The transportation team usually collects specimens on a preset schedule of every hour or two. It may be possible for some specimens to wait for the periodic scheduled pickup to the laboratory, whereas other specimens must be taken to the laboratory immediately after collection. In that case the transportation team would be notified of a special pickup. Many large health care facilities have a pneumatic tube system for transportation of specimens, patient records, X-ray films, medications, and so forth. If a specimen is to be transported by a pneumatic tube system, the specimen should first be placed in a leak-proof plastic bag to prevent contamination of the tube or the health care worker if the specimen leaks. Then the specimen is placed in a shock-resistant container to prevent breakage during transportation in the pneumatic tube.

Off-Site

In ever-increasing numbers, laboratory specimens are being collected at sites other than the clinical laboratory where testing will take place. Many doctors' offices collect their patients' specimens rather than sending patients to the outpatient laboratory of the local hospital. Certain forms of health care coverage require that the patient have blood drawn at the drawing station of a private reference laboratory. Hospital mergers have consolidated the laboratory facilities of many clinical laboratories. For example, the laboratory at Hospital A may send all of its microbiology specimens to its sister hospital across town, Hospital B, and Hospital B may send all of its chemistry tests except stat specimen tests to Hospital A.

Courier services usually transport specimens locally from the collection center to the testing site. Specimens are placed in transport boxes that will protect the specimen from rough handling conditions. The transport boxes must be labeled with a red biohazard warning label as shown in figure 10-1. Courier services must be vigilant to protect the specimens from extreme heat and cold during transportation to the testing laboratory.

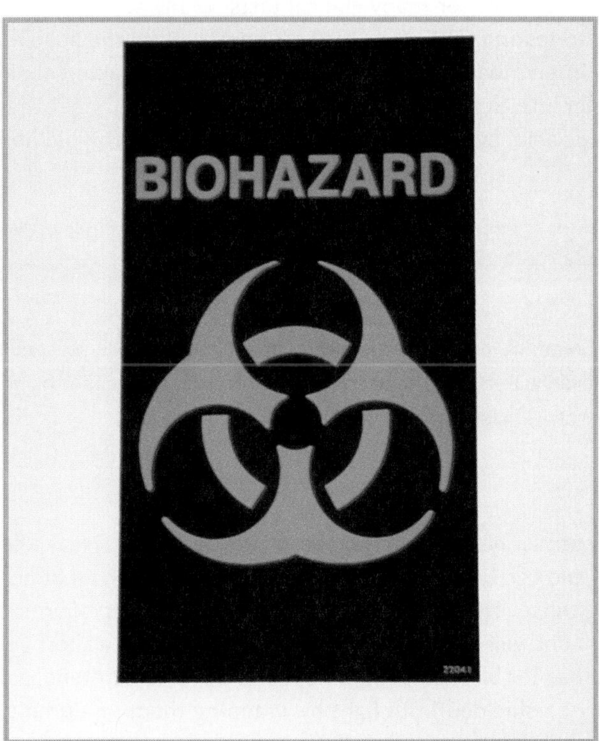

Figure 10-1
Transport boxes must be labeled with a red biohazard warning label.

Shipping Specimens

Today, many diagnostic specimens are sent across the country to specialized laboratories for rare laboratory tests. These specimens must be shipped in a manner that protects the integrity of the specimen and protects the public from possible harm if the specimen leaks. The specimens must be packaged to withstand the leakage problems and rough handling that can occur in long-distance transportation.

The specimen is collected into a primary container that is labeled with the patient's name and the specimen source and then sealed with waterproof tape. The primary container is wrapped in absorbent packing material and placed in a secondary container. The secondary container is also labeled with the patient's name and must have a leak-proof lid that screws firmly into place. The test requisition is usually placed on the outside of the secondary container. The entire package is then placed in a shipping carton. The shipping carton must be large enough to snugly hold the secondary container and any temperature control material (e.g., cold packs or dry ice). If temperature control is important to preserve the specimen, a styrofoam container is usually used. If temperature control is not important, padded envelopes are frequently employed. The outside of the shipping carton should be labeled with a biohazard sticker, and a special label is required if dry ice is used. There are currently many different transportation services available to ship diagnostic specimens ranging from the U.S. Postal Service to FedEx to commercial airlines. The receiving laboratory usually has a preferred carrier and also has shipping and packaging instructions for the sending laboratory.

Special Conditions

Many specimens require specific handling conditions to preserve the specimen for testing regardless of whether the specimen is being shipped across the country or taken down the hall from the drawing station to the laboratory.

Temperature control is an important factor for many clinical tests. Many specimens must be kept cold to preserve the specimen prior to testing. The usual procedure is to place the specimen in a mixture of ice and water. The entire specimen must be submerged in the ice-water mixture, being careful to keep the stopper or lid above the water line. Specimens that require cold include those for arterial blood gases, ammonia, catecholamine, lactic acid, pyruvate, gastrin, protime, and parathyroid hormone tests.

MED TIP

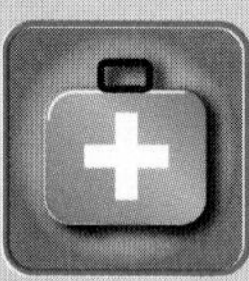

When chilling a specimen, do not use large pieces of ice because they will cause the specimen to chill unevenly. Parts of the specimen may freeze, whereas other parts may be near room temperature. Use a mixture of crushed ice and water.

Some specimens need to be kept warm or near body temperature prior to testing. Heat blocks that have depressions to hold evacuated tubes and can be set to 37°C are available. Specimens that need to remain near body temperature (37°C) include those for cold agglutinin, cryoglobulin, and cryofibrinogen tests.

Some analytes are sensitive to light and will degrade if exposed to light for even a short period of time. Light-sensitive specimens include those for bilirubin, vitamins A and B_6, beta-carotene, and porphyrin tests. Specimens for these tests may be shielded from light by wrapping them in aluminum foil or by collecting the specimen in specialized amber containers.

Laboratory Processing

Today most laboratories have a specific area called central processing, where all specimens are received. In the older method, the specimen was delivered directly to the specialized area of the laboratory where testing was to take place. For example, all specimens for complete blood counts (CBCs) went directly to the hematology laboratory, and all specimens for glucose testing went to the chemistry laboratory. This older method caused difficulties if one specimen required testing in two or more areas of the laboratory. It resulted in more blood being drawn and a delay in testing. With central processing, one specimen can be divided into several smaller portions (**aliquots**) for simultaneous testing in different laboratory areas. The central processing area is also responsible for packaging and sending specimens to outside laboratories.

MED TIP

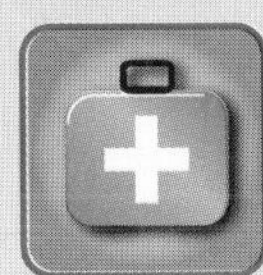

Laboratory personnel who work in central processing are required to wear protective equipment when processing specimens. The protective equipment includes gloves, spill-resistant protective laboratory coats, and eye protection with side pieces and a face mask or chin-length face shields.

The central processing area records the arrival of all specimens by logging them in, usually with a computer but sometimes by hand. Each specimen is given an accession number if one was not assigned when the requisition was generated. The process of logging in includes recording the name of the patient, specimen number, type of specimen, time it arrived in the laboratory, and ordered tests. An important function of the personnel responsible for the log-in process is to check that the patient name on the specimen matches the patient name on the requisition. If the names do not match, nothing further should be done with that specimen until the problem is resolved. If the problem cannot be resolved, the specimen should be discarded and another specimen should be obtained. Specimens that do not require further processing, such as urine, are then delivered to the appropriate laboratory area.

Laboratory tests that require plasma or serum are processed in the central processing area before distribution to the testing laboratory. Plasma specimens may be centrifuged immediately; however, serum specimens must be fully clotted (15 minutes in an evacuated tube with clot activators to 1 hour in a tube without clot activators) before **centrifugation.** Figure 10-2 illustrates a technician centrifuging a specimen. Centrifugation is the process of separating substances of different weight by spinning at high speeds. The stoppered top of a serum tube should not be removed to loosen the clot (also called rimming) because doing so may hemolyze the specimen. The rubber stopper should remain on the tube while centrifuging to prevent the formation of **aerosols** (fine mist) that could be inhaled. Most laboratories centrifuge specimens at 1,000 to 1,200 g for 10 minutes. The relative centrifugal force or g force is a calculation based on the rotating radius and the speed of rotation. Once the centrifuge has stopped spinning, the centrifuge lid may be opened and the tube removed. If the rubber stopper on an evacuated tube must be removed, the work should be done behind a safety splash shield and the stoppered top should be covered with gauze while removing it with a twisting motion. Following these guidelines will protect laboratory personnel from splatters and aerosols that can occur if the rubber stopper is popped open. The serum or plasma may have to be dispensed into aliquot tubes for distribution to different laboratory areas. Each aliquot should be labeled the same as the original sample and must be capped to prevent contamination, evaporation, and laboratory personnel exposure.

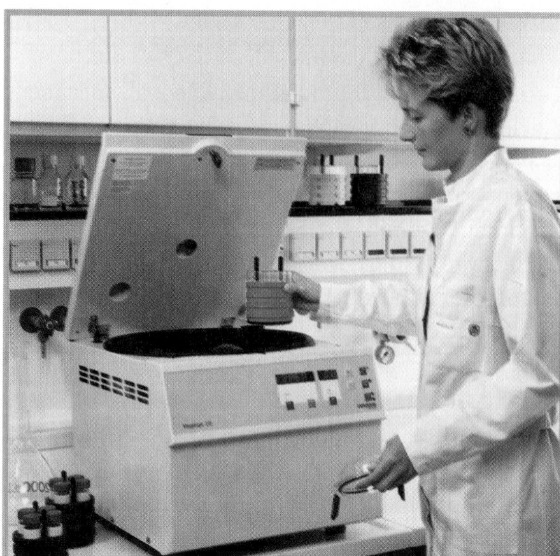

Figure 10-2
Specimens being placed in a centrifuge. (Allegiance Healthcare Corporation distributes, Kendro manufactures.)

MED TIP

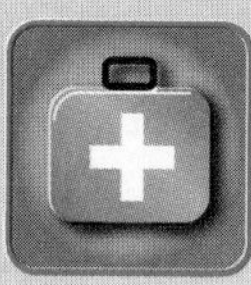

When transferring serum or plasma to aliquot tubes, never pour the specimen. Use a system such as a disposable pipette that minimizes splashes, aerosols, and droplet formation.

Specimen Rejection

Each clinical laboratory has its own criteria for rejecting specimens. The phlebotomist has the responsibility of becoming familiar with these criteria and trying to avoid collecting blood specimens that will be rejected by the laboratory. A rejected specimen means additional work for the phlebotomist, more expense for the laboratory in employee time and materials, and another venipuncture for the patient. Most clinical laboratories reject specimens for the following reasons:

- Requisition or specimen label irregularities
- Hemolyzed specimen
- Incorrect tube used
- Partially filled tube
- Improper handling conditions
- Improperly mixed tube
- Expired tube used
- Incorrect collection time

Requisition or Specimen Label Irregularities

The information on the patient requisition and the specimen label—such as the patient identification number, patient name, date of birth, type of specimen, and so forth—should be identical. If a specimen

MED TIP

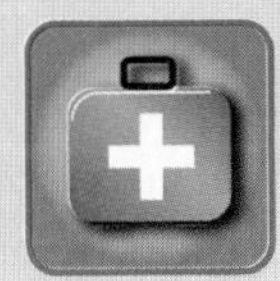

If there is any question as to the accuracy of a specimen label, discard the specimen. One of the most serious errors that can occur in the laboratory is to mislabel a patient specimen.

is received in the laboratory with the wrong label (e.g., a urine label on a blood specimen) or arrives without a label, the specimen must be rejected.

Hemolyzed Specimens

A specimen is hemolyzed when the red blood cell membranes are ruptured and hemoglobin from within the cells is released into the liquid portion of blood. Hemoglobin imparts a pink to red color to the serum or plasma. The intensity of the color depends on the number of red blood cells affected. The more red blood cells hemolyzed, the redder the color of the serum or plasma. Hemolysis affects the values of certain laboratory tests such as complete blood count (CBC), lactic dehydrogenase (LD), aspartate aminotransferase (AST), potassium (K^+), serum iron (Fe), and thyroxine (T_4). Laboratories usually discard a hemolyzed specimen if ordered for these tests, and a new specimen must be drawn. Hemolysis is usually caused by improper phlebotomy technique or the patient's physiological state. The most common reasons for hemolysis that are due to phlebotomy technique include the following:

- Rough handling of the specimen
- Vigorously mixing evacuated tubes with additives
- Using a needle that is too small
- Using a large evacuated tube with a butterfly needle
- Pulling the plunger back too rapidly when filling the syringe
- "Milking" a capillary puncture site
- Selecting a vein with a hematoma for venipuncture

If the phlebotomist notices that a specimen hemolyzes as soon as it is drawn, this fact should be noted on the requisition because it may be an indication of the abnormal physiological state of the patient.

Incorrect Tube

It is the phlebotomist's responsibility to draw the specimen into the correct evacuated tube for the ordered laboratory test. If the specimen has been drawn with the wrong tube, the specimen cannot be transferred to the correct tube. If the specimen was drawn in a plain tube and plasma was required for the laboratory test, the specimen may already have begun to clot. If the specimen was incorrectly drawn in a tube with the wrong additive, transferring the specimen to the correct evacuated tube would dilute the blood with additives from both tubes. The incorrect additive may also interfere with the testing process or cause erroneous test results.

Partially Filled Tube

If an evacuated tube is not filled to capacity, the ratio of additive to blood will be incorrect. Partially filled blue-topped evacuated tubes used for coagulation testing will not be accepted by most laboratories because the excess additive will cause erroneous test results. Plain evacuated tubes are usually accepted for testing if they are partially filled because the serum is not affected by a short draw. The other problem with partially filled tubes is that there may not be enough of the specimen to run the laboratory test. Such a specimen is referred to as **quantity not sufficient (QNS),** which should be noted on the requisition.

Improper Handling Conditions

Some laboratory tests require that specimens be transported to the laboratory under specific environmental conditions. If these conditions are not met, the specimen may be rejected because the test results would be invalid. Some analytes are extremely sensitive to light and must be shielded from light prior to testing. Temperature is another critical factor for some laboratory tests. Some specimens need to be kept cold to slow down the metabolic activity of cells. Other tests require that the specimen be transported to the laboratory in a heating block that maintains the temperature of the specimen at 37°C, or body temperature.

MED TIP

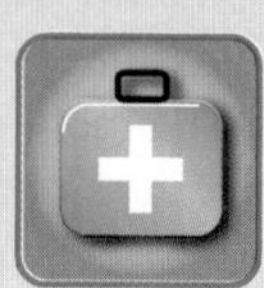

Protect all specimens from extreme heat or cold during transportation to the laboratory.

Improperly Mixed Tube

The proper protocol for handling evacuated tubes with additives is to invert them gently five to ten times as soon as they are drawn. This procedure thoroughly mixes the additive with the blood. If tubes are not mixed thoroughly, clots may form in spite of the presence of the anticoagulant. The clots render the specimen unsuitable for hematology testing because they may clog the tubing used in the hematology instruments. Vigorous shaking of the tube will cause hemolysis and should be avoided. Plain tubes used for serum do not require inverting.

Expired Tube

The phlebotomist must always check the expiration date on all expendable equipment. The expiration date is the date the manufacturer stamps on the equipment. If a product is used after the expiration date, the manufacturer will no longer guarantee that product. Additives may decompose and the vacuum may be lost in an evacuated tube that is past its expiration date. Clinical laboratories will reject specimens that are drawn in expired tubes. Expiration dates on supplies should be carefully checked, and those with short expiration dates should be used first. In the current cost-conscious health care environment, supplies should be continually rotated so that materials with long expiration dates are placed in the back and those with short expiration dates are placed in front and used first. Even though expired supplies cannot be used in patient testing, many products are still reliable after the expiration date and can be used for training or educational purposes.

Incorrect Collection Time

If a timed specimen is collected at the wrong time, the laboratory may reject it. Collecting specimens at the wrong time can lead to erroneous results in therapeutic drug monitoring, glucose testing, and other tolerance testing. If a specimen is collected at the incorrect time, the phlebotomist must always note this discrepancy on the requisition. The laboratory will then determine whether to perform the clinical testing or to reject the specimen.

CHAPTER REVIEW

Summary

The care of clinical specimens after they have been collected is just as important to the integrity of the specimen as the collection procedure. Phlebotomists must be aware of factors that can lead to poor specimen collection and specimen rejection and try to avoid those factors when collecting specimens.

Competency Review

1. Describe five physiological factors that can affect normal laboratory values.
2. Many specimens must be transported to the laboratory under specific environmental conditions. List these conditions and describe how the specimen is transported.
3. Describe the process a specimen undergoes from the time it reaches the central processing area until it reaches the specific testing laboratory.
4. Describe the protective equipment worn by laboratory personnel in central processing.
5. List five reasons why a specimen may be rejected for testing by a clinical laboratory and how rejection can be prevented.

Examination Review Questions

1. The maximum time that is permitted from drawing a specimen until the separation of serum and cells is

(A) 15 minutes
(B) 1 hour
(C) 2 hours
(D) 4 hours
(E) 30 minutes

2. Specimens that must be kept cold are

(A) immediately refrigerated after drawing
(B) put in a mixture of water and ice
(C) put on a block of ice
(D) transported to the laboratory at room temperature and then chilled
(E) drawn in an evacuated tube that has been kept in the freezer

3. To compensate for the diurnal variation of many analytes, blood should be collected

(A) in the morning
(B) after the patient has eaten
(C) when the analyte is at its highest level
(D) only when the patient is in a supine position
(E) after a 12-hour fast

4. Evacuated tubes should always be transported to the laboratory

(A) in a mixture of ice and water
(B) in a heat block
(C) covered with aluminum foil
(D) in an upright position
(E) lying on their side to promote clotting

5. Blood specimens are centrifuged to

(A) separate the cells from the serum or plasma
(B) separate the platelets from the white blood cells
(C) remove any interfering substances
(D) remove the anticoagulant
(E) separate the red blood cells from the white blood cells

6. During the log-in procedure, all of the following information is required except

(A) name of patient
(B) type of specimen
(C) time specimen arrived in the laboratory
(D) ordered tests
(E) type of evacuated tube used

7. **If a hemolyzed blood specimen arrives in the central processing area of the laboratory**
   (A) the physician must draw the patient's blood in the future
   (B) the phlebotomist is always reprimanded
   (C) the specimen can still be used because hemolysis does not affect the results of any laboratory tests
   (D) the patient's physiological state may be the cause
   (E) an expired evacuated tube was probably used

8. **When sending a specimen to a laboratory in another state**
   (A) the primary container is marked with a biohazard label
   (B) the test requisition is placed on the primary container
   (C) the shipping carton is marked with a biohazard label
   (D) it may only be sent by the U.S. Postal Service
   (E) it must always be packaged in dry ice

9. **If a laboratory test requires serum, the specimen must be**
   (A) shaken vigorously
   (B) permitted to clot and then centrifuged
   (C) centrifuged prior to clotting
   (D) kept in a mixture of ice and water
   (E) kept shielded from light

10. **Laboratory personnel should follow all of the following rules when removing a stopper from an evacuated tube except**
   (A) work with the specimen behind a safety splash shield
   (B) always wear goggles
   (C) cover the stopper with gauze
   (D) wear two pairs of asbestos gloves
   (E) wear a spill-resistant protective laboratory coat

Getting Connected

Multimedia Extension Activities

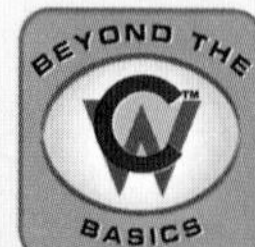

www.prenhall.com/fremgen

Use the address above to access the free, interactive Companion Website created specifically for this textbook. Enhance your studying by answering practice quiz questions, with hints and instant feedback related to chapter 10. If you would like to gain a deeper understanding of selected topics within this chapter, be sure to click on the **Beyond the Basics** feature, which provides more details for further learning. If you do not have a web connection, you may use the CD-ROM enclosed in the back of this book to take advantage of the same features off-line.

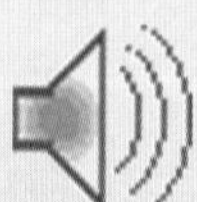

Audio Glossary

Use the CD-ROM enclosed with your textbook to hear the pronunciation of the key terms in the chapter. You may also access this material on the Companion Website www.prenhall.com/fremgen.

Bibliography

Bishop, M., J. Duben-Engelkirk, and E. Fody. *Clinical Chemistry: Principles, Procedures, Correlations,* 3rd ed. Philadelphia: Lippincott-Raven, 1996.

Burtis, C., and E. Ashwood. *Tietz: Fundamentals of Clinical Chemistry.* Philadelphia: W. B. Saunders, 1996.

Henry, J. B. *Clinical Diagnosis and Management by Laboratory Methods,* 19th ed. Philadelphia: W. B. Saunders, 1996.

National Committee for Clinical Laboratory Standards. *Procedures for the Handling and Processing of Blood Specimens* (document H18-A). Villanova, Pa.: National Committee for Clinical Laboratory Standards, 1990.

Turgeon, M. *Clinical Hematology Theory and Practice,* 2nd ed. Boston: Little, Brown, 1993.

CHAPTER 11

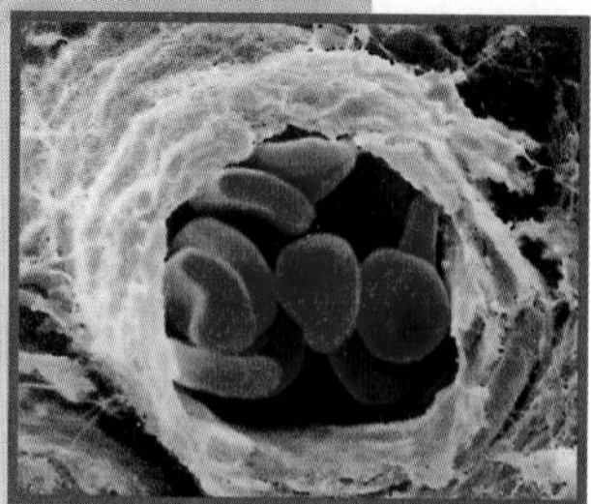

Complications and Troubleshooting

Chapter Outline

Learning Objectives

After completing this chapter, you should be able to

1. Define and spell the glossary terms listed in this chapter.
2. Discuss the proper procedure for caring for a patient who faints during venipuncture.
3. Describe the reasons for hematoma formation and how to prevent it.
4. Describe the warning signs of possible excessive bleeding during blood collection and ways to treat the patient.
5. Discuss the different types of allergies that may affect a patient during blood collection.
6. Describe the different methods of alleviating pain associated with venipuncture.
7. Discuss reasons for the inability to obtain blood.

GLOSSARY

ANAPHYLACTIC severe, sometimes fatal allergic reaction.

ANESTHETIC an agent that produces loss of feeling.

HEMATOMA swelling due to blood leaking into tissues.

LUMEN the hollow space in the center of a tube or blood vessel.

PETECHIAE small red spots on the skin due to damaged capillaries.

PROBE blindly moving the needle under the skin in the hope of finding a vein.

SYNCOPE fainting.

INTRODUCTION

Although venipuncture and dermal puncture are very common procedures, there can be complications when these procedures are performed. Phlebotomists must be aware of these complications in order to prevent them and to lessen their effect on the patient. Troubleshooting is a skill that a phlebotomist will develop with experience; however, by being aware of the possible causes of poor blood specimen collection, many problems can be avoided by even an inexperienced phlebotomist.

Complications of Blood Collection

A competent phlebotomist can avoid most of the patient complications of venipuncture. By carefully listening to and observing the patient, most problems can be avoided or their effects can be minimized by the quick action of the phlebotomist.

Fainting

Fortunately, fainting, or **syncope,** is a rare complication of obtaining a blood specimen. Some patients may feel faint at the thought of needles or at the sight of their own blood. If the phlebotomist is aware that a particular patient has a tendency to faint, special precautions must be taken to prevent harm to the patient. A phlebotomist should ask all patients if they have ever had their blood drawn and to describe their experience. If a patient has a history of fainting, he or she will usually mention it at this time. It is not a good idea to directly ask patients about fainting because doing so may cause them to think about the possibility of fainting and make them more nervous.

MED TIP

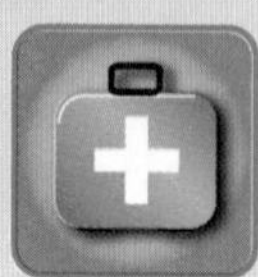

Do not directly ask patients if they have ever fainted, but direct the conversation so that patients have the opportunity to tell you if they have previously fainted during venipuncture.

If patients have a history of fainting during blood collection, place them in a position so they cannot fall during the procedure and injure themselves. If they are outpatients and normally seated in a phlebotomy chair, place them in a supine position on a bed or cot. Inpatients are already in a supine position and consequently rarely faint.

Some patients do not have a history of fainting during blood collection but may feel faint on rare occasions. The phlebotomist must be alert and carefully watch for signs of fainting. A patient may complain of feeling light-headed or nauseous, break out in a cold sweat, or suddenly turn pale. If the phlebotomist does not believe that fainting is eminent, talking to the patient may help keep him or her alert and diffuse the situation. If the patient faints, the phlebotomist's primary concern is to protect the patient from injury. The venipuncture procedure should be immediately terminated by loosening the tourniquet and safely removing the needle from the patient's arm. If the patient is not in danger of falling, the phlebotomist may momentarily leave the patient to get assistance or call for assistance. Loosening tight clothing and using smelling salts may help revive the patient. Occasionally, patients may complain of feeling light-headed after the procedure is finished. If that occurs, the phlebotomist should instruct patients to take deep breaths and, if possible, lower their head between their legs. A cold compress applied to the forehead or back of the neck and small sips of cool water may also help to revive the patients.

No patient, inpatient or outpatient, should be left alone for the first 15 minutes after recovering from a fainting episode. An outpatient should also be instructed not to drive for at least 30 minutes after recovery. The phlebotomist must follow the health care institution's policy concerning patient incidents, which usually includes reporting the incident to a supervisor and filing an incident report.

Hematoma

A **hematoma,** or bruise, is a common complication of blood collection. Hematomas, which are depicted in figure 11-1, occur when blood leaks from the vein or capillaries and collects in the tissues around the puncture site. Although hematomas are not dangerous, they may cause the patient a great deal of discomfort. Sometimes a hematoma will begin to form during the venipuncture procedure. If a phlebotomist sees swelling around the puncture site, he or she should stop the procedure immediately and apply firm pressure to the site for approximately 5 minutes. An ice pack may also be applied to the area

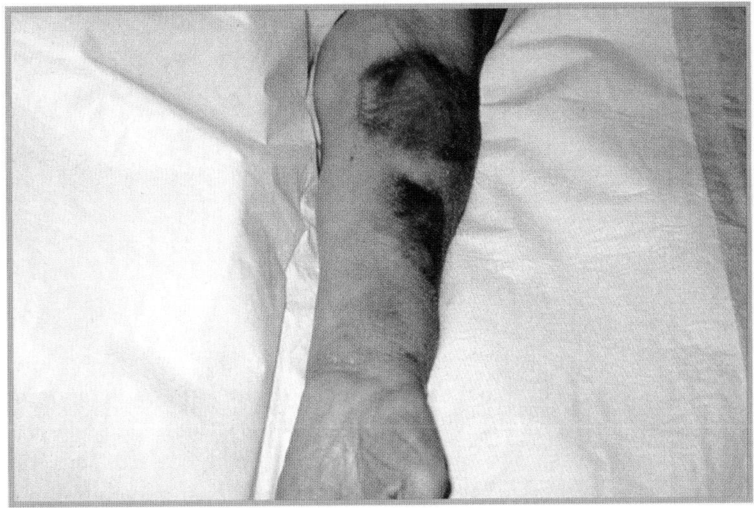

Figure 11-1
Hematomas occur when blood leaks from the vein or capillaries and collects in the tissues around the puncture site. (Johnson & Johnson Medical, Division, Ethicon Inc. 1997. Used by permission of the copyright owner.)

to help reduce swelling. Hematomas that form during the venipuncture procedure may have several causes, including the following:

- Excessive probing with the needle to find the vein
- Penetration of the needle all the way through the vein
- Partial penetration of the needle in the vein
- Removal of the tourniquet after the needle was withdrawn

Many times hematomas form after the procedure has been completed. Late-forming hematomas are due to blood leaking from the vein after the procedure has been completed. Leaking can occur in elderly patients or patients taking anticoagulation medications, because pressure was not applied for 5 minutes or because the bandage was removed too early.

MED TIP

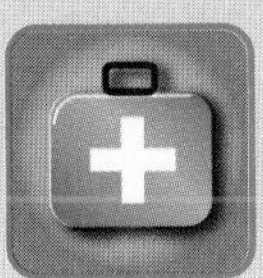

Apply firm, constant pressure to a venipuncture site until the patient has stopped bleeding to greatly reduce the incidence of hematoma formation.

PETECHIAE

Petechiae are tiny red spots that appear under the skin and are an indication of broken or bruised capillaries. They are a sign of either platelet defects or weak capillary walls. They usually occur on the skin that is under or below the tourniquet and form due to the pressure that the tight tourniquet applies to the capillaries. Petechiae are a frequent finding among geriatric patients, who may be more likely to have weak capillaries. The phlebotomist should be aware that seeing petechiae after removal of the tourniquet is a warning sign that the patient may bleed excessively from the venipuncture site and the phlebotomist should be especially careful to ensure that the patient has stopped bleeding before applying the bandage.

MED TIP

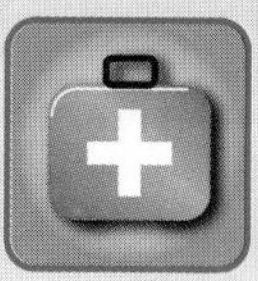

Finding petechiae on a patient's arm does not mean the phlebotomist did not follow the correct protocol but rather that the patient may have a condition that causes excessive bleeding.

Excessive Bleeding

Occasionally a phlebotomist encounters a patient who does not stop bleeding from the venipuncture site within the usual 5 minutes of pressure. These patients are usually taking anticoagulation medications such as Coumadin or heparin; they may tell the phlebotomist that they take "blood thinners." The phlebotomist should continue to apply pressure to the site until all bleeding has stopped. If it takes longer than 5 minutes, help from the nursing staff is needed. The phlebotomist is required to remain with the bleeding patient until the nursing staff takes over the patient's care.

MED TIP

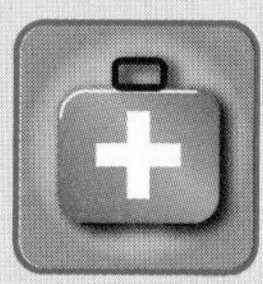

Never leave a patient alone if he or she is still bleeding from the venipuncture site.

Seizures

Seizures are a very rare complication of venipuncture. If a patient has a seizure, the tourniquet and needle should be removed immediately. The phlebotomist should dispose of the needle safely and, if possible, apply pressure to the venipuncture site without completely restricting movement of the patient's arm. The phlebotomist should call for assistance from the nursing staff or, if an outpatient, other personnel as quickly as possible but without leaving the patient unattended. Trying to keep the patient from falling and injuring himself or herself and never placing anything in the patient's mouth are two other responsibilities of the phlebotomist.

Allergies

Patients may be allergic to many of the materials used in blood collection. Allergic reactions can range from a mild skin irritation to life-threatening **anaphylactic** shock. The phlebotomist must look for signs posted on hospital room doors, beds, and patient charts warning of patient allergies. He or she should never use a product that the patient has a known allergy to without first discussing the problem with a supervisor or the patient's physician.

The most common patient allergies that a phlebotomist may encounter are to the antiseptics that are used to cleanse the puncture site. Many patients are allergic to the antiseptic iodine. If the patient has a known allergy to iodine, an alternative antiseptic should be used. Soap and water are acceptable substitutes for iodine.

Patients may also be allergic to the adhesive found in the bandages that are used to cover a venipuncture site. Sterile gauze folded into a square and held in place with hypoallergenic tape or gauze strips wrapped around the arm and taped in place may be used in place of bandages.

Due to the increasing popularity of latex products, allergies to latex are becoming more common. Most latex allergies cause very mild reactions, but some individuals are so severely affected that even being in the same room with latex products can be life threatening. A severe latex allergy should be noted on the patient's hospital room door to alert hospital staff that no latex products can be brought into the room. A phlebotomist will have to leave the phlebotomy tray or cart in the hall outside the room and bring in only the necessary equipment. It is imperative that the phlebotomist avoid using latex gloves and latex tourniquets for patients allergic to latex. Vinyl gloves and Velcro closure tourniquets or nonlatex tourniquets may be used instead of the latex products.

Infections

Infections at the site of blood collection are extremely rare. Using proper cleansing techniques at the puncture site greatly reduces the risk of infection from blood collection procedures. Arterial puncture sites are more prone to infection than venipuncture sites because if microorganisms are introduced into an artery, they are quickly circulated throughout the body. If microorganisms are introduced into a vein, they are rapidly removed by the lymphatic system because the veins are closely associated with the lymphatic ducts and nodes. Reminding the patient to keep the bandage on for a minimum of 15 minutes also reduces the risk of infection.

Pain

Blood collection, whether venipuncture or dermal puncture, usually causes minimal discomfort to the patient. A patient who is anxious about the procedure is more likely to complain of pain. The phlebotomist should calmly explain the procedure to the patient and attempt to alleviate the patient's fears. It is hoped that doing so will help the patient to relax and therefore experience less discomfort during the procedure. Arterial punctures are more painful, and many health care institutions apply a topical **anesthetic** to the site before beginning the procedure.

Children may be so afraid of needles and the hospital environment that they are unable to cooperate with the phlebotomist. The topical anesthetic EMLA (lidocaine/prilocaine cream) was approved in 1993 by the U.S. Food and Drug Administration (FDA) for relief of pain from venipuncture in pediatric patients. EMLA has proven to be quite effective (97 percent) in pain reduction, but it has one significant drawback: it must be applied to the skin and covered by gauze 1 hour before venipuncture.

The phlebotomist can prevent excessive discomfort to the patient by not blindly probing with the needle for a vein. Blind probing can be extremely painful as well as potentially damaging to the vein, nerves, and tendons. The phlebotomist must constantly be aware of the patient's body language for signs of pain that the patient may not verbalize.

MED TIP

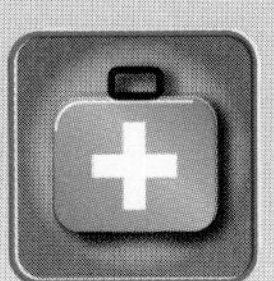

Remember to allow the alcohol to dry completely before beginning the procedure. If the alcohol is not completely evaporated, the specimen may hemolyze and the patient will feel a stinging sensation.

Damage to Veins

Occasionally puncturing a vein for blood collection will not harm the vein; however, repeated punctures to the same site over a period of time can cause scarring of the vein. A scarred vein will feel hard and gnarly on palpation and can no longer be used for venipuncture. If a patient is hospitalized for an extended stay, it is preferable to vary the venipuncture site, if possible, to avoid scarring a vein. Excessive probing with the needle may also scar veins and should be avoided.

Collapsed veins are caused by placing too much pressure on a weak or fragile vein. The pressure is caused by the vacuum of the evacuated tube or by withdrawing a syringe plunger too quickly. Once a vein has collapsed, the venipuncture should stop immediately and begin again at a new site. Collapsed veins will reopen but should be used judiciously in the future.

Troubleshooting

A phlebotomist can avoid many of the problems that can occur during a venipuncture by carefully reviewing the equipment before use and by being prepared for possible difficulties.

Inability to Obtain Blood

Most laboratories have established policies about the number of times a phlebotomist may attempt a venipuncture on a patient. The usual guideline is that a phlebotomist may try twice to obtain blood. If the second attempt is not successful, another phlebotomist should be called for that patient. Repeated attempts at venipuncture are frustrating for the phlebotomist and both frustrating and painful for the patient. If the second phlebotomist is also unsuccessful, the most experienced available phlebotomist should be sent for; if the third phlebotomist is not successful, the patient's physician should be notified.

Equipment Failure

There are many reasons for unsuccessful venipunctures besides "missing the vein." Sometimes the equipment does not work properly. An evacuated tube may lose its vacuum. To avoid this complication, the phlebotomist should check the expiration date on evacuated tubes and not use tubes that have fallen on the floor. If a tube falls to the floor, the cap may dislodge just enough to eliminate the vacuum. If the tube is punctured by the needle prior to insertion in the vein, the vacuum in the tube will be lost.

MED TIP

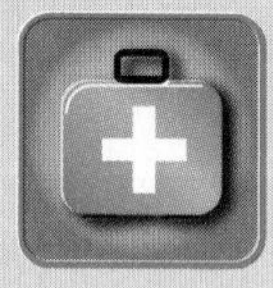

Always have extra evacuated tubes in case a tube has lost its vacuum.

Occasionally the needle may become detached from the adapter. This problem usually occurs if the needle was never tightly screwed in place. If the needle becomes loose, the phlebotomist should quickly release the tourniquet and remove the needle. A second venipuncture with new equipment will be necessary.

Needle Position

The proper positioning of the needle is the most important step in a successful venipuncture, but sometimes this step can be quite challenging. The correct position of the needle is in the center of the **lumen** (hollow space in the center) of the vein with the bevel facing upward. Sometimes the needle may not penetrate the vein completely or the needle may pass all the way through the vein. In either situation, the needle should be repositioned quickly to prevent blood from leaking under the skin and causing a hematoma. Sometimes the needle will partially enter the vein, and the evacuated tube will slowly fill as some blood leaks under the skin, forming a hematoma. If the phlebotomist sees a lump appearing under the skin at the puncture site, the tourniquet should be quickly released and the procedure should be stopped. Pressure should be placed on the site for a minimum of 5 minutes and then an ice pack is placed on the area.

Sometimes the needle is in the correct location, but the bevel of the needle is pressed against the upper or lower wall of the vein and blood is unable to enter the needle. This problem can be corrected by slowly rotating the needle until blood begins to enter the evacuated tube.

If a vein is not well anchored, it may move to one side as the needle enters. This movement causes the needle to end up on the side of the vein rather than in the lumen of the vessel. The phlebotomist may carefully reposition the needle, keeping the bevel under the skin and tightly anchoring the vein to prevent further movement. Although a small amount of careful maneuvering of the needle is acceptable, a phlebotomist must never blindly **probe** the patient's arm in the hopes of finding a vein. This type of needle movement can be quite painful and may cause nerve and tendon damage.

MED TIP

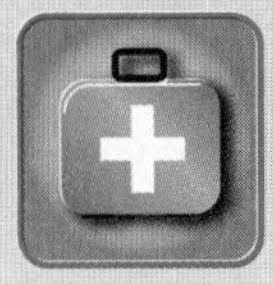

Never blindly probe with the needle in hopes of finding a vein. This practice is painful for the patient and may permanently scar the vein.

Collapsed Vein

A small or weak vein may suddenly collapse under the pressure of an evacuated tube or the pressure exerted as the plunger of the syringe is withdrawn. Collapsed veins are common in the elderly due to loss of elasticity in the wall of the vein. The phlebotomist may become aware of a vein collapse in one of two ways: as the needle enters the vein, the vein disappears or the evacuated tube or syringe suddenly stops filling with blood. Sometimes blood flow can be reestablished by tightening the tourniquet. Depending on the method of venipuncture, the evacuated tube should be removed and replaced with a smaller tube or the plunger should be withdrawn more slowly from the barrel of the syringe. If blood flow does not begin, the phlebotomist should end the procedure and try again at another site using a smaller evacuated tube, less pressure on the syringe plunger, or a winged infusion set.

CHAPTER REVIEW

Summary

In this chapter we reviewed many of the complications that can occur during a venipuncture and also gave tips on troubleshooting potential problems that may interfere with a successful venipuncture. If the phlebotomist is aware of potential difficulties, many of them can be avoided before they cause a problem.

Competency Review

1. Briefly describe the most common complications associated with blood collection.
2. Explain the appropriate precautions for performing venipuncture in a patient with a severe latex allergy.
3. Describe the procedure a phlebotomist follows when a patient does not stop bleeding within 5 minutes of a venipuncture.
4. How would a phlebotomist proceed if a vein collapsed during venipuncture?
5. Describe the procedure if a phlebotomist is unable to obtain blood from a patient.

Examination Review Questions

1. **Signs of syncope may include**
   (A) a feeling of nausea
   (B) breaking out in a cold sweat
   (C) feeling light-headed
   (D) turning pale
   (E) all of the above

2. **All of the following may cause a hematoma except**
   (A) excessive probing with the needle
   (B) removing the tourniquet before the needle
   (C) partial penetration of the needle in the vein
   (D) penetration of the needle all the way through the vein
   (E) inadequate vacuum in the evacuated tube

3. **The maximum number of times a phlebotomist may stick a patient is**
   (A) one time
   (B) two times
   (C) three times
   (D) four times
   (E) until he or she is successful

4. **Infections are rare after a venipuncture because**
   (A) there are few microorganisms on the skin
   (B) the needle has antibacterial properties
   (C) proper cleansing techniques are used
   (D) arterial blood maintains close contact with the lymphatic system
   (E) the needle has an antibacterial effect

5. **Treatment of a patient who faints includes all of the following except**
   (A) applying cold compresses
   (B) loosening tight clothing
   (C) finishing the venipuncture and then getting help
   (D) providing small sips of cold water
   (E) preventing the patient from falling

6. **If a phlebotomist is unable to obtain blood after the second attempt, he or she should**
   (A) change equipment
   (B) call the patient's physician
   (C) call another phlebotomist
   (D) send the patient to the emergency room
   (E) perform a capillary puncture

7. **Finding petechiae on skin under the tourniquet may be a sign of**
   (A) platelet defects
   (B) weak capillary walls
   (C) poor technique
   (D) a and b
   (E) all of the above

8. **The most common patient allergies that a phlebotomist may encounter are to**
   (A) plastic
   (B) cotton balls
   (C) adhesive bandages
   (D) latex
   (E) antiseptics

9. **Once a vein has collapsed**
   (A) it can never be used for venipuncture
   (B) it will be permanently scarred
   (C) it can be used for venipuncture provided the phlebotomist probes excessively
   (D) it will reopen and can be used for venipuncture
   (E) there is no circulation in the area

10. **To prevent equipment failure, all of the following precautions should be followed except**
   (A) always check expiration dates on evacuated tubes
   (B) never use an evacuated tube that has fallen on the floor
   (C) check that the needle is tightly screwed into the adapter or the syringe
   (D) a and b
   (E) all of the above

Getting Connected

Multimedia Extension Activities

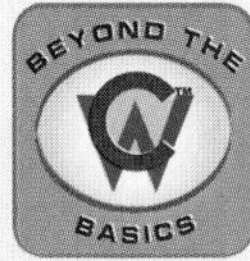

www.prenhall.com/fremgen

Use the address above to access the free, interactive Companion Website created specifically for this textbook. Enhance your studying by answering practice quiz questions, with hints and instant feedback related to chapter 11. If you would like to gain a deeper understanding of selected topics within this chapter, be sure to click on the **Beyond the Basics** feature, which provides more details for further learning. If you do not have a web connection, you may use the CD-ROM enclosed in the back of this book to take advantage of the same features off-line.

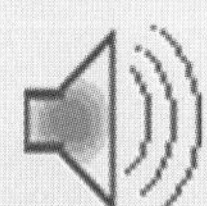

Audio Glossary

Use the CD-ROM enclosed with your textbook to hear the pronunciation of the key terms in the chapter. You may also access this material on the Companion Website www.prenhall.com/fremgen.

Bibliography

Farber, V. "Mastering Pediatric Phlebotomy." *Advance for Medical Laboratory Professionals*, January 27, 1997.

Henry, J. B. *Clinical Diagnosis and Management by Laboratory Methods*, 19th ed. Philadelphia: W. B. Saunders, 1996.

Lehman, C. A. *Saunders Manual of Clinical Laboratory Science*. Philadelphia: W. B. Saunders, 1998.

National Committee for Clinical Laboratory Standards. *Procedures for the Collection of Diagnostic Blood Specimens by Venipuncture*, 3rd ed. (document H3-A3). Villanova, Pa.: National Committee for Clinical Laboratory Standards, July 1991.

National Institute for Occupational Safety and Health. *NIOSH Alert: Preventing Allergic Reactions to Natural Rubber Latex in the Workplace*. DHHS (NIOSH) Publication No: 97-135, June 1997.

van Kan, H. J., A. C. Egberts, W, P. Rijnvos, N. J., ter Pelkwijk, and A. W. Lenderink. "Tetracaine versus Lidocaine-Prilocaine for Preventing Venipuncture-Induced Pain in Children." *American Journal of Health System Pharmacy* 54, no. 4 (1997): 388–392.

MARY FREEMAN IS working alone during the lunch hour in Dr. Williams's office laboratory. Sean Harrington, a 30-year-old construction worker, comes in to have his blood drawn for an insurance physical. He seems to be very nervous about having his blood drawn, and Mary tries to calm him down by asking him to sit down in the waiting room to relax. He says that he does not want to wait because he is on his lunch break from work and to "just get it over with." Mary decides to go ahead with the blood draw, and as soon as she begins Sean slumps over, hitting his head on the floor as he falls out of the chair. He appears to be unconscious.

How should Mary respond?

1. What is the first thing that Mary needs to do?
2. Was Mary negligent in drawing the blood sample when it appeared that Sean was nervous?
3. Is Sean at all to blame in this situation?
4. Would the situation be different if Mary had not been alone?
5. Does an incident report need to be filled out?

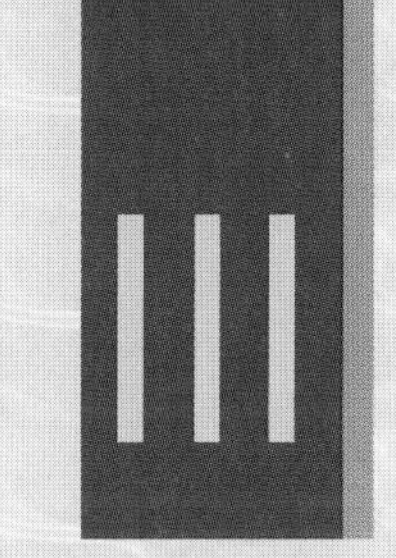

SECTION III

Basic Laboratory Values

CHAPTER 12

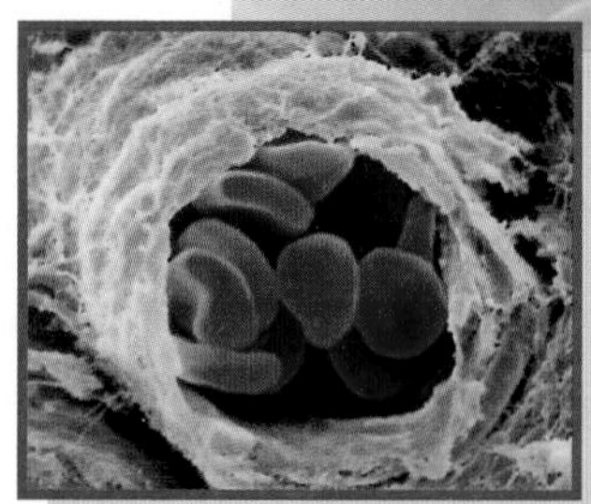

Hematology

Chapter Outline

- Introduction
- Components of Blood
- The Microscope
- Routine Hematology Tests
- Hemostasis
- Summary
- Competency Review
- Examination Review Questions
- Bibliography

Learning Objectives

After completing this chapter, you should be able to

1. Define and spell the glossary terms listed in this chapter.
2. Describe the components of blood.
3. Explain the parts of a microscope and how to use this equipment.
4. Describe the hematology tests routinely included in a complete blood count.
5. Discuss the information that can be obtained from a differential smear.
6. Describe the four tests that are used to evaluate hemostasis.

GLOSSARY

ACTIVATED PARTIAL THROMBOPLASTIN TIME (APTT) a coagulation test used to test the extrinsic coagulation system.

AGRANULOCYTE leukocytes that do not have cytoplasmic granules (e.g., lymphocytes and monocytes).

ANEMIA a condition in which there is a below normal red blood cell count or hemoglobin level.

COMPLETE BLOOD COUNT (CBC) commonly performed group of hematology tests.

DIFFERENTIAL a test that determines the number of each type of leukocyte as compared to the total white blood cell count.

ERYTHROCYTE red blood cell.

ERYTHROCYTOSIS increase in the normal number of red blood cells.

FIBRINOGEN a plasma protein that plays a role in hemostasis.

GRANULOCYTE leukocyte with cytoplasmic granules (e.g., neutrophils, eosinophils, and basophils).

HEMATOCRIT a test that compares the volume of erythrocytes to the volume of whole blood.

HEMATOLOGY the study of blood and blood-forming tissues.

HEMATOPOESIS the process of formation and development of blood cells.

HEMOGLOBIN protein in red blood cells that transports oxygen and carbon dioxide.

HEMOSTASIS the process in which bleeding is stopped.

IN VITRO outside the body.

IN VIVO within the body.

LEUKOCYTE white blood cell.

LEUKOCYTOSIS increase in the normal number of white blood cells.

LEUKOPENIA decrease in the normal number of white blood cells.

MORPHOLOGY the shape and structure of a cell.

PHAGOCYTE a cell that engulfs and digests foreign material.

PLASMA straw-colored liquid portion of blood.

PROTHROMBIN TIME (PROTIME OR PT) a coagulation screening test used to test the intrinsic coagulation system.

Reticulocyte an immature red blood cell.

Serum liquid portion of blood after it has clotted and fibrinogen is gone.

Thrombocyte platelet.

Thrombocytopenia a decrease in the normal number of platelets.

Thrombocytosis an increase in the normal number of platelets.

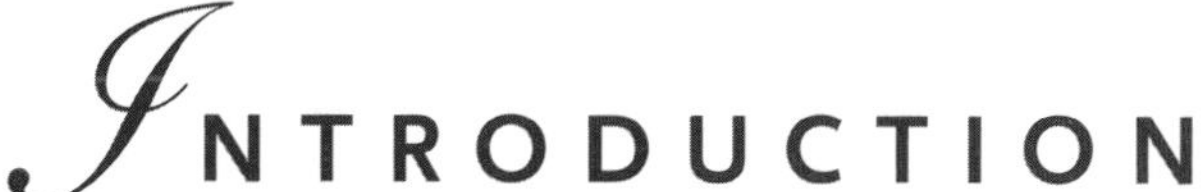

INTRODUCTION

Hematology is the study of blood and blood-forming tissues. The clinical hematology laboratory examines blood to detect disease in blood-forming tissues and the cells produced by these tissues. Clinical hematology laboratories also include the area of hemostasis or coagulation, which is the process by which bleeding stops.

Components of Blood

The average size adult has approximately 5.5 to 6 L of blood. Blood is composed of two basic parts, a liquid portion called plasma and a cellular portion. There are three main types of cells found in blood—**erythrocytes,** or red blood cells; **leukocytes,** or white blood cells; and **thrombocytes,** commonly known as platelets.

Plasma

Plasma is a straw-colored liquid that makes up about 55 percent of the total blood volume. It is composed of approximately 90 percent water and 10 percent solid materials. The solid materials are plasma proteins such as albumin, globulin, and plasma proteins (such as **fibrinogen**) that play a role in hemostasis; electrolytes such as sodium, potassium, and chloride; nutrients such as glucose, amino acids, carbohydrates, and lipids; metabolic waste products such as urea, lactic acid, and creatinine; hormones; antibodies; enzymes; vitamins; and mineral salts. **Serum** has all of the same components as plasma, with the exception of fibrinogen. Serum is the liquid portion of blood after it has clotted, and fibrinogen is used up in the clotting process. Plasma is obtained by drawing a blood sample in an evacuated tube that contains an anticoagulant and centrifuging the tube to separate the plasma from the cells. Serum is obtained by drawing a blood sample into a red-topped or gold-topped evacuated tube that does not contain an anticoagulant, allowing the specimen to clot, and then centrifuging the specimen to separate the cells from the serum.

Cellular Components

The largest cellular portion of blood consists of erythrocytes, or red blood cells (RBCs), as depicted in figure 12-1. Erythrocytes are formed and develop in the bone marrow in a process called **hematopoesis.** As red blood cells are released from the bone marrow into the bloodstream, they lose their nuclei and appear as biconcave discs. The biconcave shape provides for greater flexibility in circulating through tiny capillaries and for greater surface area that allows an increased oxygen-carrying capacity.

Figure 12-1
Red blood cells.

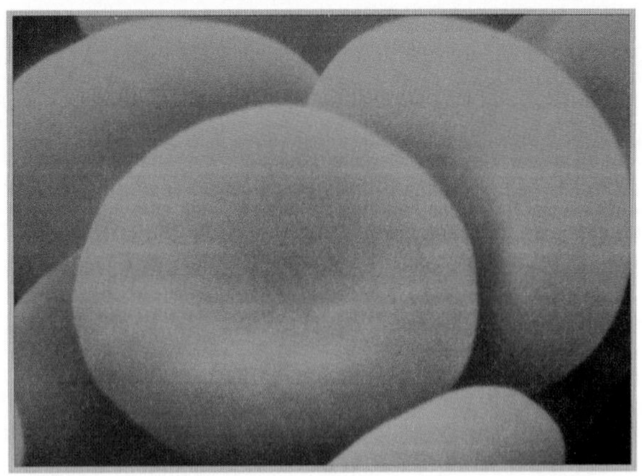

Most of the erythrocyte is composed of a large protein, called **hemoglobin,** that transports oxygen and carbon dioxide. The function of hemoglobin is twofold. First it carries oxygen from the lungs to the tissues; then it carries carbon dioxide, a waste product, from the tissues to the lungs to be expelled from the body by exhalation. When oxygen combines with hemoglobin in the lungs, oxyhemoglobin, a red-colored substance, is formed. Arterial blood has a high concentration of oxygen, hence the bright red color. In contrast, venous blood has low levels of oxygen and has a deep red-brown color.

The second largest cellular components found in blood are the leukocytes, also called white blood cells (WBCs). Leukocytes are divided into two main categories: **granulocytes,** which have granules in their cytoplasm, and **agranulocytes,** which do not have granules in their cytoplasm. There are three types of granulocytes—neutrophils (also called polymorphonuclear leukocytes, or "polys" for short), basophils, and eosinophils—and two types of agranulocytes—lymphocytes and monocytes.

The primary function of leukocytes is to defend the body against disease, and each type of leukocyte plays a specific role in the process. Neutrophils and monocytes are phagocytic cells that engulf foreign material such as bacteria and dead tissue cells. The process of phagocytosis is depicted in figure 12-2. A **phagocyte** is a cell that engulfs and digests foreign material. Eosinophils and basophils play an important role in allergic reactions. Lymphocytes produce antibodies against substances the body recognizes as foreign.

The third type of blood cell is a **thrombocyte,** or platelet; it is not a true cell but a cell fragment. Platelets play a major role in the clotting process by forming the platelet plug that seals breaks in blood vessels. Platelets also provide substances that are necessary for formation of a blood clot.

The Microscope

The microscope plays an integral role in many laboratory tests. A typical laboratory microscope is shown in figure 12-3. It can be found in many different areas of the clinical laboratory, such as hematology, microbiology, and urinalysis. This optical instrument magnifies structures unseen by the naked eye for the purpose of counting, naming, or differentiating various structures. Instructions for using a microscope are found in procedure 12-1.

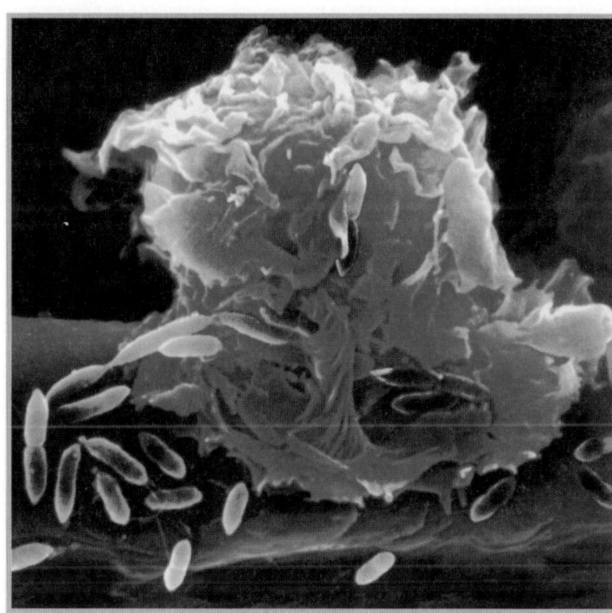

Figure 12-2
Process of phagocytosis.

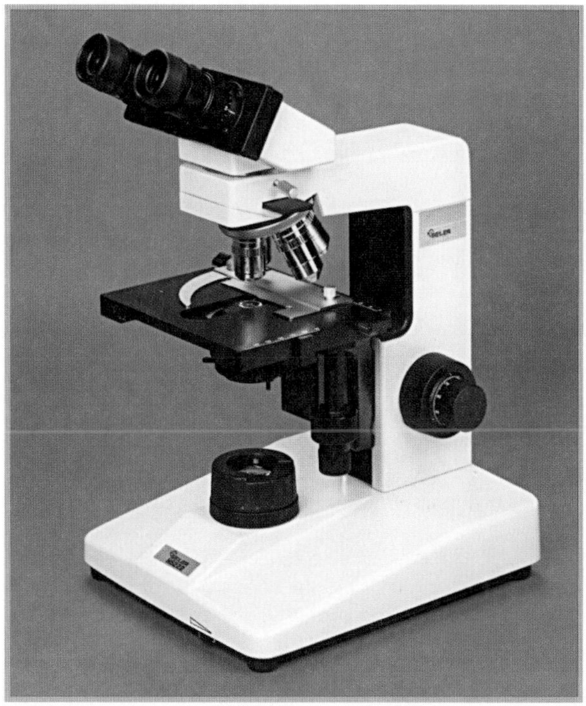

Figure 12-3
A typical laboratory microscope.

PROCEDURE 12•1

USING THE MICROSCOPE

Purpose:

To be able to properly use a microscope to perform diagnostic tests.

Terminal Performance Competency:

Observe a slide under the microscope at 10×, 40×, and 100× magnification using the correct procedure.

Equipment:

Microscope, lens paper, and immersion oil.

Procedure:

1. Lower the stage to its lowest position.
2. Place the prepared slide on the stage.
3. Turn on the light.
4. Rotate the nosepiece until the 10× objective locks into place directly over the slide.
5. Viewing the slide from the side, raise the stage using the coarse focus knob until the objective is close to the slide.
6. Look through the eyepiece and continue to move the coarse focus knob until the slide begins to come into focus.
7. Adjust the fine focus knob until the image is clear.
8. Make adjustments for the proper amount of light by adjusting the rheostat and the condenser. *Hint: Lower magnification needs lower light and greater magnification requires more light.*
9. Observe the image.
10. Raise the objective slightly and rotate the nosepiece until the 40× objective clicks into place. *Hint: If the object is not raised, the 40× objective may hit the slide and the slide or the objective may be damaged.*
11. Readjust the light and refocus.
12. Observe the image.
13. Move the 40× objective aside.
14. Place a drop of immersion oil on the slide.
15. Carefully rotate the 100× objective until it clicks into place.
16. Readjust the light and refocus.
17. Observe the image.
18. When finished, lower the stage and remove the slide.
19. Turn off the light.
20. Using lens paper, clean eyepieces and all objectives.
21. Unplug the electric cord and wrap around the base.
22. Cover the microscope with a dust cover.

The components of a microscope are as follows:

1. Eyepiece(s) (monocular or binocular) with power of magnification printed on the side
2. Adjuster for eye width
3. Body tube (directional light source)
4. Arm (used to carry the microscope)
5. Revolving nosepiece (holds objectives and rotates for selection)
6. Objectives (magnification printed on each objective)

   10× = low power

   40× = high dry

   100× = oil immersion
7. Mechanical stage (movable device that holds slide)
8. Stage (platform that slide rests on)
9. Mechanical stage adjustment (two knobs that control vertical and horizontal movement of slide)
10. Coarse and fine adjustment knobs (small knob atop larger knob that adjusts stage up and down for focusing)
11. Substage condenser (lens system used to increase light for sharper focus)
12. Diaphragm (adjustable aperture similar to a camera shutter that controls the amount of light)
13. Light source (illuminator set in base)
14. Rheostat (regulates intensity of the light)
15. Base (holds illuminator, rheostat, and microscope upright and used to carry the microscope)

It is important to use the correct objective (lens) for the type of microscope work to be done. The magnification of an object is calculated by multiplying the magnifying power of the objective times the magnification of the eyepiece. For example, using the low-power objective the magnification would be 10× (the objective) times 10× (the eyepiece) equaling 100× magnification.

Microscopes are delicate instruments that will last for many years if maintained properly. The following rules must be adhered to:

1. Follow cleaning requirements during mandatory daily cleaning.
2. Always use two hands to carry a microscope: one hand to hold the arm of the microscope, and the other hand to support the base.
3. Clean oculars, objectives, and stage using only lens paper and lens cleaner.
4. Keep extra lightbulbs on hand.
5. Document inspections and repairs in the log book.
6. Store with the electrical cord wrapped loosely around the base.
7. Cover the microscope with a dust cover when it is not in use.

Routine Hematology Tests

One of the most common blood tests ordered is a **complete blood count (CBC).** The CBC is a group of tests that usually includes a red blood cell count, white blood cell count, platelet count, hemoglobin, hematocrit, and differential leukocyte count. Blood for a CBC is drawn into a lavender-topped evacuated tube that has ethylenediaminetetraacetic acid (EDTA) as an anticoagulant. EDTA causes fewer changes in blood cells than other anticoagulants. Cell morphology will remain stable in the EDTA tube for up to 72 hours if the specimen is refrigerated.

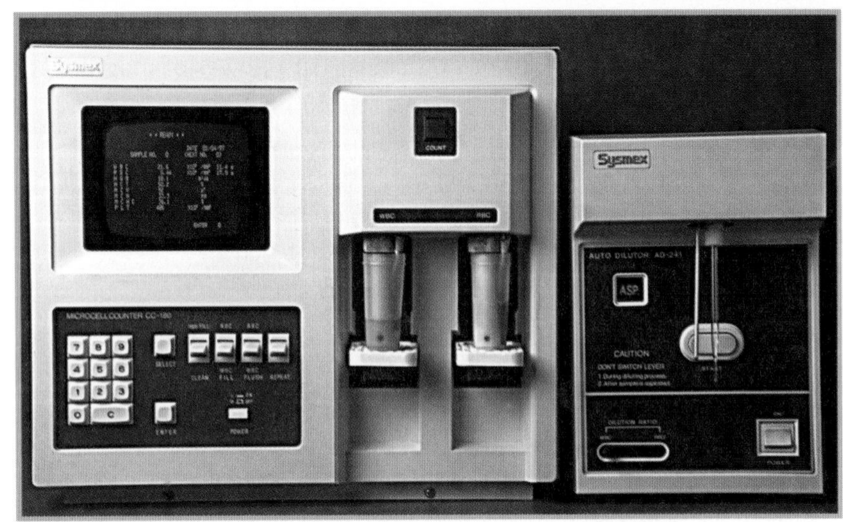

Figure 12-4
Automatic blood analyzer. (Analyzer from B. Warling.)

MED TIP

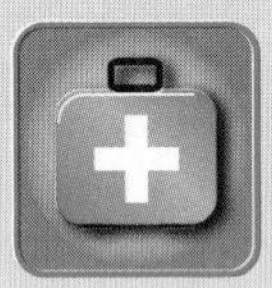

EDTA evacuated tubes must be gently inverted immediately after the specimen is drawn because clots will interfere with the hematology instruments used in clinical testing.

Routine **hematology** tests, such as those included in the CBC, are usually performed using an automated blood analyzer. Examples of automatic blood analyzers are found in figures 12-4 and 12-5. Blood analyzers range from those that perform only a single test on one sample at one time to those used in large clinical laboratories that can perform multiple tests on hundreds of samples daily. Today, the manual methods are used only if the analyzer is not working. Manual methods are slower and more costly in terms of employee time than automated methods. A manual test result may be less accurate than an automated test result if the employee is not proficient in performing the technique for the manual method.

Red Blood Cell Count

The red blood cell count determines the number of circulating red blood cells. The main function of red blood cells is to carry oxygen and carbon dioxide. If the number of erythrocytes is reduced, less oxygen will be able to get to tissues. This condition, called **anemia,** occurs when there is a below normal red blood cell count or hemoglobin level. Symptoms of anemia may include fatigue, headache, and a pale appearance. An increase in the normal number of erythrocytes is called **erythrocytosis.** It is a normal physiological response in people who live at high altitudes. It is also found in those with a condition called polycythemia. The normal red blood cell count is $3.8–5.2 \times 10^6/mm^3$ for women and $4.4–5.9 \times 10^6/mm^3$ for men. Newborns are born with high erythrocyte counts that drop in the first year of life. The normal count is $4.0–5.8 \times 10^6/mm^3$ for newborns and $3.8–5.5 \times 10^6/mm^3$ for children under 12 years of age.

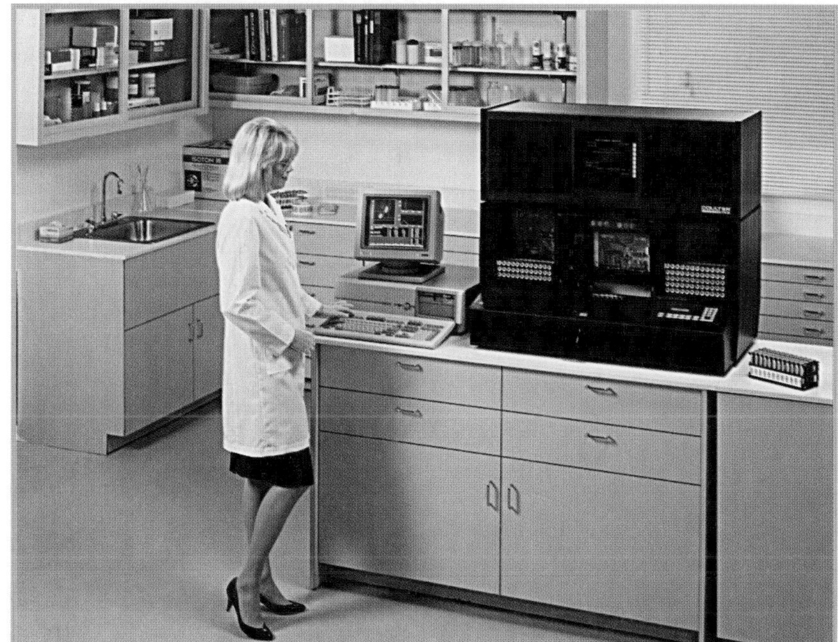

Figure 12-5
Automatic blood analyzers. (The COULTER (R) STKS Hematology Analyzer System, courtesy of Beckman Coulter, Inc., Fullerton, California.)

White Blood Cell Count

The white blood cell count determines the total number of leukocytes without determining the number of each type of leukocyte. Leukocyte counts increase due to infections, inflammation, and disease. An increase in the normal number of leukocytes is called **leukocytosis.** A decrease in the normal number of leukocytes is called **leukopenia.** Leukopenia may occur with certain viral infections such as HIV and excessive exposure to radiation or chemotherapy drugs. The normal white blood cell count varies with age. Newborns have a high white blood cell count of 9,000–30,000/mm^3 that drops within the first few months of life. Children under 12 years of age have a count of 6,000–14,000/mm^3, and adults have leukocyte counts ranging from 4,500 to 11,000/mm^3.

Platelet Count

The platelet count determines the number of platelets in the peripheral blood. This information is needed to diagnose bleeding disorder and to monitor anticoagulant therapy. Platelets have a tendency to clump together and are difficult to count. Consequently, manual platelet counts are rarely performed today; most platelet counts are performed by a multitest hematology analyzer. The normal platelet count is between 150,000 and 400,000/mm^3 of blood. **Thrombocytosis,** an increase in the normal number of platelets, can occur after a splenectomy or with certain diseases characterized by overactive bone marrow. **Thrombocytopenia,** a decrease in the normal number of platelets, can occur with some leukemias, bone marrow damage due to radiation or chemotherapy, and chronic alcoholism.

Hemoglobin

Hemoglobin is the oxygen-carrying protein found in red blood cells. A hemoglobin determination, which is a simple test, can provide the physician with valuable information. A low hemoglobin value may indicate anemia, while an elevated result may occur with severe burns. Normal values are 12–16 g/dL for women and 14–18g/dL for men.

TABLE 12-1 Normal Microhematocrit Values

Patients	Percentage
Men	40-52
Women	35-47
6-year-old children	34-42
1-year-old children	32-38
Newborns	51-61

There are many different methods for performing a hemoglobin determination. Hemoglobin determinations are included in the standard test parameters of multitest hematology analyzers. Smaller doctors' offices may have an instrument that just performs hemoglobin tests called a hemoglobinometer. The specific gravity method of measuring hemoglobin is a manual method used at many traveling blood donor centers. It is a simple test that requires no instrumentation but only provides an estimate of the hemoglobin value. Hemoglobin is a large molecule, and the more hemoglobin a red blood cell has, the heavier the cell. A drop of capillary blood is dropped into a copper sulfate solution. If the blood drop falls to the bottom of the copper sulfate container within 15 seconds, that means that it is denser than the copper sulfate due to the hemoglobin concentration and the blood may be used for blood donation. If the drop of blood floats on the top of the copper solution or floats to the bottom after 15 seconds, the hemoglobin level is low. In the latter case, the person's blood is low in hemoglobin, and it would not be safe for that person to donate blood.

HEMATOCRIT

The **hematocrit** (Hct, or "crit") is a test that compares the volume of erythrocytes with the volume of whole blood. A guide for performing a hematocrit is found in procedure 12-2. It provides the physician with reliable information about the patient's red blood cell volume. For example, a low hematocrit value may indicate anemia or hemorrhage, whereas an elevated hematocrit value may indicate dehydration or polycythemia. The test determines the percentage of whole blood that is made up of erythrocytes. The hematocrit is also sometimes referred to as the packed cell volume. Table 12-1 lists normal microhematocrit values. Figure 12-6 depicts the usual equipment, capillary tube and sealant, used in performing the microhematocrit test.

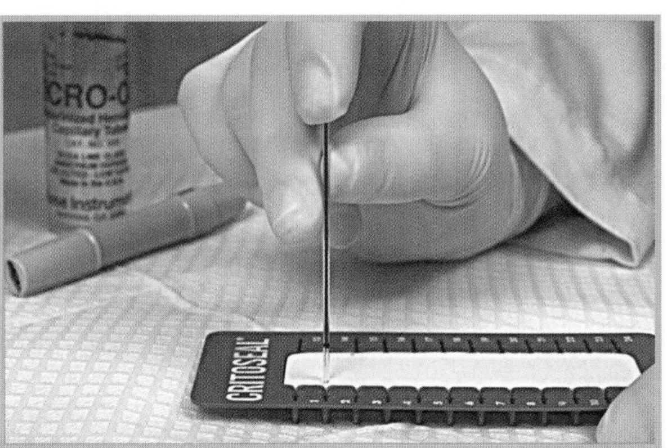

Figure 12-6 Equipment used in a manual hematocrit test.

PROCEDURE 12•2

A GUIDE FOR PERFORMING A MICROHEMATOCRIT TEST

Purpose:

To determine the percentage of red blood cells versus whole blood; used to diagnose anemia.

Terminal Performance Competency:

Perform a microhematocrit test using proper aseptic technique without error.

Equipment:

Disposable gloves, biohazard sharps container, microhematocrit tubes, microhematocrit centrifuge, sealing clay, pen, and laboratory coat.

Procedure:

1. Wash hands and put on disposable gloves.
2. Blood for this test may be capillary blood drawn directly into a heparinized microhematocrit tube or venous blood drawn into an EDTA evacuated tube. If venous blood is used, a nonheparinized microhematocrit tube is used. Make sure there are no air bubbles in the tubes.
3. Fill the tube by capillary action two-thirds to three-fourths full.
4. If the tube is not self-sealing, seal one end of the tube with clay so that the blood does not leak out.
5. Place the capillary tubes in the microhematocrit centrifuge with the sealed end on the outside against the rubber gasket.
6. Record the number of the slot in which you placed the tube.
7. Follow the manufacturer's directions to lock the centrifuge and lid and for centrifuging times and speed. Most centrifuges spin for 5 minutes at 10,000 rpm. The components of blood will separate based on weight. The heaviest components, found at the bottom of the tube, are the erythrocytes, followed by the leukocytes and platelets together in one layer called the buffy coat. This layer is followed by the plasma layer.
8. Once the centrifuge stops, place the tube in a special reader.
9. Place the end of the clay and the beginning of the red cells at the zero mark. Place the 100 mark at the top of the plasma. Read the line at the top of the red cells and record as a percentage.
10. Discard tubes in the biohazard container.
11. Remove gloves and wash hands.

TABLE 12-2 Normal Values for a Differential Leukocyte Count

Leukocytes	Percentage
Neutrophils	55-62
Eosinophils	1-3
Basophils	0-1
Lymphocyte	20-40
Monocyte	4-10

Multitest hematology instruments also determine the hematocrit value. Sometimes a physician does not want all of the tests found in a CBC and will order just a hemoglobin and hematocrit (H & H).

Differential Leukocyte Count

A **differential** white blood cell count, or a "diff," determines the number of each type of leukocyte as compared with the total white blood cell count. Results are reported as a percentage (i.e., counting one hundred leukocytes and 50 percent were neutrophils, 40 percent were lymphocytes, 8 percent were monocytes, and 2 percent were eosinophils). In addition to observing leukocytes, the red blood cell and platelet **morphology** (or shape) and structure of a cell are examined for abnormalities, and an estimate of the number of platelets is possible. Information from the differential is used to aid in the diagnosis of leukemias, anemias, and other diseases. Table 12-2 shows the normal values in a differential leukocyte count.

The differential smear can be prepared from capillary blood at the patient's side or from an EDTA collected venous specimen stored at room temperature. The smear should be made within 1 hour of collection to prevent changes in the cell morphology. See chapter 10 for the procedure on making a blood smear. After the smear is well dried, it should be stained with a hematology stain (e.g., Wright's stain). The process of performing a Wright's stain is found in figures 12-7 through 12-9. Using a bright light, the blood cells should be observed using 100× (oil immersion) under the microscope. The focus should be near the feathered edge, where the cells are one cell layer thick. Cells will appear distorted if viewed in an area where the cells overlap.

When looking at a Wright-stained differential under the microscope, the most numerous cells are erythrocytes. They should appear round with a slightly pale center and no nuclei or inclusions. If a red blood cell appears larger than normal and has gray cytoplasm, it is an immature red blood cell, called a **reticulocyte.** Platelets are the smallest of all the formed blood elements and are much smaller than erythrocytes. They appear as purple-stained structures with a rough outer edge and contain many small granules. They may appear singly or clumped together. Normally there are between five and twenty platelets in one microscopic field of view. If five to ten fields are counted and the average platelet count is between five and twenty, then there is an adequate number of platelets.

Leukocytes have distinct characteristics when stained with Wright's stain. These stained blood cells are shown in figures 12-10 through 12-14. The neutrophil is the most numerous of the leukocytes. Characteristics of a neutrophil include small pink or lilac cytoplasmic granules and a purple multilobed nucleus. A band or stab is an immature neutrophil in which the nucleus appears nonsegmented. An eosinophil has a segmented nucleus with large reddish-orange granules in the cytoplasm. Basophils

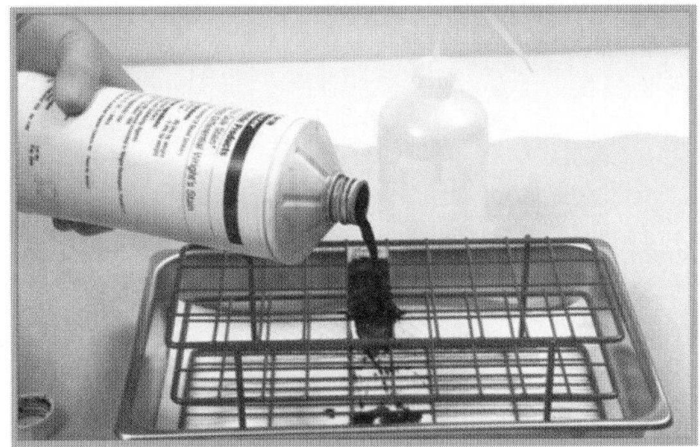

Figure 12-7
Applying stain to the differential slide.

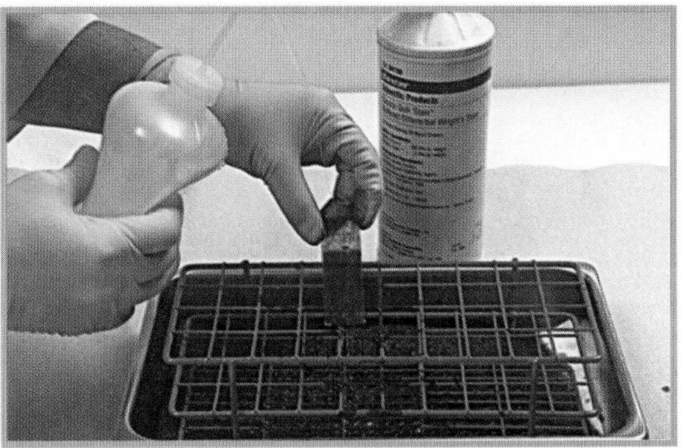

Figure 12-8
Giving the stain time to penetrate the cells.

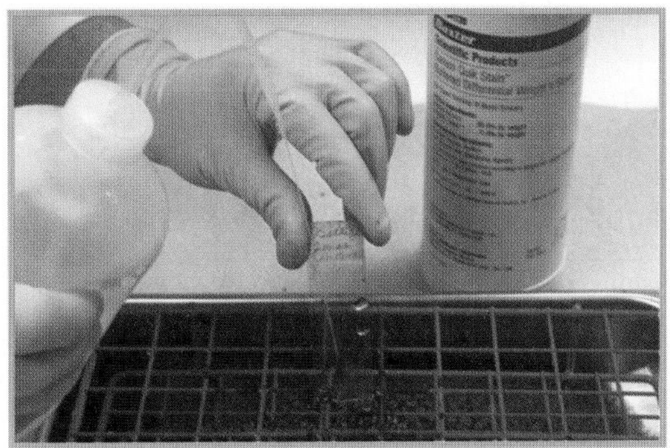

Figure 12-9
Washing off the stain.

have large purple granules that almost cover the nucleus. Lymphocytes are the smallest leukocytes. They have a single round or indented nucleus with clear pale blue cytoplasm. Monocytes are the largest leukocytes and have a large kidney-bean–shaped nucleus with clear grayish-blue cytoplasm.

Erythrocyte Sedimentation Rate

The erythrocyte sedimentation rate (ESR, or sed rate) measures the rate at which erythrocytes fall to the bottom of a tube under controlled laboratory conditions. The directions for this test are found in procedure 12-3. The sedimentation rate is affected by the number and size of the erythrocytes and the amount of protein in the plasma. This test is a nonspecific test used to monitor the extent of inflammation and tissue injury. The sedimentation rate may be elevated in patients with diseases such as rheumatoid arthritis, tuberculosis, hepatitis, and cancer. The two types of erythrocyte sedimentation rates are the Wintrobe and Westergren methods. National Committee for Clinical Laboratory Standards (NCCLS) recommends the Westergren method, which is shown in figure 12-15. The difference between these two methods is the size of the tube used to measure the rate of erythrocyte falling. The normal values for these tests are found in table 12-3.

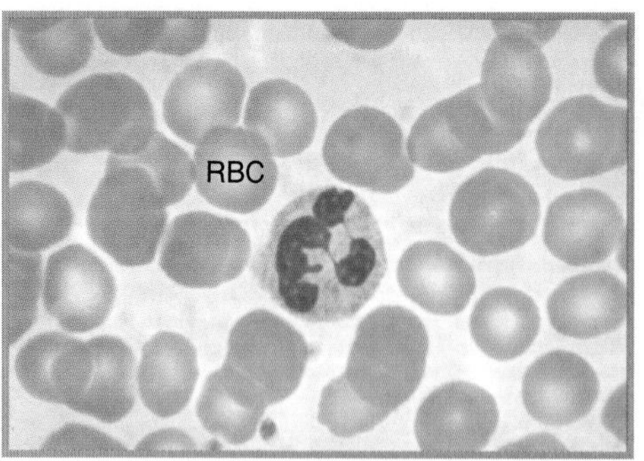

Figure 12-10
Neutrophil.

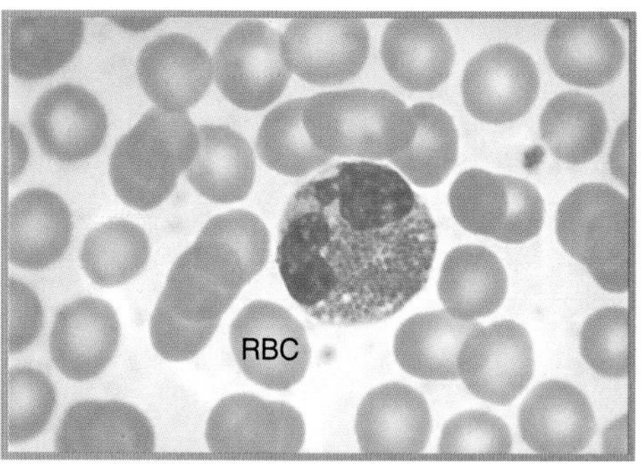

Figure 12-11
Eosinophil.

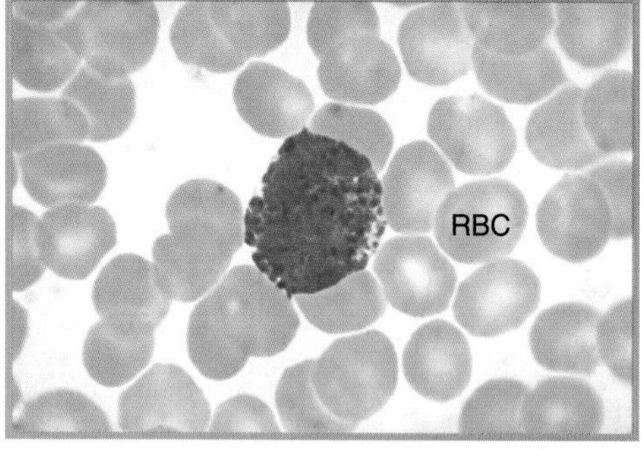

Figure 12-12
Basophil.

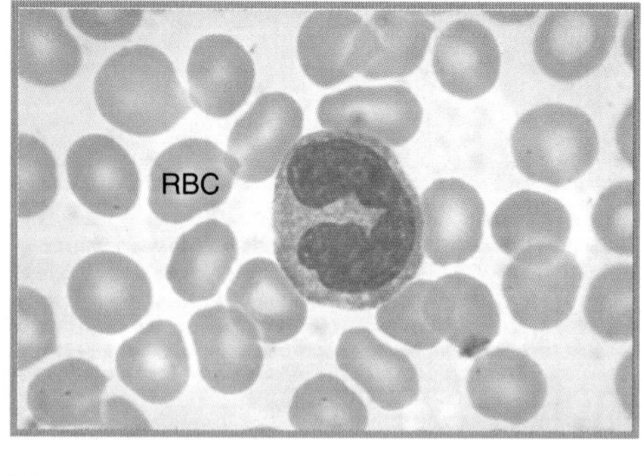

Figure 12-13
Monocyte.

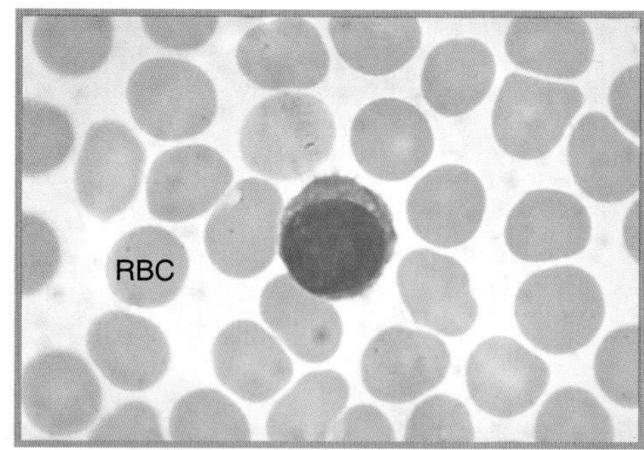

Figure 12-14
Lymphocyte.

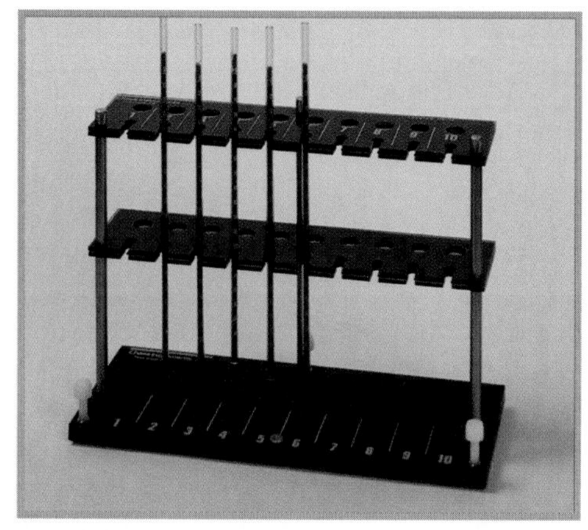

Figure 12-15
Westergren Method.

PROCEDURE 12 • 3

THE SEDIMENTATION RATE TEST (WESTERGREN METHOD)

Purpose:

To determine if red blood cells fall faster than normal, which is an indication of inflammation.

Terminal Performance Competency:

Perform an ESR using the Wintrobe method and aseptic technique without error.

Equipment:

Disposable gloves, whole blood (EDTA) or sodium citrate, Wintrobe tube, Wintrobe rack, biohazard sharps container, pen, and laboratory coat.

Procedure:

1. Wash hands and put on disposable gloves.
2. Assemble equipment.
3. Mix anticoagulated evacuated tube well. The ratio of blood to anticoagulant (4:1) is very important; therefore, the tube must be filled completely. For accurate results, blood should be kept at room temperature and be no more than 2 hours old.
4. Fill the Westergren tube with blood, avoiding air bubbles. If an air bubble occurs, discard that tube and start over.
5. Adjust the meniscus of the specimen to the zero line at the top of the tube if tube does not self-adjust to zero.
6. Place the tube in the rack, making sure it is completely vertical.
7. Set a timer for 1 hour.
8. Immediately after the timer rings, read the distance the red blood cells have fallen.
9. Record the distance in millimeters per hour.
10. Dispose of tubes in biohazard container.
11. Dispose of gloves and wash hands.

TABLE 12-3 Normal Values for the Erythrocyte Sedimentation Rate

Wintrobe	Men = 0-9 mm/hr	Women = 0-20 mm/hr
Westergren	Men <50 years = <10 mm/hr	Women <50 years = <13 mm/hr
	Men >50 years = ≤13 mm/hr	Women >50 years = ≤20 mm/hr

Hemostasis

Hemostasis is the process by which bleeding is stopped. This process is controlled by the coordination of the vascular system, platelets, and the coagulation factors. The coagulation factors are all plasma proteins with the exception of one factor, calcium. These three systems work together **in vivo** (within the body) to stop bleeding within a damaged blood vessel, and **in vitro** (outside the body) the platelets and coagulation factors work together to cause blood to clot in a red- or gold-topped evacuated tube.

The coagulation section of the hematology laboratory performs tests to help in the diagnosis of hemostatic disorders. Blood for coagulation studies is drawn in a blue-topped evacuated tube that contains the anticoagulant 0.109 M sodium citrate. It is very important that the evacuated tube fill completely because the ratio of blood to anticoagulant (9 parts blood to 1 part anticoagulant) is critical for accurate test results.

MED TIP

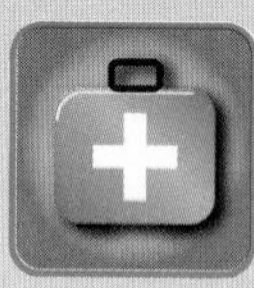

If only a blue-topped evacuated tube is needed, first draw a small amount of blood into a red-topped tube so that the blood sample is not contaminated with tissue fluid.

Specimens for coagulation studies must be drawn with minimal trauma to the area. Tissue thromboplastin, released by tissues when they are damaged, will adversely affect the specimen. It is also very important that no clots form in the specimen. If there is a clot of any size, the specimen is no longer suitable for coagulation testing. Specimens for coagulation testing may be kept at room temperature if they are going to be tested within 2 hours of collection.

MED TIP

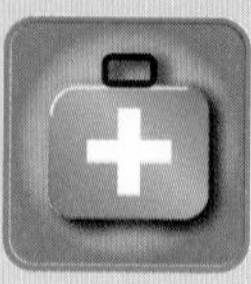

Gently invert the blue-topped evacuated tube several times as soon as the blood is drawn to prevent clots from forming in the specimen.

Coagulation Studies

The four main tests that are performed to test the body's hemostatic function are a platelet count (discussed on page 205), the bleeding time test (see chapter 8), the prothrombin time test, and the activated partial thromboplastin time. These tests are part of the usual presurgical screening because it is very important for the surgeon to know whether the patient has a prolonged bleeding time.

The **prothrombin time** (also known as protime, or PT) is one of the most commonly ordered coagulation tests. It is used not only to evaluate the patient's hemostatic ability but also to monitor the effectiveness of coumadin therapy. Coumadin is an anticoagulant medication used to prevent the formation of intravascular blood clots. Patients who have phlebitis, a stroke, or an artificial heart valve may take coumadin. The dosage must be strictly monitored because the patient should not easily form intravascular clots and yet hemostasis should occur if there is trauma to a blood vessel. The normal value of a protime is less than 10 to 15 seconds; for those taking coumadin the protime should be less than 16 to 18 seconds. The range of times for the normal value is due to differences in coagulation analyzers used in the laboratory.

The **activated partial thromboplastin time (APTT)** is one of the most useful tests to assess a patient's hemostatic ability, to detect circulating anticoagulants or inhibitors such as may be found in systemic lupus erythematosus, and to monitor the effectiveness of heparin therapy. The blood specimen should be drawn into an evacuated tube containing sodium citrate (blue top) with as little trauma as possible. The tourniquet should be removed as quickly as possible to prevent hemoconcentration. During hemoconcentration, platelets and certain coagulation factors can be activated and cause erroneous test results. After the plasma has been removed from the centrifuged evacuated tube, it should be refrigerated until testing. The normal value of an APTT varies with the testing instrument used by the laboratory but is usually less than 35 seconds.

CHAPTER REVIEW

Summary

Phlebotomists who are employed in physician offices or freestanding outpatient laboratories may be required to perform some simple hematology procedures. In this chapter we reviewed the basic hematology laboratory test and gave step-by-step procedures for tests that may be performed by phlebotomists. We also introduced the microscope, which is an essential instrument in the laboratory.

Competency Review

1. Explain how both serum and plasma are obtained.
2. Describe the cellular components of blood.
3. List some of the differences between manual hematology tests and automated hematology tests.
4. Describe the function of hemoglobin.
5. Describe the types of specimens that can be used to make a differential smear.

Examination Review Questions

1. **All of the following is found in serum except**
   (A) water
   (B) plasma proteins
   (C) fibrinogen
   (D) electrolytes
   (E) nutrients

2. **The most numerous of the cellular components of blood are**
   (A) erythrocytes
   (B) granulocytes
   (C) agranulocytes
   (D) platelets
   (E) leukocytes

3. **The ________ determines the relative percentages of the different types of leukocytes.**
   (A) hematocrit
   (B) hemoglobin
   (C) differential
   (D) sedimentation rate
   (E) leukocyte count

4. **The coagulation test that can be used to monitor the effectiveness of coumadin therapy is**
   (A) protime
   (B) activated partial thromboplastin time
   (C) platelet count
   (D) hematocrit
   (E) erythrocyte sedimentation rate

5. **The test that gives information about the red blood cell volume is the**
   (A) hemoglobin
   (B) hematocrit
   (C) erythrocyte sedimentation rate
   (D) activated partial thromboplastin time
   (E) protime

6. **Plasma is obtained by**
   (A) drawing the sample into a red-topped evacuated tube
   (B) centrifuging a red-topped evacuated tube
   (C) drawing the sample using a winged infusion set
   (D) drawing the sample into an evacuated tube with an anticoagulant
   (E) using only capillary blood

7. **One type of white blood cell that acts as a phagocytic cell is the**
   (A) erythrocyte
   (B) neutrophil
   (C) basophil
   (D) platelet
   (E) eosinophil

8. **The ________ plays a role in hemostasis.**
   (A) erythrocyte
   (B) neutrophil
   (C) monocyte
   (D) lymphocyte
   (E) thrombocyte

9. **Microscopes can be used to**
   (A) count erythrocytes
   (B) identify leukocytes
   (C) count platelets
   (D) determine cell morphology
   (E) all of the above

10. **If a physician wants information about a patient's erythrocytes, all of the following tests might be ordered except a**
    (A) red blood cell count
    (B) differential
    (C) hemoglobin level
    (D) hematocrit
    (E) packed cell volume

Getting Connected

Multimedia Extension Activities

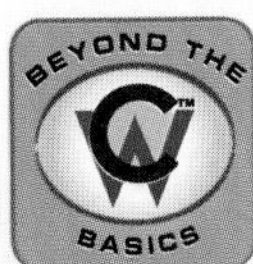

www.prenhall.com/fremgen

Use the address above to access the free, interactive Companion Website created specifically for this textbook. Enhance your studying by answering practice quiz questions, with hints and instant feedback related to chapter 12. If you would like to gain a deeper understanding of selected topics within this chapter, be sure to click on the **Beyond the Basics** feature, which provides more details for further learning. If you do not have a web connection, you may use the CD-ROM enclosed in the back of this book to take advantage of the same features off-line.

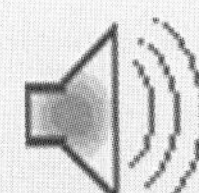

Audio Glossary

Use the CD-ROM enclosed with your textbook to hear the pronunciation of the key terms in the chapter. You may also access this material on the Companion Website www.prenhall.com/fremgen.

Bibliography

Brown, B. *Hematology: Principles and Procedures*, 6th ed. Baltimore, Md.: Williams & Wilkins, 1993.

Marshall, J. *Fundamental Skills for the Clinical Laboratory Professional.* Albany, N.Y.: Delmar, 1993.

Turgeon, T. *Clinical Hematology Theory and Procedures*, 2nd ed. Boston: Little, Brown, 1993.

Walters, N., B. Estridge, and A. Reynolds. *Basic Medical Laboratory Techniques*, 3rd ed. Albany, N.Y.: Delmar, 1996.

CHAPTER 13

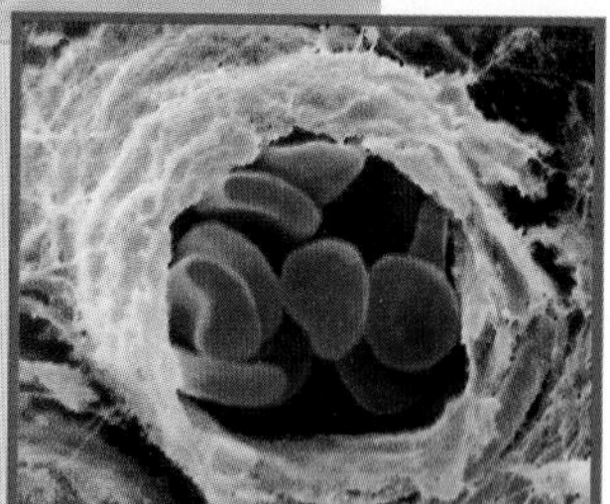

Urinalysis, Chemistry, and Related Specimen Collection

Chapter Outline

- Introduction
- Urinalysis
- Routine Analysis
- Clinical Chemistry
- Summary
- Competency Review
- Examination Review Questions
- Bibliography

Learning Objectives

After completing this chapter, you should be able to

1. Define and spell the glossary terms listed in this chapter.
2. Describe the different types of urine specimens.
3. Describe the characteristics of a physical examination of urine.
4. List the analytes tested on a reagent strip and describe their importance.
5. Describe the type of structures that can be seen during a microscopic examination of urine.
6. Explain the procedure for obtaining serum for chemical testing.
7. Explain the purpose of batching specimens.
8. Describe a chemistry profile.
9. Describe the information that can be obtained from a general chemistry profile.
10. Describe the types of testing performed in a toxicology laboratory.

GLOSSARY

CATHETER sterile flexible tube inserted into the bladder or a vein to withdraw fluid.

CAST a cylindrical protein structure formed in a kidney tubule and found in urine.

ELECTROLYTES term for four serum ions (sodium, potassium, chloride, and bicarbonate).

GLUCOSURIA the presence of sugar (glucose) in the urine.

HEMATURIA the presence of red blood cells in the urine.

HYPOGLYCEMIA low blood glucose level.

ICTERIC having a yellow color due to excess bilirubin.

LIPEMIC having a cloudy or milky white appearance due to excess lipids.

pH measurement of the degree of acidity or alkalinity of a substance.

POSTPRANDIAL after eating.

PROFILE group of chemistry tests.

PROTEINURIA the presence of protein in the urine.

SPECIFIC GRAVITY a measure of the density of a substance as compared with the density of water.

TURBIDITY having a cloudy appearance.

UTI urinary tract infection.

INTRODUCTION

One of the most common laboratory procedures is the routine urinalysis. This simple test can give the doctor valuable information about many body systems, especially kidney function. The clinical chemistry laboratory studies the level of many different chemical substances in body fluids, predominantly serum. The physician uses the information from both the urinalysis and chemical analysis to diagnose and treat many disease states.

Urinalysis

Urine is one type of specimen that can be easily collected from a patient, although many times, special instructions must be given to the patient to collect the specimen in the proper manner. Figure 13-1a and b shows many different types of urine collection containers. Large clinical laboratories may have a separate laboratory for urinalysis; in smaller facilities urinalysis may be part of the hematology or chemistry laboratory. Table 13-1 lists the different types of urine specimens.

Specimen Collection

A *random specimen* is a urine sample that is collected any time during the day. The patient is given a nonsterile collection container and instructed to void in the container. A random specimen is used only for routine screening because the composition of urine changes throughout the day.

A *first voided specimen* is also referred to as a first morning specimen. The patient is given a urine container to take home and instructed to collect a sample of the urine the first time he or she urinates in the morning. A first voided specimen is the most concentrated and is the preferred specimen for pregnancy testing, bacterial cultures, and microscopic examinations. Because urine is not stable, the specimen should be examined within 1 hour of collection. If that is not possible, the specimen should be refrigerated until it can be tested.

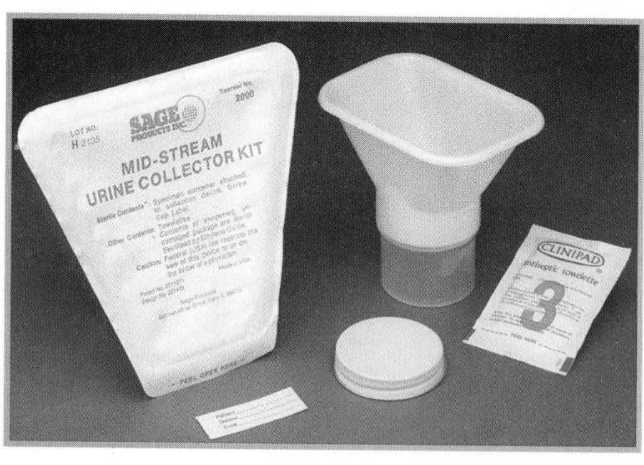

(a)

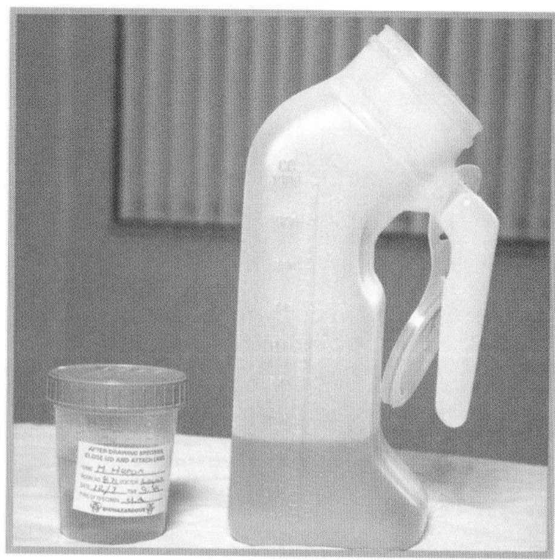

(b)

Figure 13-1
Many different types of urine collection containers.

TABLE 13-1 Types of Urine Specimens

1. Random sample
2. First voided specimen
3. Timed specimen
4. Two-hour postprandial specimen
5. Clean-catch midstream specimen
6. Catheterized specimen
7. Suprapubic aspirate

Timed specimens are used when the physician requires urine samples taken at specific intervals during the day. Twenty-four-hour urine specimens are required for creatinine clearance tests and hormone studies. The patient must be given careful instructions to collect the specimen properly (see table 13-2). Incorrect collection can make the testing invalid.

A *2-hour* ***postprandial*** urine specimen is collected 2 hours after the patient eats. This type of specimen is usually used for diabetes testing.

A *clean-catch midstream* specimen is ordered if the urine is going to be examined for microorganisms or cultured for bacterial growth. Patient instructions for collecting a clean-catch midstream specimen are found in chapter 14.

A *catheterized specimen* is obtained by inserting a **catheter** or sterile flexible tube into the bladder via the urethra to withdraw urine. This procedure is done only by specially trained personnel. Reasons for catheterization include the need for a sterile urine specimen, to determine the amount of urine remaining in the bladder after the patient has voided, to relieve urinary retention, and to empty the bladder completely before surgery or diagnostic tests.

TABLE 13-2 Instructions for a 24-Hour Urine Collection

1. The patient is given a large container (approximately 1 gallon) that is labeled with the patient's name and date; space is provided to write the time the collection begins and ends. The urine container may contain a preservative to stabilize the urine for the 24-hour period. The urine may also have to be refrigerated during the collection period.
2. The test usually begins in the morning. The patient is told to empty his or her bladder and discard the urine in the toilet and record the time on the label of the urine container. For the next 24 hours, all urine must be collected in the container. The next day at the same time the test began the patient empties his or her bladder, collects the urine in the container, and records the time the test ended. The patient should be instructed to avoid fecal contamination of the specimen.
3. The 24-hour urine sample is brought to the laboratory as soon as the 24-hour period is over.

A *suprapubic aspirate* is obtained by inserting a needle directly into the bladder and withdrawing urine. Because the specimen bypasses the urethra it is free of bacterial contamination. A suprapubic specimen is used for bacteriologic and cytology studies.

Routine Urinalysis

Urinalysis refers to the testing of urine for the presence of infection or disease. There are three parts to a routine urinalysis: physical examination (also called the macroscopic examination), chemical analysis, and microscopic examination.

Physical Examination

The physical characteristics observed in urine include appearance (clarity or turbidity), color, odor, and specific gravity.

The appearance of a urine specimen may range from clear to cloudy. **Turbidity,** or cloudiness, may be caused by a bacterial infection or excess cells. Turbidity also can be caused by crystals that form when the specimen is refrigerated. These crystals may disappear as the specimen warms to room temperature.

MED TIP

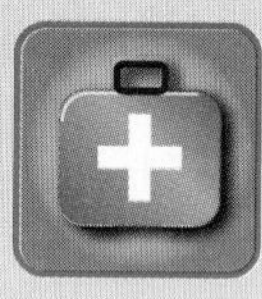

When performing a urinalysis, always have the specimen at room temperature, because specimens still cold from refrigeration may give erroneous results.

The normal color of urine varies from a pale straw to an amber color. The color of urine depends on the concentration of the specimen and the patient's diet. A dilute specimen is pale in color, whereas concentrated urine has a dark color. Some foods, such as beets, give urine a distinct color. Sometimes the color of urine indicates a serious disease process. For example, a red color may indicate bleeding in the genitourinary tract, and a greenish-brown or deep amber color may indicate a liver disorder such as hepatitis.

A normal urine specimen has an aromatic odor. An abnormal odor to urine may indicate disease. Patients with uncontrolled diabetes may have a fruity or sweet odor to their urine due to the presence of ketones (products of fat metabolism). A foul or ammonia-like odor to urine may indicate a bacterial infection. The ingestion of some foods, such as asparagus, can also result in urine with a strong odor.

Specific gravity, or density, is the weight of a substance as compared with the weight of the same amount of distilled water. The normal specific gravity of urine varies between 1.010 and 1.030 depending on how concentrated or dilute the specimen is. The specific gravity is an indicator of the kidneys' ability to concentrate the urine. A very dilute urine with a low specific gravity is found in patients with diseases such as diabetes mellitus. A high specific gravity may be a sign of dehydration. The clinical laboratory has three different methods of measuring the specific gravity of urine: urinometer, refractometer, and reagent strips.

MED TIP

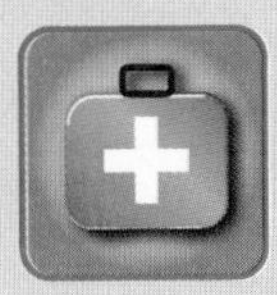

The concentration of urine changes during the day depending on fluid intake. The first morning specimen is the most concentrated and has the highest specific gravity.

Chemical Analysis

Chemical testing of urine provides information on carbohydrate metabolism, liver and kidney function, possible bacterial infection, and the body's acid-base balance. The most commonly used techniques are reagent strips, which are also called dipsticks. Reagent strips are plastic strips that have chemicals implanted on small pads on one end. The strips are then dipped into the urine and the color change on the pads is compared to a chart with normal and abnormal values. Reagent strips range from having only one pad for a single chemical determination to having ten or more pads for multiple chemical testing. Reagent strips are available for pH, protein, glucose, ketones, blood, bilirubin, urobilinogen, nitrites, leukocytes, specific gravity, and others. Table 13-3 lists the normal values for chemical testing of urine.

The reagent strips are used once and then discarded into a hazardous waste container. In the manual method, the strip is dipped into the sample and excess urine is removed by touching the back of the strip to the rim of the specimen container as it is withdrawn. Holding the strip horizontally, the pads are observed

TABLE 13-3 Normal Values for Chemical Testing

Color	Pale straw to amber
Odor	Aromatic
Appearance	Clear
Specific gravity	1.002-1.030
pH	4.5-7.5
Protein	Negative to trace
Glucose	Negative
Blood	Negative
Ketones	Negative
Bilirubin	Negative
Urobilinogen	Less than 1.0 Ehrlich unit or 1 mg/dL
Nitrites	Negative

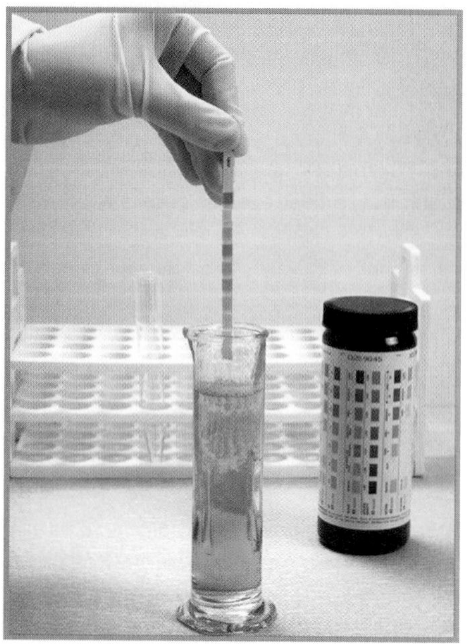

Figure 13-2
Dipstick procedure.

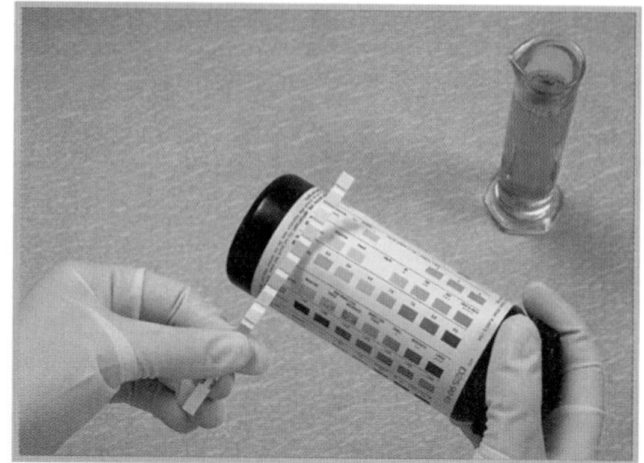

Figure 13-3
The process of comparing colors on the dipstick with the color chart.

for color change at specified time intervals. Figures 13-2 and 13-3 describe the dipstick procedure and the process of comparing colors on the dipstick with the color chart. Color changes on the pads are compared with the color chart on the reagent strip container. Some laboratories have automated strip readers (as shown in figure 13-4) that detect the color change on the reagent pad electronically.

MED TIP

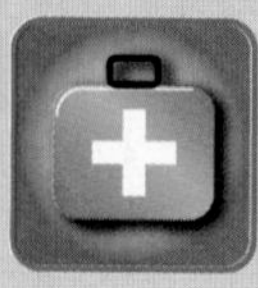

Remember that the reagent strip must not touch the side of the reagent strip container when comparing it with the color chart. Touching the container with the urine-soaked strip will contaminate the container.

The **pH** of a solution indicates acidity or alkalinity. This reaction is measured on a scale ranging from 0 to 14, with 7 representing neutrality. On this scale, 0 represents the highest level of acidity and 14 represents the highest level of alkalinity. Patients on a normal diet have urine that is slightly acidic at around pH 6. Normal kidneys can produce urine with a pH ranging from 4.5 to 8. Acidic urine is found in patients with metabolic or respiratory acidosis and high-protein diets. Alkaline urine is common in patients with fever, vomiting, diets high in fruits and vegetables, and respiratory alkalosis.

Under normal conditions, the reagent strip should be negative for protein. **Proteinuria,** the presence of protein in the urine, is one of the first signs of kidney disease. Proteinuria is also a sign of preeclamp-

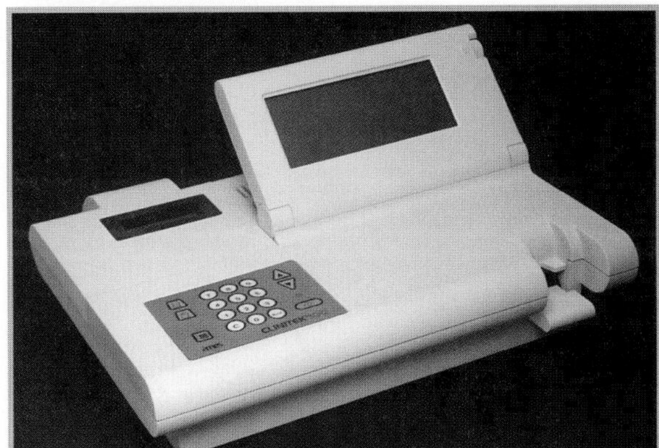

Figure 13-4
Automated strip reader that detects the color change on the reagent pad electronically. (Courtesy: Bayer Diagnostics, Tarrytown, NY 10598.)

sia (toxemia) in pregnant women and congestive heart failure. Proteinuria can also be a normal physiological response to exposure to cold, strenuous activity, or having a high-protein diet.

Small amounts of glucose may be present in urine shortly after eating a meal high in carbohydrates. The glucose will quickly disappear if there is normal carbohydrate metabolism. **Glucosuria** refers to the presence of sugar in the urine, mainly seen in patients with diabetes mellitus. Glucose will begin to "spill" into the urine when the blood glucose level exceeds 160 to 180 mg/dL. Glucosuria can also be seen with pregnancy, stress, the use of some medications, infections, and Cushing's disease. A false-negative test for glucose may result with the reagent strip if the patient consumes large amounts of vitamin C.

Normally, the reagent strip is negative for blood, although a few red blood cells may be seen during a microscopic examination. **Hematuria,** the presence of red blood cells in the urine, is usually a sign of bleeding from the urinary tract or of an infection. Free hemoglobin from lysed red blood cells will also cause a positive reaction for blood on the reagent strip. If the reagent test is positive for blood and no red blood cells are seen on microscopic examination, the most common explanation is that hemoglobin is present in the urine.

Ketone bodies are not normally excreted in urine. The finding of ketones in the urine indicates abnormal fat metabolism. Conditions associated with ketonuria are poorly controlled diabetes, dehydration, starvation, ingestion of large amounts of aspirin, and a side effect of receiving general anesthesia.

Bilirubin is a product of the breakdown of hemoglobin. Hemoglobin is converted to bilirubin in the liver and then to urobilinogen in the intestines. Bilirubin is not generally found in the urine. Its presence may be one of the first signs of liver disease. A large amount of bilirubin in the urine will cause a change in color ranging from a yellowish brown to a greenish orange.

A small amount of urobilinogen is normally found in urine (less than 1 mg/dL). However, the level may increase as a result of excessive red blood cell destruction and/or liver disease. An absence of urobilinogen in urine may mean an obstruction of the bile duct.

Nitrites in the urine indicate a possible **urinary tract infection (UTI).** Nitrates are normally found in urine, and the types of bacteria that most frequently cause urinary tract infections are able to convert nitrates to nitrites. Not all bacteria have this ability, so a false-negative reaction can occur. A false-negative result means that the patient has a UTI, but it is caused by a bacterium that does not have the ability to convert nitrates to nitrites. A false-positive result can occur if a specimen remains too long at room temperature. During that time, bacteria from skin contamination, but not from an infection, can multiply and convert the nitrates to nitrites. If a specimen cannot be tested within 2 hours of collection, refrigeration will help to eliminate the problem.

Normally there should be very few leukocytes in urine. Their presence indicates either infection or inflammation.

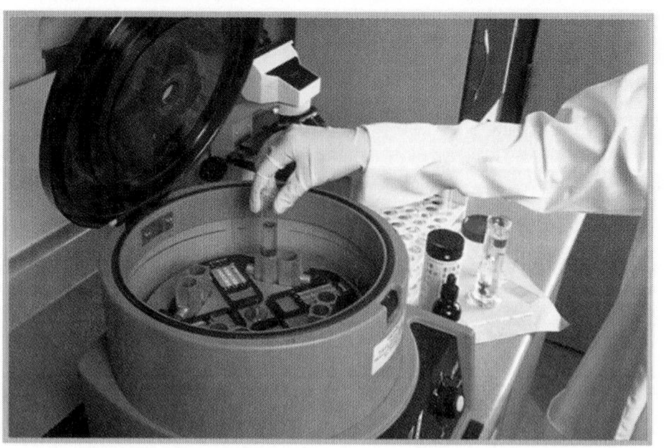

Figure 13-5
Approximately 10 mL of urine is centrifuged at 1,500–2,000 rpm for 5 minutes.

Microscopic Examination

Microscopic examination is the third part of a routine urinalysis. It can provide the physician with information used to diagnose and monitor the progress of disease. In an effort to reduce costs, many clinical laboratories will not perform the microscopic examination if the physical and chemical examinations are normal.

The first voided specimen is the preferred specimen for microscopic examination because it is the most concentrated and contains the most cellular material. The specimen is well mixed, and approximately 10 mL of urine is poured into a tube and centrifuged at 1,500–2,000 rpm for 5 minutes, as illustrated in figure 13-5. All but approximately 0.5 mL of supernatant is poured off, and the remainder is resuspended with the sediment. A drop of the sediment is placed on a clean microscope slide, covered with a cover slip, and viewed under the microscope. Urine sediment may be composed of cells, casts, crystals, and microorganisms.

Normal urine may contain a few red blood cells and a few white blood cells per high-power microscopic field. A finding of more than a few blood cells is an indication of bleeding, an infection, or inflammation. Epithelial cells may also be found in urinary sediment. These cells are continually being replaced in the lining of the urinary tract, and old cells are found in urine. Squamous epithelium is the most commonly found cell and comes from the lining of the vagina and the lower portion of the male and female urethras. Transitional epithelial cells come from the lining of the bladder, renal pelvis, and upper urethra. The third type of epithelial cell is the renal tubule epithelium cell. These cells are the most significant, and finding large numbers of these cells may indicate tubular necrosis or the rejection of a transplanted kidney.

Casts are cylindrical protein structures that are formed in the kidney tubules and found in the urine. Casts are classified according to the type of cells embedded in the protein. For example, a hyaline cast is composed solely of protein, whereas a red blood cell cast has red blood cells embedded in the protein. Sometimes the cells degenerate and it is not possible to identify them. In that case, the casts are called granular casts. A few hyaline casts are a normal finding, but the finding of other casts signifies serious renal pathology.

Crystals are a common urinary finding, and most are insignificant. They are urinary salts that precipitate out of solution due to changes in pH and temperature. The main reason to identify crystals is to detect the few abnormal crystals that may appear.

MED TIP

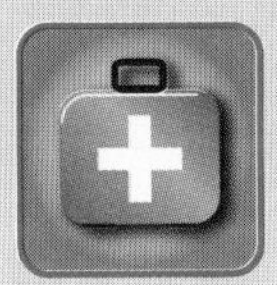

If a refrigerated urine specimen is allowed to come to room temperature before analysis, most of the normal crystals may disappear, making the microscopic examination much easier to read.

Microorganisms are not normally found in urine, and their presence in large numbers usually indicates an infection. The types of microorganisms that can be found in urinary sediment include bacteria, yeast, and the parasite, *Trichomonas spp.* A few bacteria may be seen in urine if the specimen was not collected under sterile conditions. These bacteria are from skin that contaminated the urine during specimen collection.

Clinical Chemistry

Clinical chemistry laboratories range in size from a simple instrument that performs a single analysis such as glucose testing and that might be found in a doctor's office to a large private reference laboratory in which the chemistry area is divided into several subdivisions, each with large, multiparameter analyzing instruments. An example of a multiparameter analyzing instrument is found in figure 13-6. The division of the chemistry laboratory is based on either the test methodology or the type of analyte (e.g., enzymes) being measured. The chemistry subdivisions might include general chemistry, toxicology, immunochemistry, and the electrophoresis laboratory. In a typical hospital, the chemistry laboratory is the largest and busiest area of the clinical laboratory. The chemistry laboratory receives the most specimens and performs more tests than any other area in the clinical laboratory.

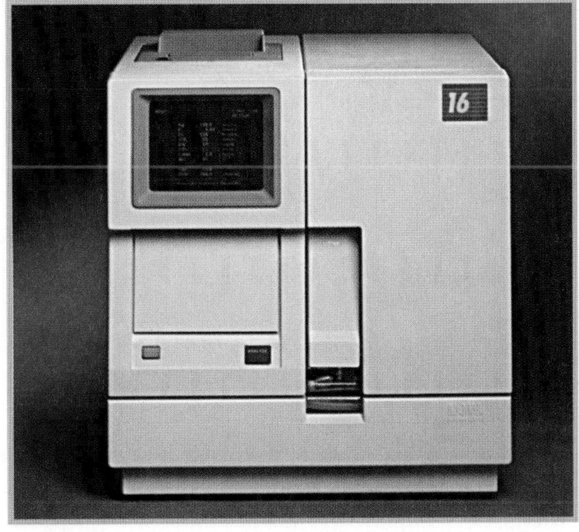

Figure 13-6 Multiparameter chemistry instrument. (Nova 16 Analyzer photograph supplied by Nova Biomedical, Waltham, MA 02454, USA.)

Specimen Collection

Most chemical analysis is performed on serum. Specimens are usually collected in red- or gold-topped evacuated tubes with a serum separator. These tubes contain a gel-like substance that separates the cells from the serum during centrifugation. Blood should be completely clotted before being centrifuged (approximately 20 to 30 minutes) to prevent products from cells from being incorporated into the serum. Most chemical analytes remain stable in serum, but if analysis will be delayed by more than 2 hours, the serum should be refrigerated. Some conditions may affect serum and make it unsuitable for testing. These conditions include hemolyzed specimens, **icteric** specimens (which have a yellow color due to large amounts of bilirubin), and **lipemic** specimens (which have a cloudy or milky white color due to excess lipid material). Many chemical analyses rely on photometric readings because many conditions impart an abnormal color to the serum. Specimens that are hemolyzed, icteric, or lipemic may give erroneous results by giving the serum a color that will interfere with the photometric readings.

Organization of the Chemistry Laboratory

The clinical chemistry laboratory is almost completely automated with large instruments that are able to perform multiple tests on a patient specimen at the same time. Groups of tests are usually organized by body system and are called **profiles.** For example, a cardiac profile would analyze various enzymes that are released if cardiac muscle is damaged. A physician usually orders a profile rather than the individual tests. Because of the instrumentation in the chemistry laboratory, it may be less expensive for the laboratory to run a profile of eight tests than to perform two or three individual tests. The chemistry laboratory may also batch specimens. Batching means that all the specimens requiring the same test or tests are run together. For example, liver profiles may be run once in the morning and once in the afternoon. The batching of specimens is more efficient and saves the laboratory money because fewer control specimens and less reagents are needed. Table 13-4 lists many of the common clinical analytes tested for in the chemistry laboratory.

Chemistry Profiles

A general chemistry profile is composed of a group of tests that monitor the functioning of the major body systems. A general chemistry profile will help the physician to determine the patient's general state of health. Tests in a general chemistry profile may include those for glucose, blood urea nitrogen (BUN), sodium (Na), potassium (K), aspartate aminotransferase (AST), lactic dehydrogenase (LD), cholesterol, triglycerides, uric acid, total protein, bilirubin, calcium, and alkaline phosphatase (ALP). Some of these tests may also be grouped into smaller profiles that analyze a specific body system. The glucose test is one of the most frequently ordered chemistry tests and is used in the diagnosis and management of diabetes mellitus and **hypoglycemia,** or low blood glucose level. Total protein is a measure of all proteins found in serum including albumin, coagulation factors, and antibodies. The total protein value can provide information about nutrition and liver function. Calcium is a mineral that is needed for blood coagulation and neuromuscular responses. Abnormal levels of calcium can be found in patients with some endocrine disorders, intestinal disorders, and kidney disease. The remainder of the tests in a general chemistry profile (BUN, sodium, potassium, AST, LD, cholesterol, triglycerides, uric acid, total protein, bilirubin, and ALP) are discussed within a more specific profile.

An **electrolyte** profile measures the four serum ions: sodium, potassium, chloride, and bicarbonate. These four electrolytes are used to monitor the body's water hydration, acid-base balance, pH, and heart and muscle function. These four electrolytes are found in different concentrations in the intracellular and extracellular spaces. Changes in the concentration of these four electrolytes can occur in patients with dehydration, vomiting and diarrhea, diabetes, and renal disease.

TABLE 13-4 Common Clinical Analytes

Analyte	Significance
Alanine aminotransferase (ALT)	Increased in liver disease
Alkaline phosphatase (ALP)	Increased in liver disease or bone disorders
Aspartate aminotransferase (AST)	Increased with a heart attack or liver disease
Bicarbonate	Affected by changes in respiration
Bilirubin	Increased in liver disease or hemolytic disorders
Blood urea nitrogen (BUN)	Elevated in kidney disease
Calcium (Ca)	Decreased in kidney disease; increased in hormone disorders
Chloride	Increased in dehydration or respiratory alkalosis
Cholesterol	Increased levels associated with cardiac risk
Creatinine	Increased in kidney disease
Glucose	Increased in diabetes
Lactic dehydrogenase (LD)	Elevated after myocardial infarction
Potassium	Increased in acidosis; decreased in dehydration
Protein	Decreased in liver or kidney disorders
Sodium	Increased in dehydration; decreased in acidosis
Triglyceride	Used in determining cardiac risk
Uric acid	Increased in gout or kidney disorders

A liver function profile consists of bilirubin and a group of liver enzymes including ALP, alanine aminotransferase (ALT), AST, and LD. Bilirubin is a product of the breakdown of hemoglobin, and excess bilirubin can occur in patients with liver disease and excessive red blood cell destruction. The other tests in a liver profile (ALP, ALT, AST, and LD) are for enzymes that are normally found in the liver; their levels in serum rise if there is damage to the liver from injury or disease.

A coronary risk profile includes total cholesterol, triglycerides, and high- and low-density lipoproteins. High levels of cholesterol, triglycerides, and low-density lipoproteins are associated with an increased risk of cardiovascular disease. Conversely, a high level of the high-density lipoproteins as compared with the low-density lipoproteins indicates that most of the cholesterol will be excreted from the body and not deposited in blood vessels, thereby reducing the risk of coronary disease.

A kidney profile usually includes creatinine, BUN, and uric acid tests. Creatinine, a waste product of muscle metabolism, is normally excreted in the urine and does not accumulate in the blood. Finding increased levels of creatinine in blood serum indicates that waste products in the blood are not being properly filtered by the kidneys. Urea is a product of protein metabolism and is normally filtered from the blood by the kidneys. The BUN level also increases in serum if the kidneys are impaired. Like BUN and creatinine levels, uric acid levels rise in patients with kidney disease, but they are also used to diagnose gout. Patients with gout produce an excess of uric acid, and these increased levels can cause joint pain and kidney damage.

Specialized Chemistry Areas

The toxicology section of the clinical chemistry laboratory is divided into two main areas: therapeutic drug monitoring and testing for drugs of abuse. Therapeutic drug monitoring analyzes the amount of a prescribed medication in the patient's serum. People metabolize drugs at different rates; some of the factors that can affect this metabolism are age, liver function, and kidney function. The physician needs to know the amount of the medication in the patient's blood to achieve optimal results before reaching toxic levels of the drug. Medications that require drug monitoring include certain antibiotics, lithium, digoxin, and theophylline. Testing for drugs of abuse is becoming more and more common because many employers require drug testing as a condition of employment. This testing is usually done on urine and requires strict control if the results are to be used in legal proceedings. Some of the drugs that are tested for include alcohol, marijuana, cocaine, and barbiturates.

Testing for blood gases may be performed in either the chemistry laboratory or the respiratory therapy department. Blood gas testing requires an arterial blood specimen (see chapter 8) and provides information about the respiratory status of the patient. Arterial blood drawn for blood gas analysis should be transported to the laboratory on ice to prevent the blood gases from escaping. Arterial blood gas (ABG) testing consists of the pH of the blood, the partial pressure of oxygen (P_{O_2}), and the partial pressure of carbon dioxide (P_{CO_2}). An arterial blood gas test measures the ability of the lungs to exchange carbon dioxide and oxygen.

Chapter Review

Summary

Chemistry is the busiest area in the clinical laboratory. Hundreds of different analytes can be tested for in blood. Urinalysis is usually considered part of the clinical chemistry area, but it may be part of the hematology area or even freestanding. The testing for most clinical analytes is quite sophisticated and beyond the scope of practice for phlebotomists.

Competency Review

1. List three different types of chemistry profiles and the chemistry tests included in each.
2. Describe the manual procedure for the chemical analysis of urine using a reagent strip.
3. Explain why hemolyzed or icteric blood specimens may interfere with chemical testing.
4. Describe the two main functions of the toxicology laboratory.
5. Explain the process of obtaining serum for chemical analysis when drawn in an evacuated tube.

Examination Review Questions

1. Which is the preferred urine specimen for a microscopic analysis?

(A) random
(B) first voided
(C) 24 hour
(D) 2-hour postprandial
(E) catheterized

2. The specific gravity is a measure of

(A) the color of the urine sample
(B) the turbidity of the urine sample
(C) the concentration of the urine sample
(D) the degree of acidity or alkalinity of the urine sample
(E) the number of cells in the sample

3. Which of the following is not a cell that can be found in urine?

(A) red blood cell
(B) white blood cell
(C) epithelial cell
(D) cast
(E) all of the above

4. Most specimens for the chemistry laboratory are collected in a

(A) red-topped evacuated tube with a serum separator
(B) syringe containing heparin
(C) microcollection tubule
(D) gray-topped evacuated tube with sodium fluoride
(E) lavender-topped evacuated tube

5. _________ measures the ability of the lungs to exchange oxygen and carbon dioxide.

(A) therapeutic drug monitoring
(B) a general chemistry profile
(C) arterial blood gas testing
(D) the electrophoresis laboratory
(E) microscopic analysis

6. In the chemistry laboratory a profile is a

(A) group of analyzing instruments
(B) group of tests with similar methodology
(C) number of patient specimens with similar results
(D) drawing of the expected patient results in graph form
(E) group of tests organized by body system

7. **Which of the following specimens are unsuitable for chemical analysis?**
   (A) hemolyzed specimens
   (B) icteric specimens
   (C) lipemic specimens
   (D) specimens collected with an anticoagulant
   (E) all of the above

8. **The color of urine is**
   (A) influenced by diet
   (B) depends on the concentration of the specimen
   (C) is greatly influenced by the glucose level
   (D) a and b
   (E) all of the above

9. **Microscopic examination**
   (A) is routinely done on all specimens
   (B) may only be performed if other tests are abnormal
   (C) gives very little useful information
   (D) can only be performed on first voided specimens
   (E) is performed on the specimen before it is centrifuged

10. **Crystals in urine**
   (A) are a common finding
   (B) always indicate serious pathology
   (C) are only found in refrigerated specimens
   (D) are only found in room-temperature specimens
   (E) can be identified by chemical analysis

Getting Connected

Multimedia Extension Activities

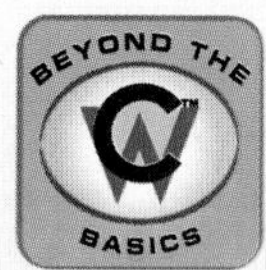

www.prenhall.com/fremgen

Use the address above to access the free, interactive Companion Website created specifically for this textbook. Enhance your studying by answering practice quiz questions, with hints and instant feedback related to chapter 13. If you would like to gain a deeper understanding of selected topics within this chapter, be sure to click on the **Beyond the Basics** feature, which provides more details for further learning. If you do not have a web connection, you may use the CD-ROM enclosed in the back of this book to take advantage of the same features off-line.

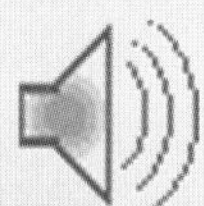

Audio Glossary

Use the CD-ROM enclosed with your textbook to hear the pronunciation of the key terms in the chapter. You may also access this material on the Companion Website www.prenhall.com/fremgen.

Bibliography

Burtis, C., and E. Ashwood. *Tietz Fundamentals of Clinical Chemistry*, 4th ed. Philadelphia: W. B. Saunders, 1996.

Lehmann, C. *Saunders Manual of Clinical Laboratory Science.* Philadelphia: W. B. Saunders, 1998.

Marshall, J. *Fundamental Skills for the Clinical Laboratory Professional.* Albany, N.Y.: Delmar, 1993.

Strasinger, S. *Urinalysis and Body Fluids*, 3rd ed. Philadelphia: F. A. Davis, 1994.

Walters, N., B. Estridge, and A. Reynolds. *Basic Medical Laboratory Techniques*, 3rd ed. Albany, N.Y.: Delmar, 1996.

CHAPTER 14

Microbiology and Related Specimen Collection

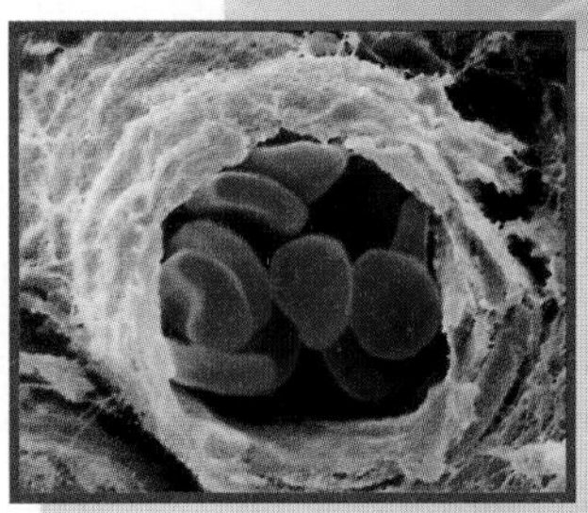

Chapter Outline

Learning Objectives

After completing this chapter, you should be able to

1. Define and spell the glossary terms listed in this chapter.
2. List the sterile body sites and those with normal flora.
3. Explain the reasons some bacteriologic specimens require special treatment during transportation to the laboratory.
4. Describe the process that a bacteriologic specimen undergoes when it is received in the microbiology laboratory.
5. Describe the information needed to identify a bacterium.
6. Describe the differences between yeast and molds.
7. Explain why parasitic infection in the United States is rare.
8. Explain why viruses cannot be cultured on the same media as bacteria.
9. Describe the type of routine testing that takes place in the immunology laboratory.

GLOSSARY

AGAR a product from seaweed that is used to solidify bacteriologic media.

ANAEROBIC without oxygen.

ANTIBIOTIC a substance produced by a microorganism that will inhibit bacterial growth.

ANTIBODY a specialized protein found in blood that reacts with an antigen.

ANTIGEN a foreign substance that causes the production of an antibody.

BACILLUS a rod-shaped bacterium.

COCCUS a spherical-shaped bacterium.

COLONY a mass of bacteria that grew from a single bacterial cell.

CULTURE the act of growing bacteria on media in the laboratory.

GRAM STAIN the primary differential stain used to classify bacteria.

HYPHAE hairlike structures of molds.

IMMUNOLOGY the study of immune processes.

INFECTION a pathological condition caused by the growth of microorganisms in a host.

MEDIA substances that will sustain bacteriologic growth in the laboratory.

MICROBIOLOGY the study of microorganisms.

MYCOSIS an infection caused by a fungus.

NORMAL FLORA microorganisms that are normally present on a host.

PARASITE an organism that lives on or in a host and causes damage to the host.

PATHOGENIC capable of causing damage in a host.

Petri dish a round covered dish used to hold agar-based media.

Serology the study of antigens and antibodies in serum.

Smear a microscope slide that has material to be stained.

Spirillus a spiral-shaped bacterium.

Tissue culture a medium of live cells used to grow viruses.

Introduction

Clinical **microbiology** is the study of microorganisms that can cause disease in humans. The main purpose of the clinical microbiology laboratory is to identify bacteria that cause infections in humans. Depending on the size of the laboratory, the clinical microbiology laboratory may also include the areas of mycology (fungi), parasitology (parasites), and virology (viruses). Some laboratories also include the area of serology and immunology with microbiology, whereas other very large, comprehensive laboratories have a separate serology and immunology area.

Bacteriology

The clinical microbiology laboratory examines specimens from patients to determine if **pathogenic** bacteria are present. Pathogenic bacteria are capable of causing damage in a host and can overcome the body's defenses and grow in tissue. This growth disrupts the normal tissue processes and is called an **infection** or a pathological condition caused by the growth of microorganisms. Some body sites are sterile and under normal conditions do not have any bacteria (see table 14-1). Other body sites have a population of bacteria that normally grow on or in the area and do not cause disease (see table 14-2). These bacteria are referred to as **normal flora.** If normal flora get into an area that is usually sterile, an infection may result, and the bacteria that cause the infection are referred to as opportunists.

TABLE 14-1 Sterile Body Sites
Blood
Body fluids
Central nervous system
Upper urinary tract
Lower respiratory tract

TABLE 14-2 Body Sites with Normal Flora
Upper respiratory tract
Lower urogenital tract
Skin
Gastrointestinal tract

TABLE 14-3	Common Types of Microbiology Specimens
Blood	Body fluids (e.g., peritoneal, synovial)
Cerebrospinal fluid (CSF)	Ears
Urine	Genitourinary tract
Nasal	Sputum
Stool	Throat
Urine	Wounds

Specimen Collection

The specimens that are received in a laboratory and are plated on media to grow are referred to as **cultures** (see table 14-3). Figure 14-1 shows the common types of microbiology specimen containers that are received in the laboratory. Some specimens for microbial culture, such as blood, may be collected by a phlebotomist (discussed in chapter 8). The phlebotomist may also provide patient instruction on the proper method to collect certain bacteriologic specimens such as clean-catch urine specimens. If the phlebotomist is employed in a doctor's office, he or she may be responsible for taking a throat culture on a patient. Other cultures are usually taken by physicians or the nursing staff and are sent to the laboratory. These cultures include specimens from wounds, body fluids such as cerebrospinal fluid (CSF) and synovial fluid, respiratory tract specimens such as sputum or bronchial washings, and genitourinary tract specimens. Two common procedures that a phlebotomist may either perform or explain to a patient are the procedure for taking a throat culture (procedure 14-1) or collecting a clean-catch urine sample (procedure 14-2).

Although in many hospitals physicians or nurses collect most specimens using equipment such as sterile cotton swabs (see figure 14-2), phlebotomists are responsible for transporting the microbiological specimens to the laboratory. Specimens must be collected in sterile containers to prevent contamination of the specimen. Extreme care must also be used in collecting specimens to prevent normal flora from contaminating the culture. Many specimens are collected on sterile swabs and then placed in a transport medium, which helps preserve the specimen until it can be cultured in the laboratory. Some

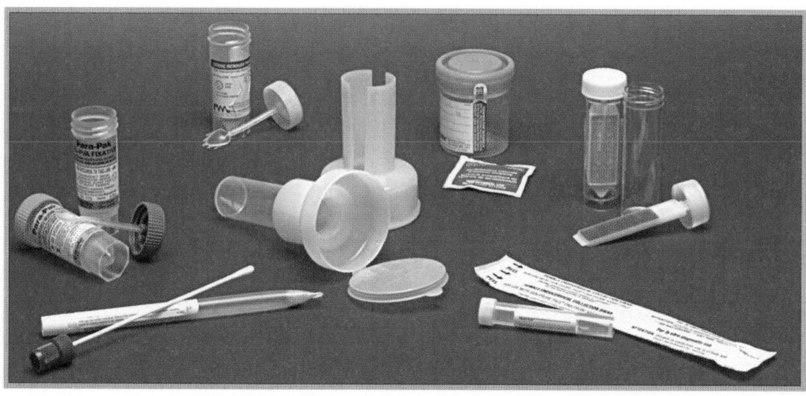

Figure 14-1 Common types of microbiology specimen containers.

PROCEDURE 14•1

TAKING A THROAT CULTURE

Purpose:

To diagnose the cause of a sore throat.

Terminal Performance Competency:

Properly collect a throat culture without contaminating the specimen.

Equipment:

Disposable gloves, tongue depressor, sterile disposable swab, transport container, and biohazard container.

Procedure:

1. Wash hands and put on disposable gloves.
2. Assemble equipment.
3. Identify patient and explain procedure to patient.
4. Using tongue depressor, hold down the patient's tongue.
5. Insert sterile disposable swab to back of throat and swab tonsillar area and any white or red areas. *Be careful not to touch the tongue, cheek, teeth, or uvula with the swab because it will contaminate the specimen.*
6. Place swab in transport container and label the container.
7. Attach the requisition to the container.
8. Wash hands and dispose of gloves and tongue depressor in biohazard container.
9. Transport the specimen to the laboratory.

bacteria are fastidious and require special conditions to remain viable. **Anaerobic** bacteria cannot live and grow in the presence of oxygen. If a physician suspects that an infection is caused by anaerobic bacteria, special collection and transportation materials are available to limit the bacteria's exposure to oxygen. Some specimens, such as urine cultures, should be refrigerated if they cannot be transported to the laboratory shortly after collection. Other specimens, such as CSF and genitourinary tract specimens, should not be refrigerated, because the cold will destroy the bacteria that usually cause infections in those areas. It is the responsibility of the health care personnel who take the specimens and those who transport the specimens to ensure that they are properly handled. The work the microbiology laboratory does in identifying the cause of an infection depends on the quality of the specimen received.

PROCEDURE 14 • 2

COLLECTING A CLEAN-CATCH URINE SPECIMEN

Purpose:

To obtain a clean-catch urine specimen to culture for bacteria to diagnose the cause of a urinary tract infection.

Terminal Performance Competency:

Properly explain to male and female patients the proper procedure for collecting a clean-catch urine specimen.

Equipment:

Sterile urine container with lid, sterile cotton balls or cleaning towelettes, mild antiseptic soap, and water.

Procedure:

1. Wash hands.

Females

2. Separate the labia and cleanse the area by using one towelette or one cotton ball wet with the antiseptic soap on each labia and one down the middle using a front to back motion.
3. Rinse the area with a cotton ball soaked in water.
4. Dry the area with a fresh cotton ball.
5. Hold the labia apart. (Go to Step 6.)

Males

2. Pull foreskin back if not circumcised.
3. Cleanse head of penis with towelette or cotton ball wet with antiseptic soap.
4. Rinse with a cotton ball soaked in water.
5. Dry area with fresh cotton ball. (Go to Step 6.)

6. Begin urinating in toilet and then catch a portion of the specimen in the container.
7. When the container is two-thirds full, finish urinating in the toilet.
8. Put lid on container.
9. Label specimen.

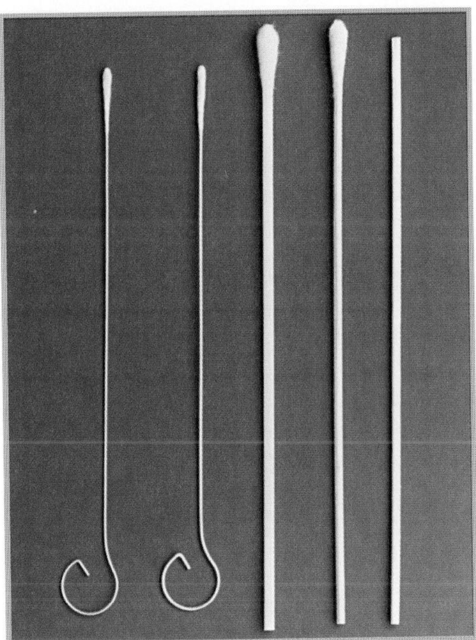

Figure 14-2
Cotton swabs for collecting microbiological specimens.

The Bacteriologic Culture

After the specimen is received in the laboratory, it is necessary to determine if pathogenic bacteria are present. This process begins by transferring the specimen from the transport container to growth **media** (substances that will sustain bacteriologic growth in the laboratory) in a process called plating. Culture media contain various nutrients that are required for bacterial growth. Table 14-4 lists common culture media. These nutrients may include proteins, carbohydrates, vitamins, and salts. Culture media may be liquid, semisolid, or solid. Media are usually solidified by the addition of 3 percent **agar** (a product from seaweed used to solidify bacteriologic media) to the heated nutrients and poured into **petri dishes.** A petri dish is a round covered dish used to hold agar-based media. As the nutrients cool, the agar changes from a liquid to a solid. Agar is very similar to gelatin in that it is a liquid when heated and a solid when cool. Blood agar is a commonly used medium. Microbiologists have learned that by changing the formula of a culture medium, some characteristics of bacteria can be determined. Enriched media inhibit certain types of bacteria from growing. Selective media enhance the growth of some bacteria while inhibiting the growth of others. Differential media can indicate certain biochemical characteristics of some bacteria.

TABLE 14-4 Common Media Used in Bacteriology

Blood agar	Chocolate agar
MacConkey agar	Eosin Methylene Blue (EMB) agar
Thayer-Martin agar	Thioglycolate broth
Selenite F broth	Phenylethyl alcohol (PEA) agar
Brucella agar	Lowenstein-Jensen agar

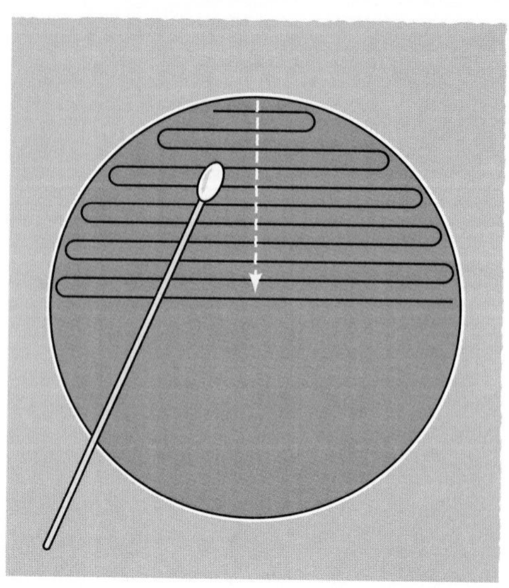

Figure 14-3
Streaking an agar plate for isolation.

Specimens are transferred to the culture media by using sterile swabs and inoculation loops. They are plated on the media using a technique called "streaking for isolation." Streaking for isolation creates areas on the surface of the agar where there will be heavy bacterial growth and areas where single isolated colonies can be viewed. One step in the process of streaking for isolation is illustrated in figure 14-3. A **colony** is the mass of bacteria on the surface of an agar plate that is visible to the naked eye and has originated from a single bacterial cell. It has been estimated that there must be at least one million bacteria for a colony to be visible.

After the specimen has been plated on the culture media it has to be incubated under the proper conditions for the bacteria to grow. Most human pathogens grow best at 35 to 37°C and will produce visible growth in 24 to 48 hours. The optimal atmospheric conditions for human bacteria vary. Aerobic bacteria require oxygen for growth, whereas anaerobic bacteria cannot grow in the presence of oxygen. Facultative anaerobes can grow either with or without oxygen. Capniophilic bacteria prefer an environment with increased carbon dioxide. To ensure that the specimen is incubated under the optimal conditions for growth, it must be streaked on multiple plates and incubated under a variety of atmospheric conditions.

The Identification Process

Once bacterial growth is visible on the culture medium, the identification process can begin. The microbiologist will note the type of medium and the atmospheric condition that produced the best bacterial growth. The colonial morphology on various media will be recorded. The shape of the bacteria is also extremely important. Bacteria can have one of three basic shapes: **coccus, bacillus,** or **spirillus.** Cocci are spherical-shaped bacteria that can be found in singles, pairs (diplococci), chains (streptococci), or clusters (staphylococci). Bacilli are rod-shaped bacteria that can also occur in singles or chains (streptobacilli). Spirilla are spiral-shaped bacteria. Because bacteria are microscopic organisms, their shape can only be seen by using a microscope. A tiny amount of material from the growth on the culture medium is placed on a clean glass slide and air dried. The result is called a **smear.** The procedure for making a smear is found in procedure 14-3. Smears can also be prepared directly from the original specimen, which provides the physician with some information about the culture without having to wait for the bacteria to grow. Once the smear has dried, it is stained with dye to increase the visibility of the bacteria.

PROCEDURE 14•3

MAKING A SMEAR

Purpose:

To properly place bacteria on a glass slide to be viewed under a microscope.

Terminal Performance Competency:

Prepare a smear for microscopic examination without error.

Equipment:

Glass slide, wax pencil, specimen swab or bacterial culture and inoculation loop, sterile water, bunsen burner, forceps, biohazard waste container, and disposable gloves.

Procedure:

1. Wash hands and put on gloves.
2. Assemble equipment.
3. Use the wax pencil to label the slide with the patient's name.
4. a. Specimens: Roll the specimen swab evenly over the surface of the slide.
   b. Cultures: Using an inoculating loop, immerse a small amount of bacterial growth in a drop of sterile water that has been placed on the slide.
5. Allow the slide to air dry.
6. Using the forceps, hold the end of the slide with the patient's name and quickly pass the rest of the slide through the flame of the bunsen burner two or three times. This process is called heat fixing, and it adheres the bacteria to the slide.
7. Let the slide cool before staining.
8. Dispose of contaminated materials in a biohazard waste container.
9. Remove gloves and wash hands.

The most common stain used in the microbiology laboratory is called the **gram stain.** The gram stain procedure can be reviewed in procedure 14-4, and step-by-step photos of the procedure are found in figures 14-4 through 14-9. The gram stain is the primary differential stain used to classify bacteria. Besides making the bacteria visible microscopically, the gram stain divides bacteria into two main groups based on the composition of the bacterial cell wall. Bacteria with a more complex cell wall are called gram positive and will stain purple. Gram-negative bacteria have a simpler cell wall composed of more lipid material and will stain pink.

The stained slide is read using the oil immersion objective of the microscope. After observing the slide, a trained microbiologist will know the shape of the bacterium and whether it is gram positive or gram negative.

PROCEDURE 14•4

GRAM STAIN

Purpose:

To classify bacteria as either gram positive or gram negative.

Terminal Performance Competency:

Prepare a smear for microscopic examination without error.

Equipment:

Heat-fixed slide, staining rack and tray, crystal violet, iodine, decolorizer, safranin, bibulous paper, wash bottle filled with water, and disposable gloves.

Procedure:

1. Wash hands and put on gloves.
2. Place heat-fixed slide on staining rack, smear side up.
3. Flood slide with crystal violet.
4. Wash off with water after 1 minute. Shake off excess water.
5. Cover slide with iodine solution.
6. Wash off with water after 1 minute. Shake off excess water.
7. Tilt slide with forceps and apply decolorizer until no more purple color washes off (no more than 10 seconds).
8. Quickly wash decolorizer off slide with water and shake off excess.
9. Flood slide with safranin.
10. Wash off with water after 1 minute.
11. Lightly blot slide with bibulous paper to dry. Back of slide may be wiped to remove excess stain, but be careful not to wipe side with specimen.
12. After slide is completely dry, it may be viewed under the microscope.

More information is still required to identify the bacteria. The biochemical properties of the bacteria are useful in the identification process of many bacteria. Biochemical testing used to be very cumbersome, with a test tube for each biochemical test. Some identifications required twenty or more test tubes. Now the biochemical tests have been miniaturized and grouped together by manufacturers in small, easy-to-inoculate packages. These newer biochemical test packages have reduced inoculation and reading times as well as the amount of space used in the incubator. Some of the newer systems

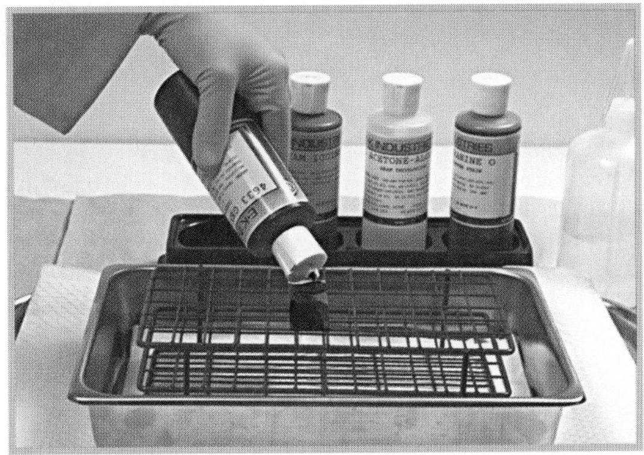

Figure 14-4
Crystal violet

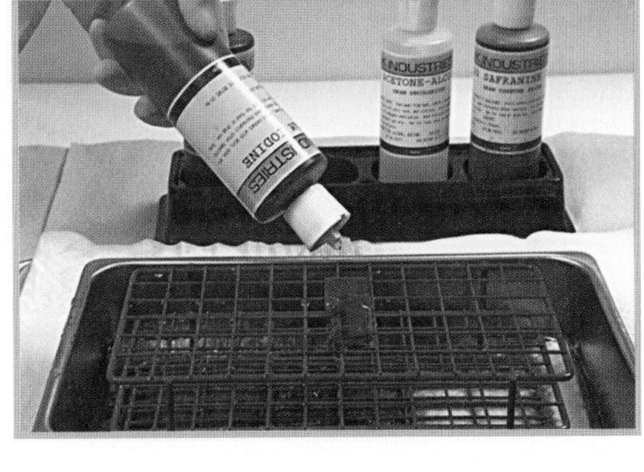

Figure 14-5
Iodine

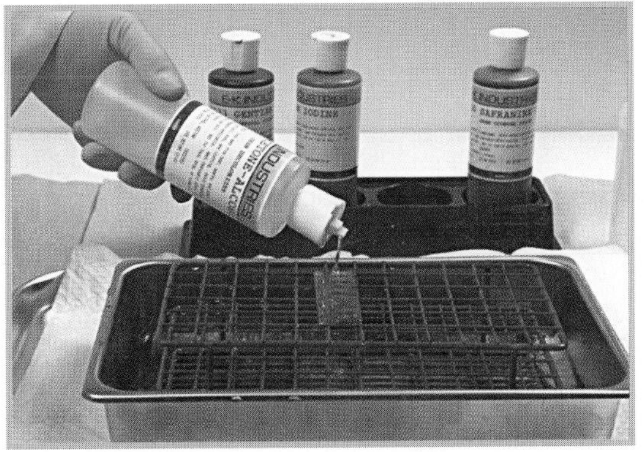

Figure 14-6
Decolorize

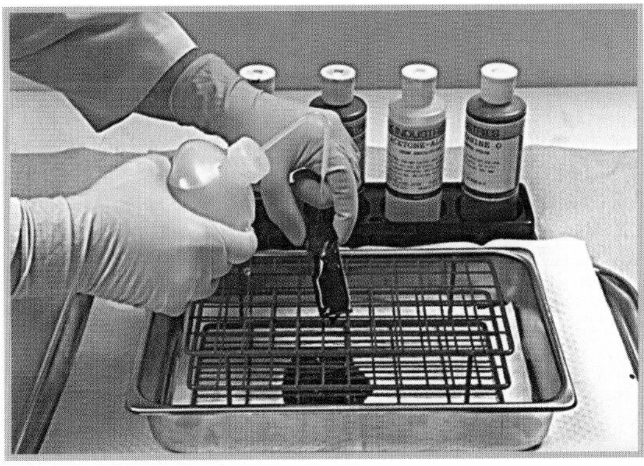

Figure 14-7
Rinse

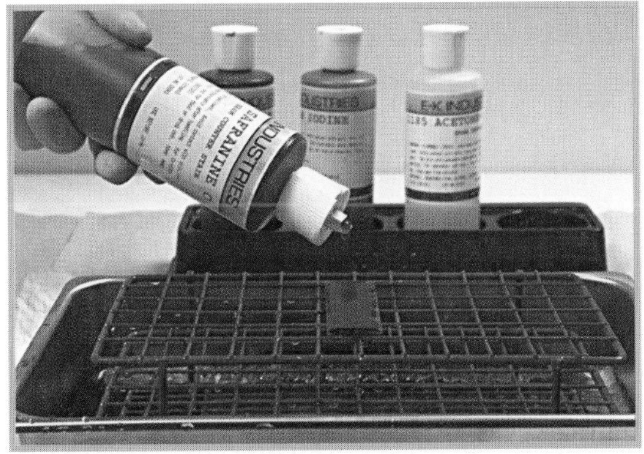

Figure 14-8
Safranin

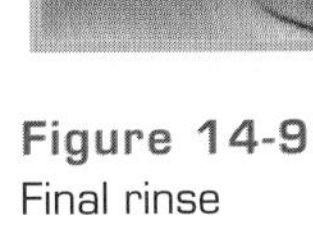

Figure 14-9
Final rinse

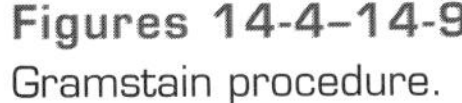

Figures 14-4–14-9
Gramstain procedure.

Figure 14-10
Rapid test kit.

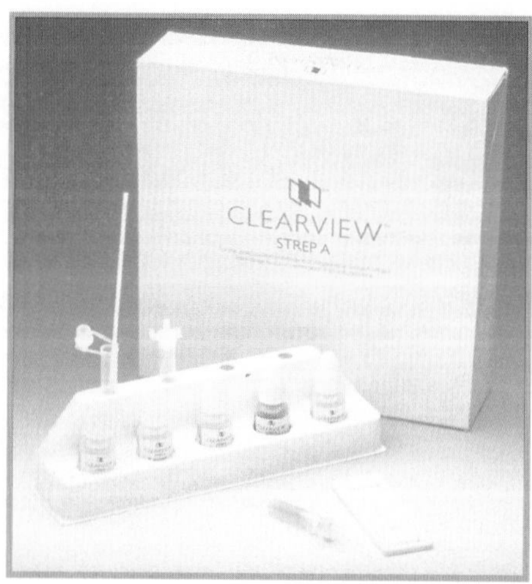

have also reduced the incubation time from 18 hours to 4 hours. Therefore, the physician can learn the cause of the patient's infection and begin antibiotic therapy sooner.

Biochemical testing is not the only means available to identify bacteria. Newer methods of identification include DNA probes and antibody testing. Manufacturers have developed these two testing methodologies as a rapid means of bacterial identification. An example of a rapid test kit is found in figure 14.10. Many pediatricians' offices use kits based on one of these two new methods to rapidly identify patients with strep throat. A throat swab is taken in the doctor's office, and within 10 to 15 minutes the doctor will know if he or she has to treat the patient for a sore throat caused by the bacterium *Streptococcus pyogenes.* Clinical microbiology laboratories are using these methods to rapidly identify pathogens such as *Neiserria meningitides* or to screen large numbers of stool specimens for *Clostridium difficile,* a bacterium that can cause colitis. Manufacturers have developed instruments in which the bacteria can be identified from the specimen swab without having to culture the bacteria. The turnaround time (the period from the time the specimen is received in the laboratory until the laboratory report is generated) is decreasing due to these advances in clinical microbiology.

After a pathogenic bacterium has been identified from a patient's specimen, the microbiology laboratory must test which **antibiotics** can be used to treat the infection. An antibiotic is a substance produced by a microorganism that will inhibit bacterial growth. This test is called an antibiotic susceptibility test. The antibiotic susceptibility test uses the bacterium from the patient's specimen and determines how it is affected by different antibiotics. The physician receives a laboratory report detailing the bacterium's resistance or susceptibility to a group of antibiotics.

Mycology

Mycology is the study of fungi. Fungi consist of two groups—yeasts and molds. Most fungi live in soil or plant matter and do not cause human infection; however, a few fungi are pathogenic in humans and can cause **mycosis** (an infection caused by a fungus). Most human mycoses are superficial infections of the skin, hair, and nails. A few fungi can cause serious systemic infections in humans, and patients with impaired immune systems are much more susceptible to these infections than those with healthy immune systems. Most clinical microbiology laboratories do not perform extensive fungal identification procedures. The majority of laboratories limit their mycology studies to looking at the specimen with a simple stain and perhaps performing one simple test to identify *Candida albicans,* the most common fungus that infects humans. Usually only large reference laboratories or the microbiology laboratories in large teaching hospitals perform fungal cultures.

Yeast are round, unicellular organisms that are similar in appearance to bacteria when grown on media. Microscopically, yeast are much larger than bacteria; if stained with gram stain they will be purple. The most common yeast infection is caused by *Candida albicans. C. albicans* may be part of the normal flora in the gastrointestinal tract and genitourinary tract. Infections caused by this yeast are usually mild, but the yeast may cause severe infection in an immunocompromised patient. Although most yeasts will grow on bacteriologic media, growth is better at a slightly lower pH. Sabouraud's dextrose agar is one media commonly used for yeasts. The pH is a measure of the degree of acidity and alkalinity of a substance, and a lower pH refers to more acidic conditions. Like bacteria, yeasts are identified by their appearance and biochemical characteristics.

Molds are large, fuzzy organisms composed of hairlike structures called **hyphae.** Each mold has its own unique arrangement of hyphae and spores. Molds grow much more slowly than bacteria and are usually cultured on media that contain antibiotics to inhibit bacterial growth. Sabouraud's dextrose agar with antibiotics is a common medium used to culture molds. Although there are thousands of species of molds in nature, very few cause infections in humans. A group of molds called the dermatophytes cause superficial infections of skin, hair, and nails. A common dermatophyte infection is tinea pedis, or athlete's foot. If the spores of some molds are inhaled, a serious systemic mycosis can result. Molds are identified by their macroscopic and microscopic appearance.

Parasitology

Clinical parasitology is the study of human parasites and the diseases they cause. A **parasite** is an organism that lives on or in another organism or host and causes damage to the host. There are two main types of human parasites—protozoa, which are one-celled organisms, and parasitic worms. Fortunately in the United States serious parasitic infections are rare, but in developing countries they are responsible for considerable morbidity and mortality. Parasitic infections are spread by insects, improper disposal of sewage, impure water supply, and intimate contact. The most common human parasite in the United States is *Trichomonas vaginalis,* a urogenital parasite.

Most smaller clinical microbiology laboratories do not test for many parasites but transport specimens to larger reference laboratories for identification. If a blood parasite is suspected, thick and thin blood smears should be sent to the reference laboratory. Fecal specimens must be placed in a preservative such as polyvinyl alcohol (PVA), or formalin before transporting to the reference laboratory. Most small laboratories and doctors' offices examine urogenital specimens for *Trichomonas vaginalis* by making a wet mount and looking for the characteristic "fluttery" movement of the *Trichomonas* parasites. This procedure is detailed in procedure 14-5.

Virology

Clinical virology is the study of human viruses and the diseases they cause. Viruses are much smaller than bacteria and cannot replicate independently. They require another living cell for replication and therefore cannot be cultured in the standard media used to grow bacteria. Specimens for viral culture are inoculated on either chick embryos or **tissue cultures.** A tissue culture is a medium of live cells that are used to grow viruses. These techniques are very costly in terms of time, resources, and personnel; therefore, most virology work is performed at reference or government laboratories. Recently, diagnostic test kits using antibodies have become available. These kits do not identify the virus but look for antibodies that are produced in response to a viral infection. Many less comprehensive clinical laboratories use these kits in either the microbiology section or the serology section of the laboratory to diagnose viral infections.

PROCEDURE 14•5

WET MOUNT

Purpose:

To use wet mount cultures to identify *Trichomonas* parasites.

Terminal Performance Competency:

Successfully perform a wet mount.

Equipment:

Specimen swab, clean glass microscope slides, normal saline, cover slips, disposable gloves, wax pencil, and biohazard waste container.

Procedure:

1. Wash hands and put on disposable gloves.
2. Label glass slide with patient's name.
3. Roll specimen swab over the surface of the glass slide.
4. Add one drop of normal saline.
5. Immediately place cover slip on slide and observe under microscope for characteristic movement of *Trichomonas* parasites.
6. Dispose of contaminated materials in biohazard waste container.
7. Remove gloves and wash hands.

Serology/Immunology

Immunology is the study of the immune processes and immunity. **Serology** is the study of **antigens** and **antibodies** in serum and is the older name for this branch of the laboratory. An antigen is a foreign substance that causes the production of an antibody; an antibody is a specialized protein found in blood that reacts with an antigen. In this section of the laboratory, all of the laboratory tests were performed on serum, thus the name serology. The size of the immunology laboratory also varies a great deal from hospital to hospital. Larger laboratories may have a separate immunology laboratory, whereas in smaller facilities it may be part of the microbiology laboratory, blood bank, or chemistry laboratory.

The immunology laboratory identifies antibodies that are produced in response to disease. Antibodies are found in serum. Blood for immunology testing is drawn into a red-topped evacuated tube, allowed to clot, and then centrifuged. The serum is then removed for clinical testing. Most serologic tests are based on the reaction of an antibody and an antigen. The differences in most test procedures are the methods that are used to make the antibody-antigen reaction visible. The most common test performed in the immunology laboratory is the rapid plasma reagin (RPR), a screening test for syphilis. Other common diseases that are tested for in the immunology laboratory are rheumatoid arthritis, infectious mononucleosis, hepatitis A, B, and C, and lupus erythematosus.

Chapter Review

Summary

The phlebotomist's main responsibilities in regard to microbiology specimens are collecting simple specimens such as throat cultures and giving patients instructions to collect clean-catch urine specimens. In the microbiology laboratory, the phlebotomist may prepare a smear of a specimen on a glass slide and then stain the slide with gram stain.

Competency Review

1. Define the term *normal flora* and describe where in the body normal flora can be found.
2. Describe the procedure for obtaining a clean-catch urine specimen from both a male and a female patient.
3. Explain the principle of streaking for isolation.
4. Explain the principle of the gram stain.
5. Explain the reasons why bacteria, molds, and viruses cannot be grown on the same media.

Examination Review Questions

1. **Which of the following is not correct?**
   (A) coccus = spherical shaped
   (B) bacillus = rod shaped
   (C) strepto = arranged in clusters
   (D) spirillus = spiral shaped
   (E) streptococci = cocci arranged in chains

2. **Most human bacteria grow best at an incubation temperature of**
   (A) near freezing (5°C)
   (B) room temperature (20°C)
   (C) body temperature (37°C)
   (D) boiling (100°C)
   (E) below freezing (−10°C)

3. **All of the following are used to identify bacteria except**
   (A) biochemical testing
   (B) DNA probes
   (C) antibody identification
   (D) tissue culture results
   (E) antibiotic sensitivity patterns

4. **The study of mycology includes**
   (A) yeast
   (B) molds
   (C) parasites
   (D) a and b
   (E) all of the above

5. ***Trichomonas vaginalis*, a parasite, is diagnosed by performing a(n)**
   (A) wet mount
   (B) gram stain
   (C) thick blood film
   (D) antibiotic sensitivity test
   (E) biochemical test

6. **Which of the following specimens should not be placed in the refrigerator before plating to microbiological media?**
   (A) throat
   (B) wound culture
   (C) CSF
   (D) skin cultures
   (E) all of the above

7. **The most frequently used bacteriologic stain is**
   (A) Wright stain
   (B) hemotoxylin stain
   (C) gram stain
   (D) saline
   (E) trichrome stain

8. **Which of the following statements about viruses is not true?**
   (A) Viruses are smaller than bacteria.
   (B) Viruses can grow on the same media as bacteria.
   (C) Viruses can only grow in living cells.
   (D) Viruses cannot replicate independently.
   (E) All statements are true.

9. **The immunology laboratory deals principally with identifying __________ found in __________.**
   (A) bacteria, blood
   (B) antibodies, plasma
   (C) antigens, plasma
   (D) antibodies, serum
   (E) antigens, serum

10. **To determine the shape of a bacterium, one must**
   (A) use a microscope
   (B) prepare a smear
   (C) stain the smear
   (D) use the oil immersion objective on the microscope
   (E) all of the above

Getting Connected

Multimedia Extension Activities

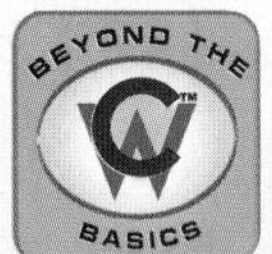

www.prenhall.com/fremgen

Use the address above to access the free, interactive Companion Website created specifically for this textbook. Enhance your studying by answering practice quiz questions, with hints and instant feedback related to chapter 14. If you would like to gain a deeper understanding of selected topics within this chapter, be sure to click on the **Beyond the Basics** feature, which provides more details for further learning. If you do not have a web connection, you may use the CD-ROM enclosed in the back of this book to take advantage of the same features off-line.

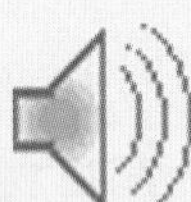

Audio Glossary

Use the CD-ROM enclosed with your textbook to hear the pronunciation of the key terms in the chapter. You may also access this material on the Companion Website www.prenhall.com/fremgen.

Bibliography

Delost, M. *Introduction to Diagnostic Microbiology: A Text and Workbook.* St. Louis: Mosby–Year Book, 1997.

Koneman, E., S. Allen, W. Janda, P. Schreckenberger, and W. Winn. *Introduction to Diagnostic Microbiology.* Philadelphia: J. B. Lippincott, 1994.

Leaventhal, R., and R. Cheadle. *Medical Parasitology: A Self-Instructional Text.* Philadelphia: F. A. Davis, 1996.

Marshall, J. *Fundamental Skills for the Clinical Laboratory Professional.* Albany, N.Y.: Delmar, 1993.

Walters, N., B. Estridge, and A. Reynolds. *Basic Medical Laboratory Techniques,* 3rd ed. Albany, N.Y.: Delmar, 1996.

CASE STUDY FOR END OF PART III

Anne Smith, a 35-year-old female patient, is seen in the urologist's office with a diagnosis of a kidney infection and the following complaints: temperature of 102°F, chills, flank pain, anorexia, and generalized fatigue. Her urine is cloudy and has a fishy odor. She is experiencing an urgent and frequent need to urinate, painful urination (dysuria), and gross hematuria. The physician ordered the following tests: clean-catch urine and culture and sensitivity.

The laboratory tests reveal the following findings: pyuria with the urine sediment containing leukocytes singly, in clumps, and in casts. A few RBCs are present. The urine culture reveals more than 100,000 organisms per millimeter of urine. Escherichia coli bacteria are present as the causative organisms. There is a low specific gravity and a slightly alkaline urine pH. Proteinuria, glycosuria, and ketonuria are also present.

What is your response?

1. Why was a culture and sensitivity ordered?
2. What is the most likely reason that *Escherichia coli (E. coli)* was found to cause the infection?
3. Define the following. (You may wish to use a medical dictionary.)
   a. Ketonuria ______________________________
   b. Glycosuria ______________________________
   c. RBCs ______________________________
   d. Pyuria ______________________________
   e. Leukocytes ______________________________
   f. Gross hematuria ______________________________

SECTION IV

Medical Terminology, Anatomy, and Physiology

CHAPTER 15

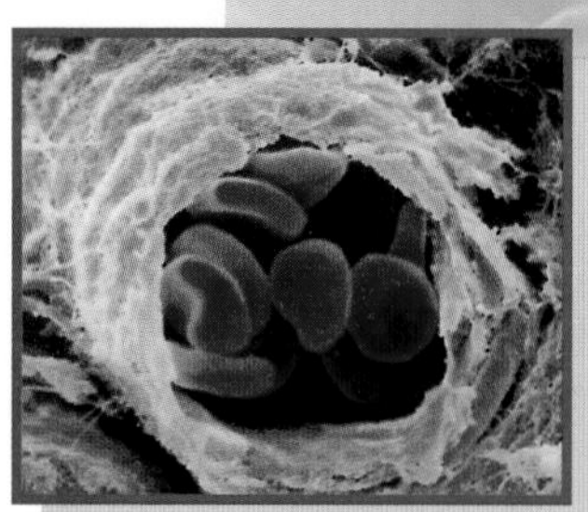

Medical Terminology

Chapter Outline

- Introduction
- Word Building
- Pronunciation
- Spelling
- Abbreviations
- Word Roots
- Combining Vowel or Form
- Prefixes
- Suffixes
- Summary
- Competency Review
- Examination Review Questions
- Bibliography

Learning Objectives

After completing this chapter, you should be able to

1. Define the glossary terms and abbreviations for this chapter.
2. Describe the four components of word building.
3. State and define fifteen common word roots that relate to body systems.
4. State and define fifteen common prefixes.
5. State and define fifteen common suffixes.

GLOSSARY

COMBINING FORM a word component that consists of a word root and a vowel, usually *o*.

PREFIX a word component added to the front of a word root that then forms a new medical term.

SUFFIX a word component added to the end of a word that adds meaning.

WORD ROOT the main portion of the word; it represents the body system or part of the body being discussed.

INTRODUCTION

To communicate effectively with other health care professionals the phlebotomist must know and understand medical terminology because it is considered the language of medicine.

The essentials of medical terminology consist of building words using four elements: word roots, prefixes, suffixes, and the combining form (usually *o*). Once the basic word roots have been mastered, it is possible to distinguish the meaning of a word by analyzing the prefix and suffix.

Word Building

Word building begins with a word root, such as *cardi* (meaning heart), adding a prefix and/or a suffix to further clarify the word, and including the vowel *o* for ease of pronunciation. See the example in table 15-1.

Pronunciation

There are differing pronunciations of medical terms depending on where people were born or educated. As long as it is clear what term people are discussing, differing pronunciations are acceptable.

TABLE 15-1 Word Building

Word Building	Part	Definition	Example
1. Word root	*cardi-*	heart	cardial
2. Prefix	*peri-*	around	pericardial
3. Combining form	*cardi/o-*	heart	cardiology
4. Suffix	*-itis*	inflammation	pericarditis

When the four components are put together, the word pericarditis is formed, meaning inflammation of the area surrounding or around the heart.

MED TIP

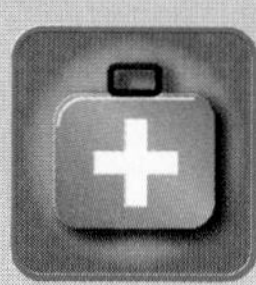

A few terms have the same pronunciation but different meanings, such as *ileum,* meaning part of the small intestine, and *ilium,* meaning part of the hipbone.

Spelling

Although there are differing pronunciations of the same term, there is only one correct spelling. If there is any doubt about the spelling, it should be looked up in a medical dictionary. For example, confusing the spelling of *ileum,* or small intestine, with *ilium,* or hipbone, could cause major problems for the patient.

Abbreviations

When working with medical terms it is often a practice in hospitals, medical offices, medical records, and laboratory reports to use abbreviations for commonly used terms. Because some medical terms are quite long, this practice can save time. However, only acceptable abbreviations can be used. Incorrect abbreviations can cause problems for the patient and with insurance records and processing. If there is concern that an abbreviation is confusing, then the word should be spelled out completely.

MED TIP

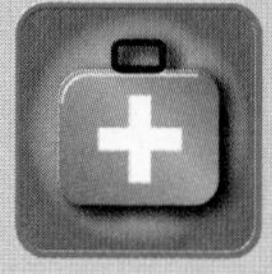

The abbreviation for complete blood count is CBC. If an abbreviation such as BC is used instead, then an insurance company may reject payment for this laboratory test because BC is not an accepted abbreviation.

The use of capital versus lowercase letters in an abbreviation can also cause confusion. For example, the abbreviation SM stands for *simple mastectomy* whereas sm represents the word *small.* Abbreviations commonly used in phlebotomy are listed in table 15-2.

Word Roots

Building words is the underlying premise of medical terminology. Words are built or constructed around the main part of the word, or word root. The **word root** represents the body system or part of the body that is being discussed. It is the fundamental part of the word, such as *cardi-*, meaning heart.

TABLE 15-2 Commonly Used Abbreviations in Phlebotomy

Abbreviation	Definition	Abbreviation	Definition
Aq	Water	NPO	Nothing by mouth, non per os
ASAP	As soon as possible	Path	Pathology
AST	Serum glutamic-oxaloacetic transaminase	pH	Hydrogen ion concentration
BUN	Blood urea nitrogen	PKU	Phenylketonuria
Bx	Biopsy	p.o.	*Per os* (orally)
cc, cm^3	Cubic centimeter	PO_2	Pressure of oxygen in blood
CBC	Complete blood count		
CK	Creatine kinase	post-op	After surgery
CPR	Cardiopulmonary resuscitation	pre-op	Before surgery
		PRN	As necessary
Crit, Hct	Hematocrit	PT	Prothrombin time, protime
DOA	Dead on arrival	pt	Patient
DOB	Date of birth	PTT	Partial prothrombin time
Dx	Diagnosis	q	Every
Eos	Eosinophil	qh	Every hour
ESR	Erythrocyte sedimentation rate	qid	Four times a day
		QNS	Quantity not sufficient
FBS	Fasting blood sugar	R	Right
g, gm	Gram	RBC	Red blood cell
Hb, Hgb	Hemoglobin	req	requisition
IM	Intramuscular	R/O	Rule out
IV	Intravenous	Rx	Prescription/treatment
K	Potassium	Sed rate	Erythrocyte sedimentation rate (ESR)
Kg, kg	Kilogram		
lymphs	Lymphocytes	Segs	Segmented white blood cells
lytes	Electrolytes	Staph	*Staphylococcus*
m	Meter	STAT	Immediately
mg	Milligram	T&C	Type and cross match
mL	Milliliter	UA	Urinalysis
mm	Millimeter	VDRL	Venereal disease research laboratory
mono	Monocyte		
neg	Negative	WBC	White blood cell

Some words have more than one word root, which can result in very long medical terms. For example, erythroblastosis combines the word root and combining term *erythro-*, meaning red blood cell, and *blast-*, meaning early stage of development. By adding the suffix *-osis*, meaning condition, we have the entire word, meaning a condition of early-developing red blood cells.

Combining Vowel or Form

To make it possible to pronounce long medical terms and to combine several word roots, a combining vowel, usually *o*, is used. A **combining form** for a word consists of a word root and a vowel, usually *o*, such as in *cardi/o-*. For example, in the word *thrombocytopenia*, the combining vowel is the *o* between the word roots *thromb/o-*, meaning blood platelet, and *cyto-*, meaning cell. The suffix *-penia* means few. Therefore, *thrombocytopenia* means an abnormal decrease in the number of blood platelets.

A word root can be joined with another word root and/or a suffix. If the suffix begins with a vowel (a, e, i, o, u), such as *-itis*, a combining vowel is usually not used. For example, *carditis* is correct rather than *cardioitis*. The combining vowel is kept between two word roots and can make pronunciation easier. See table 15-3 for examples of common word roots with the combining form.

TABLE 15-3 Combining Form of Word Roots with Meanings

Word Root	Meaning	Example	Word Root	Meaning	Example
aden/o-	gland	adenitis	ile/o-	ileum	ileum
arthr/o-	joint	arthritis	leuk/o-	white	leukocyte
carcin/o-	cancer	carcinoma	lingu/o-	tongue	lingual
cardi/o-	heart	cardiogram	nephr/o-	kidney	nephrologist
cephal/o-	head	cephalic	neur/o-	nerve	neuritis
cerebr/o-	cerebrum	cerebrum	onc/o-	tumor	oncology
cholecyst/o-	gallbladder	cholecystectomy	ophthalm/o-	eye	ophthalmology
col/o-	colon	colon	oste/o-	bone	osteomyelitis
cyst/o-	bladder	cystitis	path/o-	disease	pathology
cyt/o-	cell	cytology	ped/o-	children	pediatrics
derm/o-	skin	dermatology	pharyng/o-	pharynx	pharyngitis
encephal/o-	brain	encephalogram	phleb/o-	vein	phlebitis
enter/o-	intestines	enteritis	rect/o-	rectum	rectum
erythr/o-	red	erythrocyte	ren/o-	kidney	renal
esophag/o-	esophagus	esophagitis	rhin/o-	nose	rhinoplasty
gastr/o-	stomach	gastritis	splen/o-	spleen	splenectomy
gloss/o-	tongue	glossitis	thromb/o-	clot	thrombophlebitis
gynec/o-	female	gynecology	trache/o-	trachea	tracheotomy
hem/o-	blood	hematology	ur/o-	urinary tract	urology
hemat/o-	blood	hematemesis	vas/o-	vessel	vasoconstriction
hepat/o-	liver	hepatitis	ven/o-	vein	venipuncture
hyster/o-	uterus	hysterectomy			

Prefixes

A new medical term is formed when a **prefix** is added in front of the word root. The prefix frequently gives information about the location of the organ, the number of parts, or the time (frequency). For example, the prefix *bi-* stands for two of something, such as in *bilateral.* Table 15-4 contains some of the most common prefixes in medical terminology. In some cases both the prefix and the combining form are given. See table 15-5 for a list of prefixes pertaining to number and measurement.

TABLE 15-4 Common Prefixes

Prefix	Meaning	Prefix	Meaning
a-	without, away from	in-	not, into
ab-	away from, absent	infra-	under, below, beneath
ad-	toward	inter-	among, between
ambi-	both, both sides	intra-	within
an-	without	later/o-	side
ante-	before, in front of	leuk/o-	white
anter/o-	before, in front of	macr/o-	large
anti-	against	mal-	bad, ill, poor
ar-	without	medi-	middle
auto-	self	mes/o-	middle
bi-	two	micro-	small
brady-	slow	mid-	middle
circum-	around	pan-	around
contra-	against	peri-	around
dextr/o-	right	ploy-	many, much
dia-	through, across	post-	after
diplo-	double	poster/o-	after, behind
dors/o-	back	pre-	before
dys-	painful, different	pro-	before, in front of
ec-, ecto-	out, out from	pseudo-	false
endo-	within	re-	back
epi-	upon	retro-	after, behind
ex-	out from	sinistro-	left
exo-	out	sub-	below, under
hemi-	half	super-	above
heter/o-	different	supra-	above
homo-	same	syn-	together
hydro-	water	tachy-	rapid, fast
hyper-	over, above	trans-	through, across
hypo-	under, below	ultra-	beyond, excess

TABLE 15-5 Prefixes Pertaining to Number and Measurement

Prefix	Meaning	Prefix	Meaning
bi-	two	mono-	one
di-	two	multi-	many
diplo-	double	poly-	many
hemi-	half	quad-	four
macro-	large	semi-	partial, half
micro-	small	tri-	three

Suffixes

A **suffix** is a word part attached to the end of a word to add meaning, such as a condition, disease, or procedure. Not all words have suffixes, but when a word does, the suffix is added at the end of the combining form of the word. See table 15-6 for a list of common suffixes in medical terminology.

When learning medical terminology, it is important to break down each word into its components (prefix, word root/combining form, and suffix). Instead of trying to memorize every medical term, it is best to figure out how the word is formed from its components. Table 15-7 contains word parts that relate to the study of phlebotomy.

MED TIP

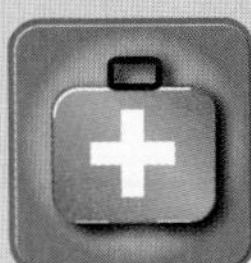

To gain a quick understanding of the term, read the term from the end of the word (or the suffix) to the beginning (prefix) and then pick up the word root.

Example: *pericarditis.*

Suffix = *-itis,* meaning inflammation of

Prefix = *peri-,* meaning the area surrounding or around

Word root = *cardi-,* meaning the heart

Therefore, *pericarditis* is an inflammation of the area surrounding the heart.

TABLE 15-6 Common Suffixes

Suffix	Meaning	Suffix	Meaning
-ac	pertaining to	-ize	removal
-al	pertaining to	-lysis	destruction
-algia	pertaining to pain	-malacia	softening
-blast	early development stage	-megaly	enlargement
-cele	swelling, hernia, protrusion	-oid	resembling, like
-centesis	surgical puncture	-ology	study of
-cide	kill	-osis	state of
-cise	cut	-ostomy	surgical opening
-cle	small	-otomy	cutting into
-cyte	cell	-parous	giving birth
-dyne, -dynia	pertaining to pain	-pathy	disease
-ectasis	dilation, stretching	-penia	few
-ectomy	surgical removal	-pexy	fixation
-ectopy, ectopic	displacement	-phasia	speech
-emia	condition of blood	-phobia	abnormal fear
-genic	produced by	-plasty	surgical repair
-gram	record or picture, film	-pnea	breathing
-graph	instrument used to record or write	-ptosis	dropping, prolapse
		-rrhage	excessive flow
-graphy	process of recording	-rrhea	discharge, flow
-ia	pertaining to	-rrhexis	rupture
-iasis	presence of or condition of	-scopy	process of visualization
-ic	pertaining to	-spasm	twitch
-id	condition of	-stalsis	constriction or stoppage
-ion	small	-stenosis	abnormal narrowing
-itis	inflammation	-trophy	nourishment, development
-ium	small	-uria	pertaining to urine

TABLE 15-7 Word Parts Related to Phlebotomy

Word Root	Definition	Example
angi/o-	vessel	angioplasty
arteri/o-	artery	arteriothrombosis
cyt/o-	cell	cytology
erythr/o-	red	erythrocyte
glyc/o-	sugar	glycosuria
hem/o-	blood	hematology
leuk/o-	white	leukocyte
path/o-	disease	pathology

(continued)

TABLE 15-7 Word Parts Related to Phlebotomy *(continued)*

Word Root	Definition	Example
phleb/o-	vein	phlebitis
scler/o-	hard, sclerotic	thrombosclerosis
thromb/o-	clot	thrombophlebitis
vas/o-	vessel	vasoconstriction
ven/o-	vein	venogram
Prefix	**Definition**	**Example**
aero-	air	aerobic
cyto-	cell	cytoplasm
hemo-	blood	hemostasis
hyper-	high	hyperglycemia
hypo-	low, under	hypoglycemia
inter-	between	intercellular
intra-	within	intramuscular
macro-	large	macrocyte
micro-	small	microscope
poly-	many, much	polycythemia
Suffix	**Definition**	**Example**
-ac, -al, -ic	pertaining to	hemolytic
-centesis	surgical puncture	thoracentesis
-coccus	spherical-shaped bacteria	Streptococcus
-cyte	cell	leukocyte
-emia	condition of the blood	anemia
-gram	recording, writing	electrocardiogram
-itis	inflammation of	phlebitis
-lysis	breakdown, destruction	hemolysis
-megaly	enlargement	hepatomegaly
-ologist	one who studies	nephrologist
-ology	study of	pathology
-oid	resembling	scleroid
-oma	tumor	melanoma
-ometer	instrument to count or measure	hemacytometer
-osis	condition of	osmosis
-otomy	incision, cutting into	phlebotomy
-pathy	disease	osteopathy
-penia	deficiency, few	leukopenia
-rrhage	excessive flow	hemorrhage
-stasis	stoppage, standing still	hemostasis
-trophy	development	atrophy
-uria	pertain to urine	anuria

Chapter Review

Summary

Medical terminology is the basis for the language of medicine. The phlebotomist must be familiar with terms when he or she reads them. It is advisable to understand how words are developed—word root, combining vowel, prefix, and suffix—rather than to memorize hundreds of medical terms.

Competency Review

1. List and describe the four components of word building.
2. Make flash cards and practice the most commonly used abbreviations found in this chapter with another student.
3. Prepare flash cards for the most common word roots, prefixes, and suffixes. Place the word part on one side of the flash card and the meaning on the reverse side. Test your understanding of the word parts and meanings with another student.
4. Prepare flash cards with the most common abbreviations and meanings. Practice learning these with another student.
5. Define the following terms. Then break apart each term and indicate the prefix (P), word root (WR), combining vowel (CV), and suffix (S), if present, in each.

Term	Definition	Break-Apart Term
	(Example)	WR CV S
1. phlebotomy	cutting into a vein	phleb / o / tomy
2. leukocyte		
3. erythrocyte		
4. intramuscular		
5. intravenous		
6. hematology		
7. hemostasis		
8. leukopenia		
9. anemia		
10. hemolysis		

Examination Review Questions

1. **The abbreviation *qid* means**
   (A) every other day
   (B) every day
   (C) four times a day
   (D) three times a day
   (E) nothing by mouth

2. **The suffix *-rrhage* when added to a medical term indicates**
   (A) development of flow
   (B) excessive flow
   (C) stoppage of flow
   (D) deficiency of flow
   (E) none of the above

3. **The suffix *-centesis* when added to a medical term indicates**
   (A) stoppage
   (B) condition of
   (C) breakdown
   (D) inflammation of
   (E) surgical puncture

4. **The term *endocardium* means**
   (A) upon the heart
   (B) above the heart
   (C) below the heart
   (D) within the heart
   (E) repair of the heart

5. **The term *intramuscular* means**
   (A) between the muscle
   (B) within the muscle
   (C) outside of the muscle
   (D) opening into the muscle
   (E) abnormal condition of the muscle

6. **The medical term for hardening of an artery is**
   (A) arteriosclerosis
   (B) arteriophlebitis
   (C) thrombophlebitis
   (D) arteritis
   (E) arterioplasty

7. **The medical term for the presence of sugar in the urine is**
   (A) glycoria
   (B) hypoglycemia
   (C) hyperglycemia
   (D) glycosuria
   (E) hypoglycosuria

8. **The prefix meaning one-half is**
   (A) *diplo-*
   (B) *di-*
   (C) *hemi-*
   (D) *bi-*
   (E) *mono-*

9. **One who studies disease is called a**
   (A) phlebotomist
   (B) pathologist
   (C) hematologist
   (D) cardiologist
   (E) nephrologist

10. **A word root and combining vowel that can be used to indicate a vein or a problem with a vein are**
   (A) *phleb/o-*
   (B) *ven/o-*
   (C) *vas/o-*
   (D) *thromb/o-*
   (E) all of the above

Getting Connected

Multimedia Extension Activities

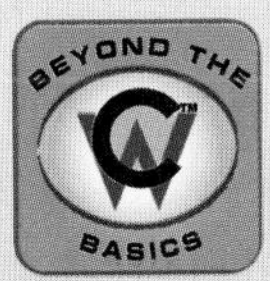

www.prenhall.com/fremgen

Use the address above to access the free, interactive Companion Website created specifically for this textbook. Enhance your studying by answering practice quiz questions, with hints and instant feedback related to chapter 15. If you would like to gain a deeper understanding of selected topics within this chapter, be sure to click on the **Beyond the Basics** feature, which provides more details for further learning. If you do not have a web connection, you may use the CD-ROM enclosed in the back of this book to take advantage of the same features off-line.

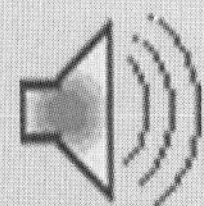

Audio Glossary

Use the CD-ROM enclosed with your textbook to hear the pronunciation of the key terms in the chapter. You may also access this material on the Companion Website www.prenhall.com/fremgen.

Bibliography

Clayman, C. *The Human Body*. New York: Dorling Kindersley, 1995.

Fremgen, B. *Medical Terminology*. Upper Saddle River, N.J.: Brady/Prentice-Hall, 1997.

Martini, F. *Fundamentals of Anatomy and Physiology*. Upper Saddle River, N.J.: Brady/Prentice-Hall, 1995.

Taber's Cyclopedic Medical Dictionary, 18th ed. Philadelphia: F. A. Davis, 1997.

CHAPTER 16

The Circulatory System and Its Relationship to Phlebotomy

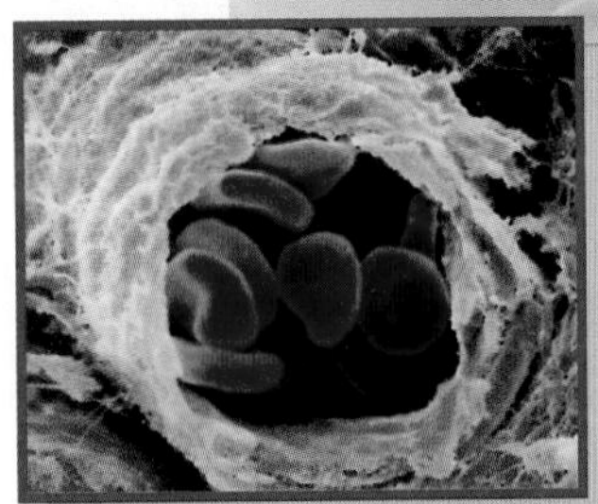

Chapter Outline

Learning Objectives

After completing this chapter, you should be able to

1. Define and spell all glossary terms.
2. Describe the difference between pulmonary and systemic circulation.
3. Identify the layers and structures of the heart and describe their functions.
4. Trace the flow of blood throughout the cardiovascular system.
5. Identify the three major types of blood vessels.
6. List and describe the major components of blood.
7. Describe the difference between red blood cells and white blood cells.
8. Locate and describe the veins that are preferred for phlebotomy procedures.
9. Discuss blood grouping and its purpose.
10. List the major blood tests relating to the circulatory system.

GLOSSARY

ARTERIOLES small branches of arteries.

ARTERIOSCLEROSIS thickening or hardening of the walls of the arteries.

ATHEROSCLEROSIS the most common cause of arteriosclerosis, it is a buildup of plaques of cholesterol on the inner walls of the arteries.

CARDIOVASCULAR SYSTEM also called the circulatory system; includes the heart and blood vessels.

COAGULATION clumping together of blood cells to form a clot.

DIASTOLE the relaxation phase of the heartbeat that occurs when the ventricles relax.

ERYTHROBLASTOSIS FETALIS condition in which antibodies in the mother's blood enter the fetus's blood and cause anemia, jaundice, edema, and enlargement of the liver and spleen; a life-threatening condition for the newborn.

HEMATOPOIESIS formation of blood cells.

HEMOGLOBIN iron-containing pigment in the blood.

LUMEN cavity or channel of a blood vessel.

OXYGENATED blood that has been exposed to oxygen in the lungs.

OXYHEMOGLOBIN a combination of oxygen and hemoglobin; carries oxygen to the tissues.

PHAGOCYTOSIS the process in which white blood cells (WBCs) ingest and digest foreign material.

SINOATRIAL NODE where the heartbeat begins; also called the pacemaker.

SPHYGMOMANOMETER blood pressure cuff.

SYSTOLE the contraction phase of the heartbeat that occurs when the ventricles contract.

INTRODUCTION

The circulatory system, also called the **cardiovascular system,** maintains the distribution of blood throughout the body. It is composed of the heart and blood vessels. All the other systems of the body are linked to the cardiovascular system through a network of nerves, tissues, and fluids.

The circulatory system provides for the transport of oxygen, electrolytes, hormones, water, nutrients, enzymes, gases, and other materials to all cells. This system also transports carbon dioxide and other waste products from metabolism to the lungs and kidneys, where they are eliminated from the body.

The circulatory system is composed of two parts: pulmonary circulation and systemic circulation. Pulmonary circulation, which involves the heart and lungs, transports blood to the lungs and back again to the heart. In systemic circulation blood is carried away from the heart to the tissues and cells in the body and then back to the heart.

The lymphatic system is closely linked to the cardiovascular system through shared vessels. The lymphatic system also produces blood cells and lymph fluid to aid in the body's immune process.

Heart

The heart is about the size of a man's fist and is shaped like an upside-down pear with the tip, or apex, pointing to the left side of the body. It beats between 70 and 80 times per minute, or about 100,000 times in one day. Actually, it is a muscular "pump" that is made up of fibers. Although the heart is located in the center of the chest cavity or mediastinum, most of it is actually to the left of the mediastinum. There are four chambers or cavities in the heart: two atrial, or upper, chambers and two ventricles, or lower, chambers. The chambers are divided into right and left sides by walls called septa. The upper chambers (atria) are the receiving chambers for all incoming blood vessels. The lower chambers (ventricles) are the pumping chambers. The right ventricle pumps blood into the pulmonary circulatory system, and the left ventricle pumps blood into the systemic circulatory system. The study of the heart is called cardiology. See figure 16-1 for an illustration of blood circulation through the heart.

Layers of the Heart

The outer double-walled sac that contains fluid to prevent friction during heartbeats is called the pericardium. The heart itself is composed of three muscle layers: epicardium, myocardium, and endocardium. The epicardium is a thin, outer heart layer that is an extension of the inner layer of the pericardium. The myocardium is the muscular, middle layer of the heart, and the endocardium is the thin inner layer of the heart.

MED TIP

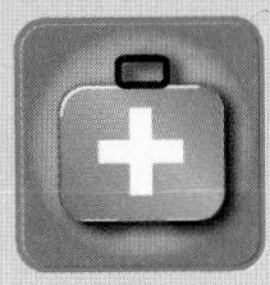

You can visualize the pericardium if you imagine placing your fist into an inflated balloon. Your fist represents the heart, and the balloon represents the pericardium.

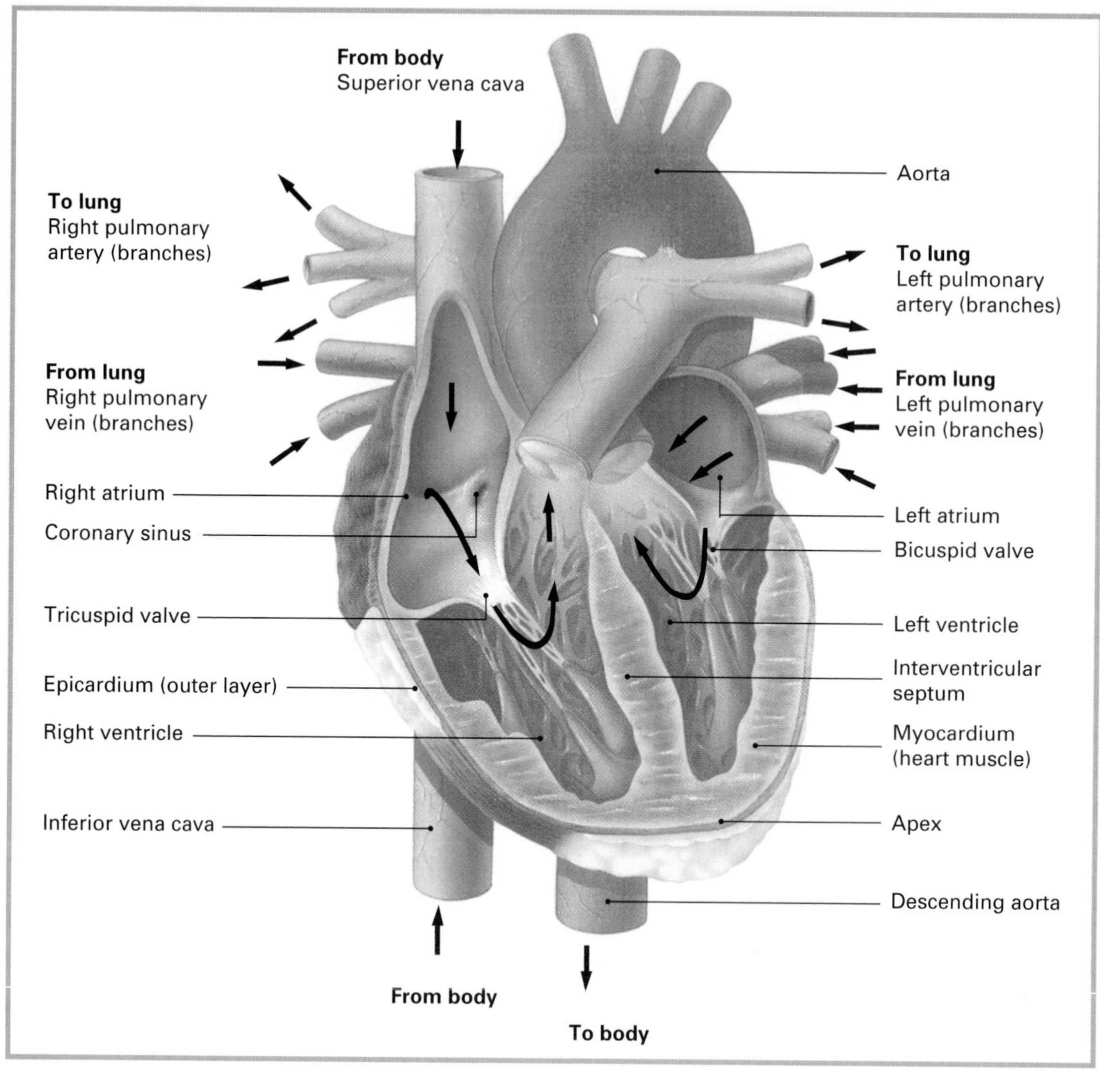

Figure 16-1
Illustration of blood circulation through the heart.

VALVES

Four valves in the heart act as restraining gates to control the direction of blood flow. They are located at both the entrances and exits to the ventricles. The valves are as follows:

1. Tricuspid valve: This valve, also known as the atrioventricular valve, controls the opening between the right atrium and the right ventricle. It is a one-way valve, which means that once the blood enters the right ventricle it cannot back up into the atrium again. It is often referred to as tricuspid because the valve has three cusps, or flaps, which enable secure closure.

2. Pulmonary semilunar valve: This valve is located between the right ventricle and the pulmonary artery. This important valve allows blood to flow from the right ventricle through the pulmonary artery into the lungs. It is named *semilunar* because of its half-moon shape.
3. Mitral valve: Blood flows from the mitral valve to the left ventricle and cannot go back up into the left atrium. This valve is also called the bicuspid valve, which indicates that it has two cusps, or flaps. The term *mitral* is derived from *mitre*—a bishop's hat—which signifies its shape.
4. Aortic semilunar valve: This valve is between the left ventricle and the aorta. Blood leaves the left ventricle through this valve.

Blood Flow through the Heart

The flow of blood through the heart is quite orderly. Blood progresses through the heart to the lungs (where it receives oxygen), back to the heart, and then out to the body tissues and organs. The normal flow is as follows:

1. Blood is received into the right atrium from all the tissues in the body (with the exception of lung tissue). It enters the right atrium through two blood vessels called the superior vena cava and the inferior vena cava. The blood then flows from the right atrium by way of the tricuspid valve into the right ventricle.
2. Blood leaving the right ventricle flows into the left and right pulmonary arteries through the pulmonary semilunar valve. The pulmonary arteries branch within the lungs, and specifically to the lungs' capillaries, where gas exchange (O_2 and CO_2) occurs. This is the pulmonary circulatory system.
3. Oxygenated blood then passes through the left and right pulmonary veins and empties into the left atrium.
4. The left atrium then receives blood that has been **oxygenated** by the lungs. This blood enters the left atrium through the four pulmonary veins. These are the only veins in the body that carry oxygenated blood.
5. The blood then flows through the mitral valve into the left ventricle.
6. Blood leaving the left ventricle enters the aortic semilunar valve and flows into all parts of the body except the lungs. This is the systemic circulatory system.

Heartbeat and Conduction System of the Heart

Since the autonomic nervous system controls the heartbeat and because of the unusual structural characteristics of the heart, humans cannot directly control the beating of their hearts. However, certain activities, such as exercise, can cause the heart rate to increase.

The pulse is a measurement of the number of times the heart beats in a minute. Pulse rate occurs as a result of pressure when the ventricles contract and blood is forced through the arteries. The pulse is usually taken by compressing the radial artery on the thumb side of the wrist. Normally the adult heart beats around 70 beats per minute (BPM), with a range of normal of 60 to 80 BPM. A rate above 100 BPM is called tachycardia; a rate below 60 BPM is called bradycardia. Children generally have a faster heart rate than adults.

MED TIP

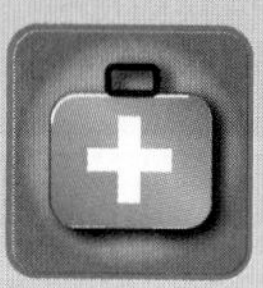

To determine a pulse rate, place your second and third fingertips on the radial artery on the thumb side of the wrist. Count the pulse beats for 1 full minute. The number should always be an even number. You can note the difference in heart rate as a result of exercise by taking your pulse while you are sitting still and then taking it again after you have run in place for 1 minute.

PULSE SITES

There are several sites in the body where the pulse can be easily measured since the artery is close to the skin. These pulse sites are radial, brachial, carotid, temporal, femoral, popliteal, and dorsalis pedis. The locations of common pulse sites are described in table 16-1.

The heart pumps about 5 L of blood per minute. This volume of blood per minute is called the cardiac output. Special tissue within the heart is responsible for the contraction impulses of the atria and ventricles and the order in which they occur. The order in which the impulses travel is as follows:

1. The **sinoatrial (SA) node,** or pacemaker, is where the heartbeat begins.
2. The pacemaker causes a wave of impulse through the muscles of the atria, which causes them to contract.
3. Next, the atrioventricular (AV) node is stimulated, which causes it to send a stimulation wave to the bundle of His and down the right and left bundle

TABLE 16-1 Location of Common Pulse Sites

Pulse Site	Location
Radial	Thumb side of the wrist approximately 1 inch below base of the thumb; this is the most frequently used site for counting pulse rate
Brachial	Inner (antecubital fossa or space) aspect of the elbow; this is where the pulse is heard and felt when taking blood pressure
Carotid	Located between the larynx and the sternocleidomastoid muscle in the side of the neck, this is the pulse used during cardiopulmonary resuscitation (CPR); it can be felt by pushing the muscle to one side and pressing gently against the larynx
Temporal	At the side of the head just above the ear
Femoral	Near the groin where the femoral artery is located
Popliteal	Behind the knee; this pulse is located deep behind the knee and can be felt when the knee is slightly bent
Dorsalis pedis	On the top of the foot slightly lateral to midline; this pulse can be an indication of adequate circulation to the feet

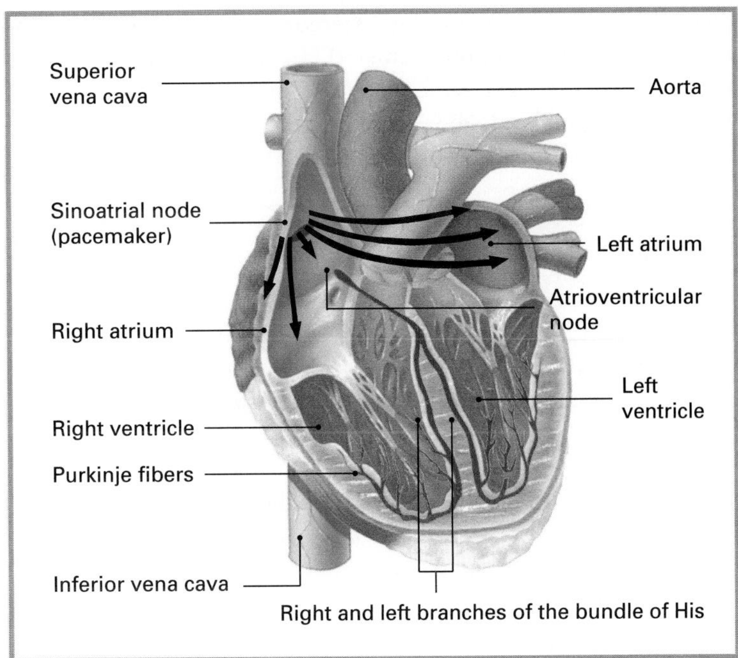

Figure 16-2
Illustration of conduction system of the heart.

branches. The wave then spreads throughout the ventricular walls along the Purkinje fibers.

4. The ventricles then contract almost simultaneously, forcing blood through the semilunar valves.
5. The atria and ventricles will then relax for a brief moment before the cycle begins again.

The cardiac cycle is one complete contraction and relaxation of the heartbeat and lasts for about 0.08 seconds. See figure 16-2, for an illustration of the conduction system of the heart. The cardiac cycle can be recorded with an electrocardiogram (ECG or EKG). The ECG/EKG is a measurement of the electrical activity of the heart.

Systole, the contraction phase of the heartbeat, occurs during ventricular contraction when blood is forced into the pulmonary artery and the aorta. **Diastole** is the relaxation phase of the heartbeat that occurs when the ventricles relax and blood flows into the heart from the pulmonary veins and the inferior vena cava and superior vena cava.

Blood Pressure

Blood pressure, which is measured using a **sphygmomanometer** or blood pressure cuff, is a measurement of the force or pressure being exerted by the blood on the walls of the artery. Blood pressure is expressed in millimeters of mercury (mm Hg). The blood pressure reading is the ratio of the systolic pressure to the diastolic pressure. The systolic pressure occurs first and is the highest reading. It occurs when the ventricles contract and send blood through the body. The diastolic pressure, or lowest reading, occurs when the heart muscles relax before the cycle begins again.

A blood pressure measurement is taken using a stethoscope placed over the brachial artery in the upper arm. A blood pressure cuff (sphygmomanometer) is wrapped around the upper arm and inflated, which compresses the brachial artery and temporarily cuts off the flow of blood. The cuff is slowly and steadily deflated until a heart sound (systole) is heard using the stethoscope. The cuff is then further deflated until a muffled heart sound is heard, which is the diastolic pressure as the ventricles relax.

MED TIP

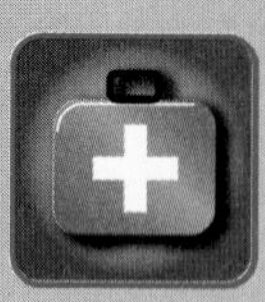

The average normal blood pressure for an adult is 120/80, in which the systolic pressure is 120 mm Hg and the diastolic pressure is 80 mm Hg.

The volume of blood in a person's system can affect the blood pressure. Abnormally low blood volume, as found when hemorrhage occurs, can result in abnormally low blood pressure readings. An excess of circulating blood (hypervolemia) can place an added burden on the heart because there is additional fluid for the heart to pump.

Blood Vessels

There are three types of blood vessels: arteries, veins, and capillaries. The arteries are the largest vessels and (with the exception of the pulmonary artery) carry the blood containing oxygen away from the heart. The pulmonary artery carries deoxygenated blood, or blood without oxygen, from the ventricles to the lungs.

A blood vessel has three layers or tunics of covering, which consist of a variety of connective tissue, endothelial cells, smooth muscle, and elastic fibers. The three layers are tunica adventitia (or outer layer), tunica media (or middle layer), and tunica intima (or inner layer).

MED TIP

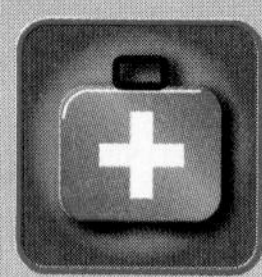

When performing venipuncture, you will actually feel the needle pierce the vessel layers. A skilled phlebotomist must be able to enter a blood vessel without piercing all the way through the vessel.

When the walls of the blood vessels have a buildup of yellowish plaques of cholesterol, as seen in **atherosclerosis,** the potential for a heart attack occurring increases. Atherosclerosis is the most common cause of **arteriosclerosis,** or hardening of the walls of the arteries. Both conditions force the heart to work harder because the **lumen,** channel or cavity of the blood vessel, becomes smaller.

Arteries

The largest artery, the aorta, begins from the left ventricle of the heart. The coronary artery then branches from the aorta and provides blood to the myocardium, or heart muscle. The small branches of the arteries are called **arterioles.** These branches carry blood to the capillaries. Arterial puncture is performed to test for arterial blood gases when determining respiratory function. See figure 16-3 for an illustration of the circulatory system.

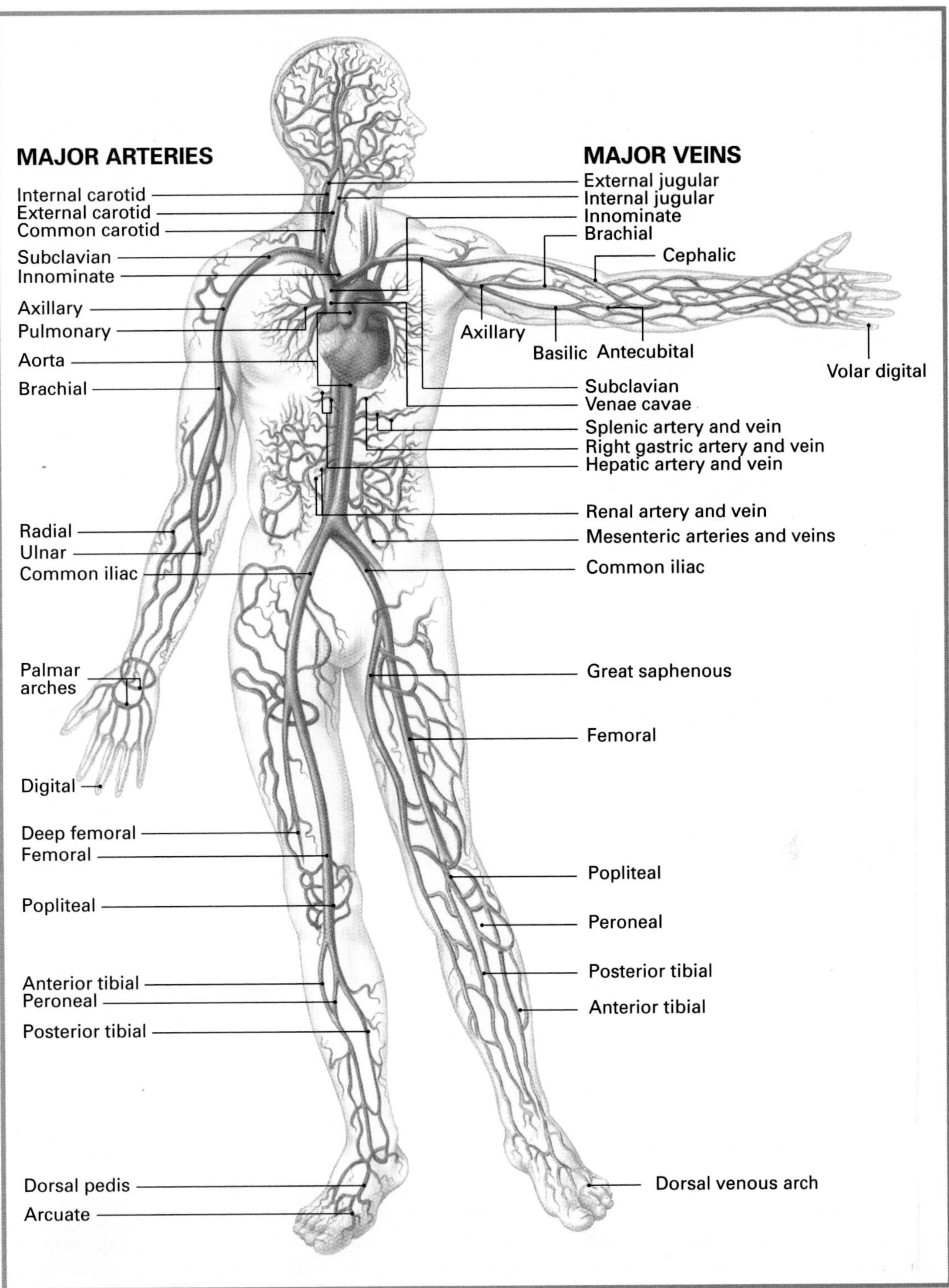
MAJOR ARTERIES
Internal carotid
External carotid
Common carotid
Subclavian
Innominate
Axillary
Pulmonary
Aorta
Brachial
Radial
Ulnar
Common iliac
Palmar arches
Digital
Deep femoral
Femoral
Popliteal
Anterior tibial
Peroneal
Posterior tibial
Dorsal pedis
Arcuate
MAJOR VEINS
External jugular
Internal jugular
Innominate
Brachial
Cephalic
Axillary
Basilic
Antecubital
Volar digital
Subclavian
Venae cavae
Splenic artery and vein
Right gastric artery and vein
Hepatic artery and vein
Renal artery and vein
Mesenteric arteries and veins
Common iliac
Great saphenous
Femoral
Popliteal
Peroneal
Posterior tibial
Anterior tibial
Dorsal venous arch

Figure 16-3
Illustration of the circulatory system.

MED TIP

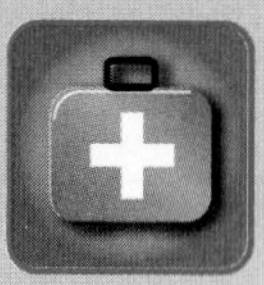

Phlebotomists should not perform arterial puncture. This procedure requires special training because the puncture could result in pain and/or excessive bleeding for the patient.

VEINS

The veins, with the exception of the pulmonary veins, carry deoxygenated blood back to the heart. Veins are smaller and much thinner than arteries, causing them to collapse easily. The veins also have valves that allow the blood to move only toward the heart. These valves prevent blood from backing away from the heart. The two large veins that enter the heart are the superior vena cava, which carries blood from the upper body, and the inferior vena cava, which carries blood from the lower body. Blood pressure in the veins is much lower than in the arteries. Muscular action within the veins helps in the movement of blood.

The major veins in the arms that the phlebotomist should know are the cephalic, basilic, and median cubital. They are located in the antecubital fossa, which is the area on the inner aspect at the bend of the elbow. These veins, which are closer to the surface, or superficial, in this area, are referred to as antecubital veins.

MED TIP

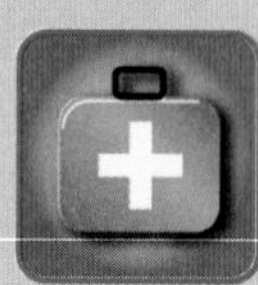

The terms *superficial* and *deep* are important concepts when studying the veins. Superficial (meaning close to the surface) veins, such as the median cephalic vein, are often easier to feel and locate for blood collection purposes. The deeper veins, such as the brachial vein, may be more difficult to locate by feel.

The major leg veins are the femoral, greater saphenous, lesser saphenous, and popliteal veins in the legs. Phlebotomists do not use the leg veins for venipuncture, but physicians may use them in special situations such as in a patient with amputations of both arms. Table 16-2 describes the locations of the major veins in the arms and legs.

When the antecubital veins are not suitable or are unavailable, such as when an arm cast is present, then veins on the back of the hand or forearm may be used. A needle with a smaller lumen (such as a butterfly needle) is generally used for these smaller veins to lessen the discomfort for the patient.

CAPILLARIES

The tiny capillaries are actually connecting units between the arteries and the veins. The capillaries are very thin and carry oxygen-rich blood from the arteries to the body cells. Because the capillaries are so small, the blood will not flow as quickly through them as it does through the arteries and veins. Consequently, the blood has time for an exchange of nutrients, oxygen, and waste material to take place between the surrounding cells and the tissue fluid.

TABLE 16-2 Major Veins in the Arms and Legs

Vein	Location
Arms	
Cephalic	Located on the lateral surface of the arm and forearm; it can be used for venipuncture.
Basilic	Found on the medial side of the arm and forearm; it divides below the antecubital fossa to form the median cubital vein and the ulnar vein and divides above the antecubital fossa to form the deep brachial vein. It can be used for venipuncture but tends to roll more than the other veins. There is also a danger of puncturing the artery when using this vein because they are in close proximity.
Median cubital	A superficial vein that lies across the antecubital fossa and serves as a link between the cephalic and basilic veins. This vein is most frequently used for venipuncture because it is large and well anchored.
Legs*	
Femoral	Found on the lateral to midline of the thigh; it is an extension of the popliteal vein.
Greater saphenous	A superficial vein that ascends along the medial aspect of the leg and thigh; it is the longest vein in the body.
Lesser saphenous	A short vein that arises from the dorsal surface of the foot and ascends along the posterior and lateral aspect of the calf.
Popliteal	A deep vein that is palpated behind the kneecap.

*These veins are not used by the phlebotomist for venipuncture. Physicians may use them in special situations.

Blood Components

The study of blood is called hematology. **Hematopoiesis,** the formation of blood cells, begins during fetal development. All blood cells originate from the hematopoietic stem cell but mature into individual cells:

- Red blood cells (RBCs)
- White blood cells (WBCs) (five types)
  - Neutrophils (segmented cell)
  - Lymphocytes
  - Monocytes
  - Eosinophils
  - Basophils
- Platelets (thrombocytes)

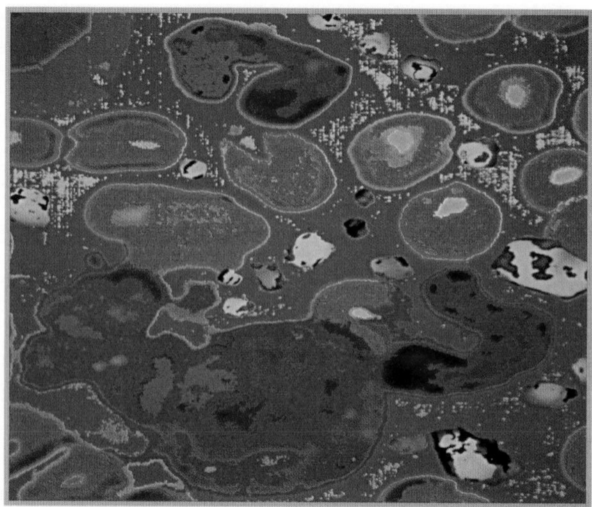

Figure 16-4
Computer visualization of RBCs and WBCs.

Blood is a specialized tissue consisting of a cellular component (red blood cells, white blood cells, and platelets) and a liquid component (plasma). The average adult has about 5.5 to 6 liters of blood, a combination of plasma and formed elements or blood cells. See figure 16-4 for computer visualization of RBCs and WBCs.

Plasma

Plasma transports substances in the blood to different parts of the body. It is the clear, straw-colored liquid portion of the blood that contains approximately 55 percent of the total blood volume and is 90 percent water. The remaining 10 percent of plasma consists of solid substances, including plasma proteins (albumin, globulin, fibrinogen, and prothrombin); electrolytes (sodium [Na], potassium [K], and chloride [Cl]); nutrients (glucose, amino acids, lipids, and carbohydrates); metabolic waste products (urea, lactic acid, uric acid, and creatinine); respiratory gases (oxygen and carbon dioxide); and miscellaneous substances (hormones, antibodies, enzymes, vitamins, and mineral salts). Fibrinogen, which converts to fibrin, and prothrombin are the clotting proteins.

There are also small amounts of inorganic substances in plasma, such as calcium, potassium, and sodium. Organic components consist of urea, uric acid, ammonia, and creatinine. Plasma carries these materials to all parts of the body. Serum is plasma after all the clotting proteins have been removed. The serum portion of blood is extracted from the liquid portion that does not contain the clot.

MED TIP

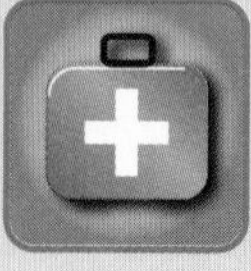

When a blood sample is centrifuged or the RBCs are allowed to settle, the RBCs will settle to the bottom of the test tube because they are the heaviest component. Platelets will form a thin white layer on top of the RBCs. This layer is called the buffy coat and consists of platelets and white blood cells. Plasma fluid will stay on the top of the tube.

There are three basic types of blood cells in the plasma: erythrocytes, leukocytes, and platelets.

Erythrocytes

The largest cellular portion of blood consists of erythrocytes, or RBCs. These are nonnucleated (no central kernel), donut-shaped, biconcave discs that live for 120 days before they are destroyed by the liver. The biconcave shape provides a greater surface area, which allows an increased oxygen-carrying capacity.

MED TIP

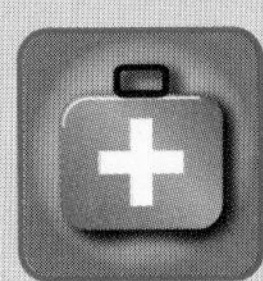

The shape of a cell and the presence of a nucleus are important factors when observing cells under a microscope. The red blood cell is readily apparent due to its rounded, concave shape and lack of a nucleus.

Red blood cells contain **hemoglobin,** which is the iron-containing pigment and gives the RBC its red color. The function of hemoglobin is twofold. First it carries oxygen from the lungs to the tissues. Then it carries carbon dioxide, a waste product, from the tissue to the lungs to be expelled from the body via expiration. When oxygen combines with hemoglobin in the lungs, **oxyhemoglobin** is formed. Therefore, hemoglobin is critical to life. A sudden decrease in red blood cells, such as occurs in a hemorrhage, can be life threatening. Arterial blood has a higher concentration of oxygen, hence the bright red color. In contrast, venous blood has low levels of oxygen and a deep red color.

There are approximately 5 million erythrocytes per cubic millimeter of blood. The total number in an average-sized adult is 35 trillion; males have more red blood cells than do females. Erythrocytes (RBCs), with an average life span of 120 days, need higher production rates to maintain their concentration in the blood. Therefore, millions of RBCs are formed and destroyed daily. Bone marrow needs an adequate supply of vitamin B complex, amino acids, and minerals including iron to form a sufficient number of RBCs. A decreased amount results in anemia.

Leukocytes

The second largest cellular portion consists of white blood cells (WBCs), or leukocytes. They are formed in the bone marrow and lymphatic tissues. WBCs provide protection for the body against the invasion of bacteria and other foreign material. They are able to leave the bloodstream and search out the foreign invaders such as bacteria, viruses, and toxins. A process called **phagocytosis** occurs when WBCs ingest and digest foreign material.

White blood cells have a spherical shape with a nucleus and number around 8,000/mm^3 of blood, with a normal range of 4,000–11,000/mm^3. WBCs are slightly larger than RBCs and live between a few hours and several days. There are five types of WBCs, all containing a distinct nucleus and having a distinct function. Also, WBCs can be divided into two categories: granulocytes, which contain granules in the cytoplasm, and agranulocytes, which do not contain granules in the cytoplasm. The various categories of white leukocytes (WBCs) are determined by a differential white cell count. Leukocyte classifications are contained in table 16-3.

TABLE 16-3 Leukocyte Classification

Leukocyte	Function
Granulocytes	
Basophils (0–1 percent)	Release histamine and heparin to damaged tissues
Eosinophils (1–3 percent)	Destroy parasites and increase during allergic reactions
Neutrophils (55–62 percent)	Most numerous of the leukocytes; important for phagocytosis
Agranulocytes	
Monocytes (4–10 percent)	Important for phagocytosis
Lymphocytes (20–40 percent)	Provide protection through an immunity activity by producing antibodies in response to an antigen

PLATELETS

Platelets, also called thrombocytes, have a round or oval disc shape or platelike appearance. Platelets, the smallest of all the formed blood elements (one-half the size of erythrocytes), have a life span of 9 to 12 days and aid in the clotting process. There are between 150,000 and 400,000/mm^3 of blood in the body. Platelets differ from erythrocytes in that they contain no hemoglobin.

Platelets play a critical role in the clotting process. They agglutinate, or clump, into small clusters when blood is shed. Platelets release thrombokinase, which, in the presence of calcium, reacts with prothrombin to form thrombin. Thrombin converts to fibrin, which eventually becomes the meshlike blood clot.

Coagulation and the Healing Process

Coagulation is the process of a clumping together of blood cells to form a clot. Injury to a small blood vessel results in bleeding or hemorrhage. When bleeding occurs the body initiates a series of steps to stop the blood loss. The first step in this process is called vasoconstriction, in which there is a decreased blood supply to the injured area and blood vessel. Platelets then clump together to form a plug or clot on the injured vessel to stop or diminish bleeding. Coagulation then occurs when a fibrin mesh or clot is formed. The clot will begin to recede or retract after the bleeding has stopped. In the final stage, the blood vessel begins to heal and regenerate as the clot slowly dissolves.

Injuries to large veins and arteries require surgical control such as suturing. Suturing is a necessary step during surgical procedures. Minor bleeding, such as occurs during venipuncture procedures, can be stopped when manual pressure is applied over the puncture site.

Serum

Serum is the watery portion of the blood after coagulation has occurred. It is the fluid that is found when clotted blood has been left standing long enough for the clot to shrink. The serum will remain separate from the fibrin clot of blood.

Blood Groupings

Blood grouping is also referred to as blood typing. The blood of one person is different from that of another due to the presence of antigens on the surface of erythrocytes. These antigens, or markers on the blood cell, stimulate the production of antibodies, which are then involved in the antigen-antibody reaction. The major antigens of blood groups are A and B. RBCs that contain both A and B antigens are found in those with group AB blood. RBCs that have neither A nor B antigens are found in those with group O blood. Patients with type A blood cannot be given type B blood and those with type B blood cannot be given type A blood, because there will be incompatibility between the two types and possibly a severe reaction.

MED TIP

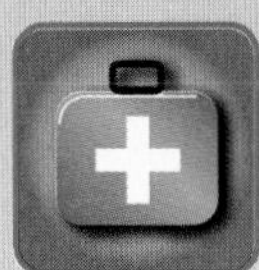

Type O is the most common blood type; around 46 percent of the population has type O blood. Type A blood is found in 40 percent of the population, type B is found in 10 percent, and type AB is found in only 4 percent. Type O negative blood is considered to be a universal donor type; in an emergency it can safely be given to anyone.

Rh FACTOR

The two types of Rh factors are Rh-positive (+), indicating the presence of the Rh factor, and Rh-negative (−), or the absence of the factor. The Rh blood type is important information when a blood transfusion is necessary. If a person with Rh− blood receives a transfusion of Rh+ blood, it will cause the formation of anti-Rh agglutination. Any transfusions *after* the first one can result in serious reactions. A pregnant woman who is Rh− may become sensitized by an Rh+ fetus. In pregnancies after the first, if the fetus is Rh+, the maternal antibodies may cross the placenta and destroy fetal cells, which will lead to **erythroblastosis fetalis.** Erythroblastosis fetalis, or hemolytic disease of the newborn, is a condition in which antibodies in the mother's blood enter the fetus's blood and cause anemia, jaundice, edema, and enlargement of the liver and spleen. Disorders relating to the circulatory system are described in table 16-4.

MED TIP

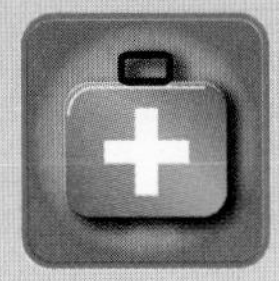

Serious conditions and even death have occurred when a patient has been given the wrong type of blood due to an error such as a mistyping of the blood or a mislabeling of the specimen. Extreme care must be taken when handling blood products.

TABLE 16-4 Disorders Relating to the Circulatory System	
Disorder	**Description**
Anemia	Reduction in the number of red blood cells, resulting in less oxygen reaching the tissues
Aneurysm	A weakness or outpouching in an arterial wall that can result in rupture and severe hemorrhage
Atherosclerosis	The formation of yellowish plaques of cholesterol building up on the inner walls of arteries
Bacterial endocarditis	Inflammation of the inner wall of the heart caused by a bacterial infection
Congestive heart failure (CHF)	Condition in which the outflow of blood from the left side of the heart is reduced, resulting in breathlessness, edema, and weakness
Erythroblastosis fetalis	Condition in which antibodies in the mother's blood enter the fetus's blood and cause anemia, edema, and enlargement of the liver and spleen; also called hemolytic disease of the newborn
Hematoma	Swelling or mass of blood caused by a break in a vessel in an organ, in a tissue, or beneath the skin
Hemophilia	Hereditary blood disease in which there is a prolonged blood-clotting time; transmitted by a sex-linked trait from females to males, it appears almost exclusively in males
Leukemia	Condition caused by an increase of white blood cells in the circulating blood and the bone marrow
Leukopenia	Abnormal decrease in the number of white blood cells
Myocardial infarction (MI)	Condition caused by the partial or complete occlusion of one or more of the coronary arteries; may be caused by a blood clot or a buildup of fatty deposits in the arterial walls; also called a heart attack
Polycythemia vera	Production of too many red blood cells by the bone marrow
Purpura	Condition in which there are multiple small hemorrhages under the skin, in the mucous membranes, and within tissues and organs
Thrombocytopenia	A marked decrease in the number of platelets in the body; may be seen in patients who are receiving chemotherapy treatments
Thrombocytosis	A marked increase in the number of platelets
Varicose veins	Swollen veins, especially in the lower limbs

Table 16-5 describes diagnostic and laboratory tests relating to the cardiovascular system and hematology.

TABLE 16-5 Diagnostic and Laboratory Tests Relating to the Cardiovascular System and Hematology

Test	Description
Arterial blood gases	Measurement of the amount of O_2, CO_2, and nitrogen in the blood
Aspartate aminotransferase (AST, SGOT)	Blood test to determine if there has been recent muscle damage such as with a myocardial infarction (MI)
Bleeding time	Blood test to measure the amount of time it takes for blood to coagulate
Cholesterol	Blood test to determine the level of cholesterol a sterol found in animal tissue
Complete blood count (CBC)	Measurement of the total number of white and red blood cells per cubic millimeter of blood
Creatinine kinase (CK, CPK)	Blood test to determine if an enzyme is present in cardiac muscle; can indicate a recent myocardial infarction (MI)
Differential	Blood test to determine the number of each variety of leukocytes
Electrocardiogram (ECG/EKG)	Test to determine the electrical activity of the heart
Electrolytes	Blood test to measure sodium (Na), potassium (K), bicarbonate (HCO_3), and chlorides (Cl) in the blood
Erythrocyte sedimentation rate (ESR)	Blood test to determine the rate at which mature red blood cells settle out of the blood after the addition of an anticoagulant
Fibrinogen	Blood test to determine the presence of fibrinogen, a protein found in blood plasma, as an indication of coagulation or a clotting disorder
Hematocrit (HCT, Hct, crit)	Blood test to measure the volume of erythrocytes in a given volume of blood
Hemoglobin (Hgb, Hb)	Measurement of iron-containing pigment of red blood cells that carries oxygen from the lungs to the tissues
Lactic dehydrogenase (LDH)	Blood test to determine the presence of the enzyme that oxidates lactate
Packed cell volume (PCV)	Blood test for hematocrit, which is the total number of erythrocytes in a given volume of blood
Platelet aggregation	Platelet (thrombocyte) count
Potassium (K)	Blood test specific for amount of potassium in blood
Prothrombin time (PT)	Blood test to measure the time it takes for a sample of blood to coagulate
Red blood cell (RBC) count	Blood test to determine the number of RBCs in a volume of blood
Reticulocyte (Retic) count	Blood test for immature red blood cells (reticulocytes)
Triglycerides	Blood test for fatty substances (lipids) in the blood
White blood cell (WBC) count	Blood test to measure the number of leukocytes in a volume of blood

Chapter Review

Summary

The heart is the major component of the circulatory system and is interrelated to all other systems and organs. An understanding of the circulatory system, with an emphasis on the blood vessels, is critical for the phlebotomist. Before performing an invasive procedure such as venipuncture the professional must understand the anatomy and physiology of the system.

Competency Review

1. Discuss the route taken as blood flows through the heart.
2. Describe the heartbeat and the conduction system of the heart.
3. Create a chart describing the leukocytes.
4. List the major blood groupings and describe their importance.
5. Discuss the role of platelets in the body.

Examination Review Questions

1. The most numerous leukocyte is the

(A) monocyte
(B) basophil
(C) neutrophil
(D) lymphocyte
(E) eosinophil

2. The pacemaker of the heart is the

(A) sinoatrial node
(B) aortic semilunar valve
(C) atrioventricular node
(D) Purkinje fiber
(E) bundle of His

3. A heart rate above 100 BPM is referred to as

(A) within a normal range
(B) systole
(C) diastole
(D) bradycardia
(E) tachycardia

4. The function of the blood is to

(A) restrict fluid loss
(B) regulate pH
(C) act as a toxin defense
(D) regulate temperature
(E) all of the above

5. The vein of choice for venipuncture is the

(A) basilic
(B) median cubital
(C) cephalic
(D) popliteal
(E) femoral

6. The largest cellular component of the blood is

(A) neutrophils
(B) leukocytes
(C) erythrocytes
(D) plasma
(E) serum

7. The chambers of the heart refer to

(A) atria
(B) ventricles
(C) aorta
(D) superior vena cava and inferior vena cava
(E) a and b only

8. Another term for thrombocyte is

(A) erythrocyte
(B) monocyte
(C) eosinophil
(D) platelet
(E) neutrophil

9. **The most common blood group is**
    (A) AB
    (B) O
    (C) A
    (D) B
    (E) Rh−

10. **A blood test to determine if immature red blood cells are present is referred to as a**
    (A) hematocrit
    (B) ESR
    (C) reticulocyte count
    (D) differential
    (E) RBC

Getting Connected

Multimedia Extension Activities

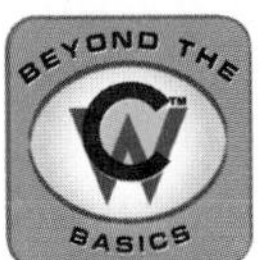

www.prenhall.com/fremgen

Use the address above to access the free, interactive Companion Website created specifically for this textbook. Enhance your studying by answering practice quiz questions, with hints and instant feedback related to chapter 16. If you would like to gain a deeper understanding of selected topics within this chapter, be sure to click on the **Beyond the Basics** feature, which provides more details for further learning. If you do not have a web connection, you may use the CD-ROM enclosed in the back of this book to take advantage of the same features off-line.

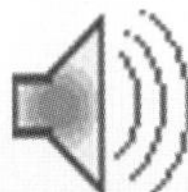

Audio Glossary

Use the CD-ROM enclosed with your textbook to hear the pronunciation of the key terms in the chapter. You may also access this material on the Companion Website www.prenhall.com/fremgen.

Bibliography

Chernecky, C., R. Krech, and B. Berger. *Laboratory Tests and Diagnostic Procedures.* Philadelphia: W. B. Saunders, 1993.

Clayman, C. *The Human Body.* New York: Dorling Kindersley, 1995.

Fishbach, F. *A Manual of Laboratory and Diagnostic Tests.* Philadelphia: Lippincott, 1996.

Fremgen, B. *Medical Terminology.* Upper Saddle River, N.J.: Brady/Prentice-Hall, 1997.

Martini, F. *Fundamentals of Anatomy and Physiology.* Upper Saddle River, N.J.: Brady/Prentice-Hall, 1995.

Palko, T., and H. Palko. *Laboratory Procedures for the Medical Office.* New York: Glencoe, 1996.

Taber's Cyclopedic Medical Dictionary, 18th ed. Philadelphia: F. A. Davis, 1997.

CASE STUDY FOR END OF PART IV

BILLY BROWN, A 2-YEAR-OLD BOY is being seen by a hematologist. The child presents with symptoms of high fever, thrombocytopenia, abnormal nosebleeds, gingival (gum) bleeding, purpura, ecchymosis, and bruising after minor traumas. The physician has ordered blood tests including a **CBC** and a bone marrow aspiration to confirm the diagnosis of acute lymphocytic leukemia (ALL).

What is your response?

1. There is usually an elevated white blood count in patients with ALL. Why did the physician order a CBC rather than just a WBC?
2. Define the following:
   a. Hematologist ______________________________
   b. Thrombocytopenia ______________________________
   c. Ecchymosis ______________________________
   d. Purpura ______________________________
   e. Lymphocytic ______________________________

APPENDICES

Appendix A • Laboratory Values

HEMATOLOGY	
Red blood cell count	F = 3.8–5.2 × 10^6/mm^3
	M = 4.4–5.9 × 10^6 mm^3
White blood cell count	4,500–11,000/mm^3
Platelet count	150,000–400,000/mm^3
Hemoglobin	F = 12–16 g/dL
	M = 17–18 g/dL
Hematocrit	M = 40–52 percent
	F = 35–47 percent
Differential leukocyte count	Neutrophils 55–62 percent
	Eosinophils 1–3 percent
	Basophils 0–1 percent
	Lymphocytes 20–40 percent
	Monocytes 4–10 percent
Erythrocyte sedimentation rate	Wintrobe M = 0–9 mm/m F = 0–20 mm/m
	Westergren M <50 years < 10 mm/m F <50 years ≤ 13 mm/m
	M >50 ≤ 13 mm/m F >50 ≤ 20 mm/m
Prothrombin time	<10–15 seconds
Activated partial thromboplastin time	<35 seconds
Bleeding time	2–9 minutes
URINALYSIS	
Specific gravity	1.002–1.030
pH	4.5–7.5
Protein	Negative to trace
Glucose	Negative
Blood	Negative
Ketones	Negative
Bilirubin	Negative
Urobilinogen	Less than 1.0 Ehrlich unit or 1 mg/dL
Nitrite	Negative
Leukocytes	Negative
CHEMISTRY*	
Alanine amino transferase (ALT)	M = 10–40 μ/L
	F = 10–28 μ/L
Alkaline phosphatase (ALP)	25–100 μ/L
Aspartate aminotransferase (AST)	M = 15–40 μ/L
	F = 13–35 μ/L
Bicarbonate	22–29 mmol/L
Bilirubin	<1.5 mg/dL
Blood urea nitrogen (BUN)	7–18 mg/dL
Calcium (Ca)	8.0–10.5 mg/dL

Chloride	98–109 mmol/L
Cholesterol	M = 114–265 mg/dL
	F = 112–280 mg/dL
Creatinine	M = 0.9–1.5 mg/dL
	F = 0.7–1.3 mg/dL
Glucose	<115 fasting mg/dL
Lactic dehydrogenase (LD)	140–280 μ/L
Potassium	3.5–5.0 mmol/L
Protein	6.4–8.3 g/dL
Sodium	135–145 mmol/L
Triglyceride	M = 30–327 mg/dL
	F = 35–262 mg/dL
Uric acid	M = 3.6–7.7 mg/dL
	F = 2.5–6.8 mg/dL

*C. Lehman. *Saunders Manual of Clinical Laboratory Medicine.* Philadelphia: W. B. Saunders, 1998.

Appendix B • Laboratory Math

Weights and Measures

Weights and measurements are used in the medical laboratory for a variety of reasons. Many items require counting, such as the number of cells present in a specimen of blood. The amount or volume of the specimen also has to be measured. These measurements can then be compared with normal values, which the physician uses to assist in determining the diagnosis and treatment. Other measurements include temperature, weight, size, time, and concentration.

Two systems of weights and measurement are used to calculate dosages: apothecary and metric. In addition, there are also common household measurements, such as teaspoon (t) and tablespoon (T), which are often used even though they are not considered medical measurements. These household units are useful when instructing patients. The metric system is very useful because small amounts such as those measured in the laboratory can be more easily calculated using this system.

The Apothecary System

The apothecary system is considered to be the oldest system of measurement. The dry weight equivalent as established in this system is 1 grain = 1 gram of wheat. The basic units of weight are grain (gr), gram (g), dram (ʒ), ounce (℥), and pound (lb). Fluid measurements using the apothecary system are called minims (mn), fluid dram (fl ʒ/dram), fluid ounce (fl ℥), pint (pt), quart (qt), and gallon (C). Some of the common household measurements (e.g., pint, quart, and gallon) are based on the apothecary system.

Roman numerals are used for numbering in this system. For example, 3 grains would be gr iii, and 4 ounces would be ℥ iv. The apothecary system also uses fractions such as 1/4 and 1/2. Therefore, three-fourths of a grain would be gr 3/4. The unit of measurement (gr) is placed before the dosage in the apothecary system.

The Metric System

The metric system, based on the decimal system, is more widely used in laboratories than the apothecary system. In the metric system, all the numbers are derived by either multiplying or dividing by the power of 10. The metric system also makes extensive use of prefixes to indicate an increase or decrease in size. For example, the prefix kilo (meaning 1,000) can be added to meter to indicate 1,000 meters (1 km = 1,000 m). Likewise, 1 kg is 1,000 g, and 1 kL is 1,000 L. Table A-1 lists commonly used prefixes in the metric system.

TABLE A-1 Commonly Used Prefixes Based on the Metric System

Prefix and abbreviation	Multiple	Length (m)	Volume (L)	Weight (g)	Example
kilo- (k)	1,000	km	kL	kg	1 kg = 1,000 g
hecto- (h)	100	hm	hL	hg	1 hg = 100 g
deca- (da)	10	dam	daL	dag	1 dag = 10 g
deci- (d)	1/10	dm	dL	dg	1 dg = 1/10 g
centi- (c)	1/100	cm	cL	cg	1 cg = 1/100 g
milli- (m)	1/1,000	mm	mL	mg	1 mg = 1/1,000 g
micro- (μ)	1/1,000,000	μm	μL	μg	1 μg = 1/1,000,000 g

TABLE A-2 Common Abbreviations for Weights and Measures in the Apothecary and Metric Systems

Apothecary System

Symbol	Abbreviation	Meaning
gt	drop	drop
minim	min	minim
dram ʒ	dr	dram
fl ʒ	fl dr	fluid dram
℥	oz	ounce
fl ℥	fl oz	fluid ounce
O	pt	pint
C	gal	gallon
	gr	grain

Metric System

Weight

Abbreviation	Meaning
mg	milligram
gm	gram

Volume

Abbreviation	Meaning
L	liter
mL	milliliter
cc	cubic centimeter
μL	microliter

Usually only the metric units for weight, volume, length, and temperature are used for measurement in the laboratory. The millimeter and the centimeter are two of the most frequently used for laboratory measurements.

In the metric system, liter means volume, gram stands for weight, and meter represents length. See table A-2 for common abbreviations for weights and measures.

See table A-3 for commonly used equivalents for the apothecary and metric systems.

For a comparison of the three systems (household, apothecary, and metric) for liquid measurement see table A-4.

MED TIP

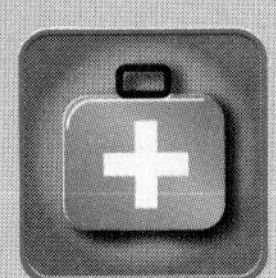

It is helpful to remember that 1 kg is equal to 2.2 lb, 1 L is equal to approximately 1 qt, and 1 m is equal to 39.37 inches, or slightly longer than a yard.

TABLE A-3 Commonly Used Equivalents for the Apothecary and Metric Systems

Apothecary System

Apothecary Measure	Metric Equivalent
1 gr	65 mg or 0.065 g
5 gr	325 mg or 0.33 g
10 gr	650 mg or 0.65 g
15 or 16 gr	1 g
15 or 16 m	1.00 mL or 1 cc
1 dram	4 mL
1 oz	30 cc, 30 mL, 8 drams
1 lb	450 g
1 lb	0.4536 kg
1 minim (min)	0.06 mL
4 minim (min)	0.25 mL
Liquid Measure	
1 fl dr	4 mL
2 fl dr	8 mL
2.5 fl dr	10 mL
4 fl dr	15 mL
1 fl oz	30 mL
3.5 fl oz	100 mL
7 fl oz	200 mL
1 pt	500 mL
1 qt	1,000 mL
60 gtt (drops)	4 mL

TABLE A-4 Comparison of Household, Apothecary, and Metric Liquid Measurements

Household	Apothecary	Metric
1 drop (gt)	1 minim (min)	0.06 mL
1 t	1 fl dr (fl ʒ)	4–5 mL
1 T	4 fl dr (fl ʒ)	15–16 mL
2 T	1 fl oz (fl ℥)	30–32 mL
1 cup or glass	8 fl oz (fl ℥)	250 mL
2 cups or glasses	16 fl oz (fl ℥) or 1 pt	500 mL
4 cups or glasses	1 qt	1,000 mL = approximately 1 L

Converting Measurement Systems

It may be necessary to convert from one system to another. You may have to convert an order written using the metric system into the apothecary system or vice versa. You would use a conversion chart such as that found in tables A-2 and A-3. In some cases, the household measurement will be used and will need to be converted to another system; for example, a patient may measure a urine sample in a household measurement such as cups. This amount would have to be converted to the metric system for purposes of documentation. In the example of 1 cup, the amount 250 mL would be noted on the medical chart.

A conversion from one system to another will result in equivalents that are only approximate. It may be necessary to round off the amounts. Guidelines for conversions include the following:

1. ***To change grains to grams, divide by 15.***
2. ***To change ounces to cubic centimeters (cc), multiply by 30.***
3. ***To change grains to milligrams (mg), multiply by 60. (Only use this rule when you have less than 1 grain.)***
4. ***To change kilograms to pounds, multiply by 2.2.***
5. ***To change cubic centimeters (cc) to ounces, divide by 30.***
6. ***To change drams to milliliters (mL), multiply by 4.***
7. ***To change cubic centimeters (cc) or milliliters to minims, multiply by 15 or 16.***
8. ***To change minims to cubic centimeters (cc), divide by 15 or 16.***
9. ***To convert drams to grams, multiply by 4.***

A simplified list of conversions that can be memorized is found in table A-5

A more common type of conversion is to change numbers within the metric system. It may be necessary to convert milliliters to liters or grams to kilograms. For example, you may have to determine how many milligrams are in a sample containing a certain number of grams. Many laboratories and medical offices have conversion charts available to handle this type of conversion within the metric system. However, conversions are not difficult to perform without a conversion chart if a few guidelines are followed:

1. ***There is no change necessary to change milliliters into cubic centimeters. They are equal to each other (1 mL = 1 cc).***
2. ***To change grams to milligrams, multiply grams by 1,000, or move the decimal point three places to the right.***

TABLE A-5 Conversion List

Apothecary	Metric
15 or 16 min	1 mL or 1 cc
1 fl dr	4 mL or 4 cc
1 fl oz	30 mL or 30 cc
1 qt	1,000 mL or 1,000 cc
1/60 gr	1 mg
1 gr	0.065 g
15 gr	1 g
2.2. lb	1 kg

TABLE A-6	Temperature Scale Conversion	
Scale	**Formula**	**Example**
Centigrade	(°F − 32) 5/9 = °C	101°F − 32 = 69 × 5/9 = 38.3 °C
Fahrenheit	(°C × 9/5) + 32 = °F	38.3 °C × 9/5 = 69 + 32 = 101 °F

3. ***To change milligrams to grams, divide milligrams by 1,000, or move the decimal point three places to the left.***
4. ***To convert liters to milliliters, multiply liters by 1,000, or move the decimal point three places to the right.***
5. ***To convert milliliters to liters, divide milliliters by 1,000, or move the decimal point three places to the left.***

Temperature Conversions

The Fahrenheit (F) scale of temperature measurement is widely used throughout the United States. Body temperature is usually calculated using the Fahrenheit scale. The centigrade (C) or Celsius scale is frequently used in the laboratory to measure boiling points, reaction, and temperatures such as for incubation purposes. Using the Celsius scale, the freezing point of water is 0 degrees and the boiling point is 100 degrees. Using the Fahrenheit scale, the freezing point of water is 32 degrees and the boiling point is 212 degrees.

To convert Fahrenheit to Celsius subtract 32, then multiply by 5/9. To convert Celsius to Fahrenheit, multiply by 9/5 and then add 32. See table A-6 for temperature scale conversion formulas and examples.

The International System of Units

The International System of Units (SI units) is a system for reporting laboratory results that is used throughout the world. This system is adapted from the metric system. In 1977 the World Health Organization (WHO) recommended adoption of SI units so there would be a standard unit of measurement throughout the world. However, some areas of the United States have been slow to adopt the system.

The phlebotomist should note the difference in the terminology when using this system. For example, a diabetic patient from Canada may be accustomed to hearing a normal glucose value expressed as 6.0 mmol/L using the SI units and may become confused when it is reported as 108 mg/dL in the United

TABLE A-7	Use of the SI Unit in Selected Cell Counts and Tests	
Test	**SI Unit**	**Metric System**
Hemoglobin	Grams per liter (g/L)	Grams per deciliter (g/dL)
Glucose	Millimoles per liter (mmol/L)	Milligrams per deciliter (mg/dL)
Hematocrit	Percentage as a decimal (e.g., 0.32)	Percentage (e.g., 32%)

States. In this example, if the glucose reference range for a normal test in the metric system is 70–110 mg/dL, then it would be 3.9–6.1 mmol/L under the SI system.

Under the metric system, blood cell counts are expressed as the number of cells per cubic millimeter (cu mm or μL). But under the SI system they are expressed as the number of cells per liter of blood (cells/L). It is important to state which system is being used when reporting test results. Table A-7 describes the use of SI units for selected cell counts and tests.

Decimals and Fractions as Equivalent Percentages

Sometimes information given in decimal or fraction form needs to be translated into its equivalent percentage form in the laboratory. To convert a decimal to a percentage, multiply by 100. Move the decimal point two places to the right and add a percent sign. For example,

0.125 = 12.5%

0.75 = 75%

Ratio

A ratio is the relationship of one quantity to another or a comparison of two quantities. The two terms of a ratio are separated by a colon that is read as "to." For example,

1:2 is read "1 to 2"

1:10 is read "1 to 10"

The ratio is also equivalent to a fraction. For example, the ratio 3:4 is equivalent to a fraction (3/4) and a percentage (75%). This can also be the same as 3:4 = 3/4 = 0.75 = 75%. A ratio is frequently stated in fractional form. The terms of the ratio, such as 1:10, become the terms of the fraction (numerator and denominator). The fraction bar then means "divided by." For example,

1:10 = 1 to 10 = 1/10 = 1 ÷ 10 = 0.1

Ratios are frequently used to express the strength of a solution. (The solution strength can also be stated as a percentage). A dilution, which is a ratio, is expressed as the relationship between a part of the solution and the whole solution. To dilute a substance is to weaken it or reduce the concentration of the solution. A 1:25 solution means that there is 1 part of solute (the substance dissolved in a solution) in 25 parts of solution. An example of a 1:1,000 solution is 1 mL of pure liquid solute contained in 1,000 mL of solution.

In a 1:20 dilution there is 1 part solute and 20 parts in total. Therefore, you would need 1 part of solute (such as serum) and 19 parts of solution (such as saline) to prepare a 1:20 dilution. A 1:10 solution of bleach means there is 1 part bleach in a total of 10 parts of solution.

Proportions

A proportion states that two ratios are equal; it is the same as two equivalent fractions. The first terms of the ratio are related to each other; likewise, the second terms are related in the same manner to each other. Proportions can be expressed in one of two ways:

1:2 :: 2:4 *or* 1/2 = 2/4

Note that the symbol (::) is read "as"; the preceding equation reads "one is to two as two is to four."

The middle terms in a proportion are called the means, and the outer terms are the extremes. In the preceding example, 1:2 :: 2:4, the means are 2 and 2, and the extremes are 1 and 4. We can prove that one side of this proportion is equivalent to the other side by cross multiplication of the means and the extremes. This proportion is equivalent because the means and extremes provide the same product when multiplied ($2 \times 2 = 4$; $1 \times 4 = 4$).

It is useful to remember this concept when searching for an unknown term (X). For example, if you have a 25% (25 parts in 100) solution and wish to know how many grams of pure solute are contained in 400 mL, then set up a proportion to solve the equation:

25 g:100 mL = *X* g:400 mL

$$\frac{25}{100} = \frac{X}{400}$$

Cross multiply 100 × *X* and 25 × 400

Multiply the means together; then multiply the extremes together to find the value of X. Cross multiply $100X = 25(400)$.

$$100X = 10{,}000$$

$$10{,}000/100 = 100$$

$$X = 100$$

Solution: If 25 g of pure solute are contained in 100 mL, then 100 g of pure solute are contained in 400 mL of solution.

Bibliography

Dawe, R. *Math and Dosage Calculations for Health Occupations.* New York: Glencoe, 1993.

Julius, E. *Rapid Math Tricks and Tips.* New York: John Wiley & Sons, 1992.

Kogelman, S., and B. Heller. *The Only Math Book You'll Ever Need.* New York: Facts on File, 1986.

Sperling, A., and M. Stuart. *Mathematics Made Simple.* New York: Doubleday, 1991.

Introductory Phrases for Patients

English	Spanish
Hello	Hola
Please	Por favor (Begin or end any request with the words *por favor* [please].)
Thank you	Gracias
You are welcome	De nada.
Good morning	Buenos días
Good afternoon	Buenas tardes
Good evening	Buenas noches
My name is . . .	Mi nombre es . . .
I work in the laboratory.	Trabajo en el laboratorio.
What is your name?	¿Cómo se llama?
What is your address?	¿Su domicilio?
Who is your doctor?	¿Quien es su doctor?
Do you understand me?	¿Me entiende?
I do not understand.	No entiendo.
How old are you?	¿Cuántos años tienes?
How do you feel?	¿Cómo se siente?
Do you have pain?	¿Tiene dolor?
Where is the pain?	¿Endonde es el dolor?
Good	Bien, bueno
Bad	Mal, malo
Speak slower, please.	Hable más despacio, por favor.
Say it again, please.	Repítalo, por favor.
I speak . . .	Hablo . . .
We are going to analyze your blood.	Vamos a analizar su sangre.
We are going to analyze your urine.	Vamos a analizar su orina.
Empty your bladder.	Orinar, orine.
Here is the bathroom.	Aqui esta el baño.
You may not eat or drink.	No coma ó bebe.
You can only drink water.	Solo puede tomar agua.
Drink fluids.	Beba liquidos.
Have you had breakfast?	¿Ya tomó el desayunó?

Early in the morning	Temprano enor la mañana
At noon	Al mediodia
At bedtime	Al acostarse
At night	Por la noche
We are going to analyze your sputum.	Vamos a analizar su esputo.
Relax, please.	Relájese, por favor.
I need to stick your finger.	Necesito pincharle un dedo.
I need to take a sample of your blood.	Necesito sacarte sangre.
I am going to . . .	Voy a . . .
Please be seated.	Sientese, por favor.
Please make a fist.	Cierre el puño, por favor.
Please roll up your sleeve.	Levántese la manga, por favor.
Please bend your arm.	Doble el brazo, por favor.
Please do not move.	No se mueva, por favor.
Cough.	Tosa.
Please open your mouth.	Abra la boca, por favor.
Grasp my hand.	Apriete mi mano.
Breathe slowly.	Respire despacio.
This will hurt a little.	Le va a doler un poquito.
It will be uncomfortable.	Será incómodo.
You will feel pressure.	Va a sentir presión.
It will sting.	Va a arder.
Do you feel faint?	¿Se siente como si se va a desmayar?
You must lie down.	Necesita acostarse.
Do you still feel weak?	¿Se siente muy débil todavia?
Do you feel dizzy?	¿Tiene usted vértigo?
Yes	Sí
No	No
Doctor	Doctor
Physician	Médico
Nurse	Enfermera
Hospital	Hospital
Midwife	Comadre
Right	Derecha
Left	Izquierda

Courtesy Titles

Mr.	Señor
Miss	Señorita
Mrs.	Señora

General Terminology Relating to Time and Day

Zero	Cero
One	Uno
Two	Dos
Three	Tres
Four	Cuatro
Five	Cinco
Six	Seis
Seven	Siete
Eight	Ocho
Nine	Nueve
Ten	Diez
Twenty	Veinte
Thirty	Treinta
Forty	Cuarenta
Fifty	Cincuenta
Sixty	Sesenta
Seventy	Setenta
Eighty	Ochenta
Ninety	Noventa
One hundred	Cien
One hundred and one	Ciento uno
Sunday	Domingo
Monday	Lunes
Tuesday	Martes
Wednesday	Miércoles
Thursday	Jueves
Friday	Viernes
Saturday	Sábado
Today	Hoy
Tomorrow	Mañana
Yesterday	Ayer

ABGs arterial blood gases.

Accreditation the process in which an institution (school) voluntarily completes an extensive self-study, after which an accrediting association visits the school to verify the self-study statements.

Acquired immunodeficiency syndrome (AIDS) a series of infections and disorders that occur as a result of infection by the human immunodeficiency virus (HIV), which causes the immune system to break down.

Activated partial thromboplastin time (APTT) a coagulation test used to test the extrinsic coagulation system.

Aerobic microorganism that is able to live only in the presence of oxygen.

Aerosol a fine mist.

Agar a product from seaweed that it used to solidify bacteriologic media.

Agranulocyte leukocytes that do not have cytoplasmic granules (e.g., lymphocytes and monocytes).

Aliquot a portion of a patient specimen used for testing.

Allen test test used to determine if an artery is safe to use for an arterial blood gas test.

Anaerobic microorganism that thrives best or lives without oxygen.

Analyte term for a substance being tested.

Anaphylactic severe, sometimes fatal allergic reaction.

Anemia a condition in which there is a below normal red blood cell count or hemoglobin level.

Anesthetic an agent that produces loss of feeling.

Antecubital fossa area formed at the inside bend of the elbow.

Antibiotic a substance produced by a microorganism that will inhibit bacterial growth.

Antibody a specialized protein found in blood that reacts with an antigen.

Antigen a foreign substance that causes the production of an antibody.

Antiseptic substance used to reduce the bacterial population of the skin.

Arterioles small branches of arteries.

Arteriosclerosis thickening or hardening of the walls of the arteries.

Arteriospasm involuntary contraction of an artery.

Asepsis germ free.

Atherosclerosis the most common cause of arteriosclerosis, it is a buildup of plaques of cholesterol on the inner walls of the arteries.

Autologous donation donating blood for one's own use.

Autopsy tests conducted on the organs and tissues of deceased persons to assist in determining the cause of death.

Bacillus a rod-shaped bacterium.

Basal state a resting metabolic state early in the morning and a minimum of 12 hours after eating.

Biological safety hood a protective cabinet that should be used when in contact with aerosols (airborne particles) to draw the particles away from the laboratory worker.

Bloodborne pathogens disease-producing microorganisms transmitted by means of blood and bodily fluids containing blood.

Breach (neglect) of duty neglect or failure to perform an obligation.

Calcaneus heel bone.

Cannula temporary surgical connection between an artery and a vein or a temporary device implanted in a vein for attachment to dialysis equipment.

Cardiovascular system also called the circulatory system; includes the heart and blood vessels.

Carrier a person who is unaware that he or she has a disease but who is capable of transmitting it to someone else.

Case law law that is based on precedent.
Cast a cylindrical protein structure formed in a kidney tubule and found in urine.
Catheter sterile flexible tube inserted into the bladder or a vein to withdraw fluid.
Caustic capable of burning or eating away tissue.
Centrifugation the process of separating substances of different weights by spinning at high speeds.
Certification the issuance by an official body of a certificate to a person indicating that certain requirements to practice have been met.
Chain of custody a specific protocol for legal specimens that documents the specimen from collection to the final test result.
Coagulation clumping together of blood cells to form a clot.
Coccus a spherical-shaped bacterium.
Collateral circulation more than one artery supplies blood to the same area.
Colony a mass of bacteria that grew from a single bacterial cell.
Combining form a word component that consists of a word root and a vowel, usually *o*.
Complete blood count (CBC) commonly performed group of hematology tests.
Consent to give permission, permit, or allow.
Consent, implied inference by signs, inaction, or silence that consent has been granted.
Consent, informed patient's consent to undergo treatment or surgery based on knowledge and understanding of the potential risks and benefits provided by the physician before the procedure is performed.
Contact isolation a form of isolation in which anyone entering the patient's room and having direct contact with the patient wears gloves and a gown.
Continuing education units (CEUs) a credit granted to a participant at the completion of a designated program.
Contract agreement between two or more persons that creates an obligation to perform or not perform some action or service.
Criminal law court action brought by the state against persons or groups of people accused of committing a crime, resulting in a fine or imprisonment if found guilty.
Criteria standards against which something is compared to make a decision or judgment.
Culture the act of growing bacteria on media in the laboratory.
Cumulative having an effect that builds over time.
Cytology area of surgical pathology that examines bodily fluids and tissues for evidence of abnormality after the histologist has prepared them.

Damages compensation for a loss or injury.
Data statistics, figures, or information.
Defendant person or group of persons who are accused in a court of law.
Delta test a comparison between the current results of a laboratory test and the previous test results for the same patient.
Diabetes mellitus a condition in which there is impaired carbohydrate metabolism due to lack of insulin.
Diastole the relaxation phase of the heartbeat that occurs when the ventricles relax.
Differential a test that determines the number of each type of leukocyte as compared to the total white blood cell count.
Diurnal daily.
Duty obligation or responsibility as a result of the physician-client relationship.

Edema an accumulation of fluid in tissues.
Electrolytes term for four serum ions (sodium, potassium, chloride, and bicarbonate).
Emancipated minors persons under the age of 18 who are free of parental care and financially responsible for themselves.
Empathy the ability to understand the feelings of another person without actually experiencing the pain or distress that person is going through.
Enteric isolation isolation used for persons with infections of the intestinal tract.
Erythroblastosis fetalis condition in which antibodies in the mother's blood enter the fetus's blood and cause anemia, jaundice,

edema, and enlargement of the liver and spleen; a life-threatening condition for the newborn.

Erythrocyte red blood cell.

Erythrocytosis increase in the normal number of red blood cells.

Ethics principles and guides for moral behavior.

Evacuated tube collection tube with a vacuum used in blood collection.

Felony a crime more serious than a misdemeanor; it carries a penalty of death or imprisonment.

Fibrinogen a plasma protein that plays a role in hemostasis.

Fistula an artificial connection between an artery and a vein.

Floor book a laboratory reference manual; also referred to as a procedure, reference, or test manual.

FUO fever of an undetermined origin.

Gauge diameter or internal size of a needle.

Geriatric pertaining to the elderly.

Glucosuria the presence of sugar (glucose) in the urine.

Glycolysis process of breaking down glucose.

Gram stain the primary differential stain used to classify bacteria.

Granulocyte leukocyte with cytoplasmic granules (e.g., neutrophils, eosinophils, and basophils).

Guardian ad litem court-appointed guardian to represent a minor or unborn child in litigation.

Hematocrit a test that compares the volume of erythrocytes to the volume of whole blood.

Hematology department department that conducts laboratory analysis testing to identify diseases of the blood and blood-forming tissues.

Hematology the study of blood and blood-forming tissues.

Hematoma swelling due to blood leaking into tissues.

Hematopoiesis the process of formation and development of blood cells.

Hematuria the presence of blood in the urine.

Hemoconcentration a condition in which plasma enters the tissues, resulting in a higher than normal concentration of the cellular components of blood.

Hemoglobin protein in red blood cells that transports oxygen and carbon dioxide.

Hemolysis the destruction of red blood cells.

Hemostasis the process in which bleeding is stopped.

Histology the study of tissues.

Human immunodeficiency virus (HIV) virus that causes AIDS.

Hyphae hairlike structures of molds.

Hypoglycemia condition in which the amount of glucose in the blood is lower than normal.

Hypothyroidism congenital condition in which the thyroid gland is impaired due to production of defective enzymes.

Iatrogenic physician induced.

Icteric having a yellow color due to excess bilirubin.

Immunology department department that runs tests on blood samples to determine the presence of an antigen-antibody reaction of the body.

Immunology the study of immune processes.

In vitro outside the body.

In vivo within the body.

Incident report a formal written description of an unusual occurrence.

Infection a pathological condition caused by the growth of microorganisms in a host.

Inpatient hospitalized patient.

Interstitial space between cells or tissue.

Isolette individual clear plastic basket used in nurseries for newborns.

Keloid thick, raised scar.

Lancet sterile, disposable, sharp instrument used in dermal puncture.

Law rules of conduct established and enforced by an authority such as the legislature.

Leukocyte white blood cell.

Leukocytosis increase in the normal number of white blood cells.

Leukopenia decrease in the normal number of white blood cells.

Libel written false statements placed about another person.

Licensure the legal permission, granted by the state where the phlebotomist will work, to engage in an occupation or activity.

Lipemic having a cloudy or milky white appearance due to excess lipids.

Luer adapter a device that tightly connects the syringe to the needle.

Lumen the hollow space in the center of a tube or blood vessel.

Lymphostasis obstruction of the normal flow of lymph.

Malpractice "bad practice"; also called professional negligence.

Mature minor person, usually under 18 years of age, who possesses an understanding of the nature and consequences of proposed treatment.

Media substances that will sustain bacteriologic growth in the laboratory.

Medical asepsis killing organisms after they leave the body.

Microbiology department department that analyzes specimens for the presence and identification of type of microorganisms.

Microbiology the study of microorganisms.

Microorganisms small living organisms that are capable of causing disease. Also called microbes.

Minor person under the age of 18.

Misdemeanor crime that is less serious than a felony; it carries a penalty of up to one year imprisonment and/or fine.

Morphology the shape and structure of a cell.

Mycosis an infection caused by a fungus.

Myeloproliferative disease chronic malignant disorder due to an abnormal proliferation of a cell line.

Negligence failure to perform professional duties in an accepted standard of care.

Neonate a newborn infant.

Nonpathogenic non-disease-producing.

Norm standard, criterion, or the ideal measure for a specific group.

Normal flora microorganisms that are normally present on a host.

Normal value the amount of a substance that is normally present.

Nosocomial infection infection that is acquired after a person has entered the hospital. It is caused by the spread of an infection from one person to another.

Occurrence any event or incident outside of the norm.

Osteomyelitis infection of bone.

Outpatient patient who is not staying in a hospital but comes to the hospital for treatment.

Oxygenated blood that has been exposed to oxygen in the lungs.

Oxyhemoglobin a combination of oxygen and hemoglobin; carries oxygen to the tissues.

Palmar palm side of the hand.

Palpation to examine by touching.

Parasite an organism that lives on or in a host and causes damage to the host.

Pathogenic capable of causing damage in a host.

Pathogens disease-producing microorganisms.

Petechiae small red spots on the skin due to damaged capillaries.

Petri dish a round covered dish used to hold agar-based media.

pH measurement of the degree of acidity or alkalinity of a substance.

Phagocyte a cell that engulfs and digests foreign material.

Phagocytosis the process in which white blood cells (WBCs) ingest and digest foreign material.

Phenylketonuria (PKU) hereditary metabolic disorder due to lack of the enzyme phenylalanine hydroxylase that can cause severe mental retardation if not detected soon after birth.

Phlebotomist a person trained to perform blood collection procedures using various techniques that include venipuncture and capillary puncture.

Phlebotomy the practice of obtaining blood samples that are used for analysis and diagnostic purposes.

Plaintiff person or group of persons who bring an action to litigation (lawsuit).

Plantar sole side of the foot.

Plasma straw-colored liquid portion of blood.

Point of care testing laboratory testing performed at the patient's bedside rather than in the laboratory.

Postprandial after eating.

Precedent law that is established in a prior case.

Prefix a word component added to the front of a word root that then forms a new medical term.

Probe blindly moving the needle under the skin in the hope of finding a vein.

Procedure manual a collection of policies and procedures for carrying out day-to-day operations in the laboratory.

Profile group of chemistry tests.

Proteinuria the presence of protein in the urine.

Prothrombin time (protime or PT) a coagulation screening test used to test the intrinsic coagulation system.

Proximate cause natural continuous sequence of events, without an intervening cause, that produces an injury. Also referred to as the direct cause.

QNS quantity not sufficient.

Quality assurance program a program in which laboratories and hospitals evaluate the services and/or tests they provide by comparing their services and/or tests with accepted standards.

Quality assurance gathering and evaluating information and data about the services or tests provided as well as the results achieved compared with an acceptable standard.

Reciprocity agreement in which one state recognizes the licensure granted to a person by another state.

Requisition physician's order to obtain a specimen for testing.

Res ipsa loquitur Latin phrase that means "the thing speaks for itself." This is a doctrine of negligence law.

Reservoir source of the infectious pathogen.

Respiratory isolation used for patients with diseases that can be spread by droplet infection. Anyone entering the patient's room must wear a mask.

Respondeat superior Latin phrase that means "let the master answer." This means the physician or employer is responsible for the acts of the employee.

Reticulocyte an immature red blood cell.

Reverse isolation isolation procedure put into effect to protect the patient from infection. Also called protective isolation.

Rule of discovery the statute of limitations begins to run at the time the injury is discovered or when the patient should have known of the injury.

Sclerosed hard, gnarled and scarred.

Septicemia bacterial infection of the bloodstream.

Serology the study of antigens and antibodies in serum.

Serum liquid portion of blood after it has clotted and fibrinogen is gone.

Sinoatrial node where the heartbeat begins; also called the pacemaker.

Slander false, malicious spoken words about another person.

Smear a microscope slide that has material to be stained.

Specific gravity a measure of the density of a substance as compared with the density of water.

Sphygmomanometer instrument for determining blood pressure.

Spirillum a spiral-shaped bacterium.

Standard of care the ordinary skill and care that medical practitioners such as physicians, nurses, and phlebotomists must use that is commonly used by other medical practitioners when caring for patients.

Stat derived from the Latin word meaning immediately.

Statute of limitations maximum time set by federal and state governments during which certain legal actions can be brought forward.

Statutes acts of a federal, state, or county legislature.

Strict isolation isolation required for patients with highly contagious diseases.

Subpoena court order for a person to appear in court. Both documents and persons may be subpoenaed.

Suffix a word component added to the end of a word that adds meaning.

Supine a reclining position on the back with face looking upward.

Surgical asepsis a technique practiced to maintain a sterile environment.

Sympathy feeling sorry for or pitying patients.

Syncope sudden loss of consciousness (i.e., fainting).

Systole the contraction phase of the heartbeat that occurs when the ventricles contract.

TAT an acronym for *turnaround time.*

TDM therapeutic drug monitoring.

Therapeutic phlebotomy drawing blood for the purpose of treating a medical condition.

Thrombocyte platelet.

Thrombocytopenia a decrease in the normal number of platelets.

Thrombocytosis an increase in the normal number of platelets.

Tissue culture a medium of live cells used to grow viruses.

Tort wrongful act (other than a breach of contract) committed against another person or property.

Tourniquet a strap or beltlike device applied to the upper arm to reduce the speed of venous blood flow.

Turbidity having a cloudy appearance.

UTI urinary tract infection.

Venules the smallest veins.

Word root the main portion of the word; it represents the body system or part of the body being discussed.

Wound or skin isolation isolation used to protect the medical worker when a patient has an open wound.

BD Indispensable to human health

BD Vacutainer™

Tube Guide

A full line of BD Vacutainer Blood Collection Needles, Needle Holders and Blood Collection Sets is also available.

BD Vacutainer™ Tubes with Hemogard Closure	BD Vacutainer™ Tubes	Additive	Inversions at Blood Collection*	Laboratory Use	Your Lab's Draw Volume/Remarks
Gold		• Clot activator and gel for serum separation	5	BD Vacutainer™ SST™ Tube for serum determinations in chemistry. Tube inversions ensure mixing of clot activator with blood. Blood clotting time 30 minutes.	
Light Green		• Lithium heparin and gel for plasma separation	8	BD Vacutainer™ PST™ Tube for plasma determinations in chemistry. Tube inversions prevent clotting.	
Red		• None (glass) • Clot activator (Plus plastic with Hemogard closure)	0 5	For serum determinations in chemistry and serology. Glass serum tubes are recommended for blood banking. Plastic tubes contain clot activator and are not recommended for blood banking. Tube inversions ensure mixing of clot activator with blood and clotting within 60 minutes.	
Orange		• Thrombin	8	For stat serum determinations in chemistry. Tube inversions ensure complete clotting which usually occurs in less than 5 minutes.	
Royal Blue		• Sodium heparin • Na_2EDTA • None	8 8 0	For trace element, toxicology and nutritional chemistry determinations. Special stopper formulation provides low levels of trace elements. (see package insert)	
Green		• Sodium heparin • Lithium heparin	8 8	For plasma determinations in chemistry. Tube inversions prevent clotting.	
Gray		• Potassium oxalate/sodium fluoride • Sodium fluoride • Sodium fluoride/K_2EDTA	8 8 8	For glucose determinations. Tube inversions ensure proper mixing of additive and blood. Oxalate and EDTA anticoagulants, will give plasma samples. Sodium fluoride is the anti-glycolytic agent.	
Tan		• Sodium heparin (glass) • K_2EDTA (Plus plastic)	8 8	For lead determinations. This tube is certified to contain less than .01 µg/mL(ppm) lead. Tube inversions prevent clotting.	

	Yellow	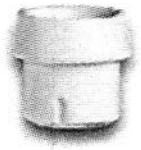	• Sodium polyanetholesulfonate (SPS) • ACD - Acid Citrate Dextrose Additives: **Solution A -** 22.0g/L trisodium citrate, 8.0g/L citric acid, 24.5g/L dextrose **Solution B -** 13.2g/L trisodium citrate, 4.8g/L citric acid, 14.7g/L dextrose	8 8 8	For blood culture specimen collections in microbiology. Tube inversions prevent clotting. For use in blood bank studies, HLA phenotyping, DNA and Paternity testing.
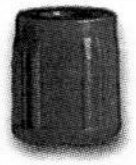	Lavender	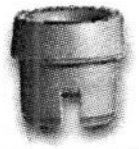	• Liquid K_3EDTA (glass) • Spray-dried K_2EDTA (Plus plastic)	8 8	For whole blood hematology determinations. Tube inversions prevent clotting.
NEW 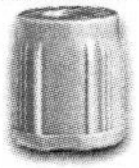	Pink		• Spray-dried K_2EDTA	8	For whole blood hematology determinations and blood banking. Tube inversions prevent clotting. Designed with special crossmatch label for required patient information by the AABB.
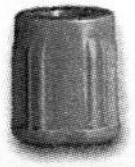	Light Blue	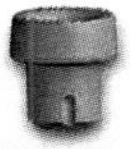	• .105M sodium citrate (≈3.2%) • .129M sodium citrate (≈3.8%)	3-4	For coagulation determinations. Tube inversions prevent clotting. NOTE: Certain tests may require chilled specimens. Follow your institution's recommended procedures for collection and transport.
Partial-draw Tubes (2ml and 3ml: 13 × 75 mm)		Small-volume Pediatric Tubes (2ml: 10.25 × 47 mm, 3ml: 10.25 × 64 mm)			
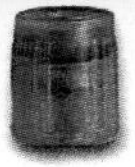	Red	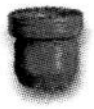	• None	0	For serum determinations in chemistry and serology. Glass serum tubes are recommended for blood banking. Plastic tubes contain clot activator and are not recommended for blood banking. Tube inversions ensure mixing of clot activator with blood and clotting within 60 minutes.
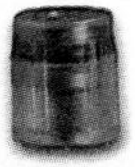	Green	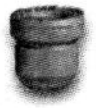	• Sodium heparin • Lithium heparin	8 8	For plasma determinations in chemistry. Tube inversions prevent clotting.
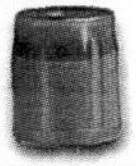	Lavender	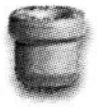	• Liquid K_3EDTA (glass) • Spray-dried K_2EDTA (Plus plastic)	8 8	For whole blood hematology determinations and blood banking. Tube inversions prevent clotting.
	Light Blue	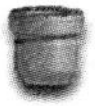	• .105M sodium citrate (≈3.2%) • .129M sodium citrate (≈3.8%)	3-4	For coagulation determinations. Tube inversions prevent clotting. NOTE: Certain tests may require chilled specimens. Follow your institution's recommended procedures for collection and transport of specimen.

BD Vacutainer Systems
Preanalytical Solutions
1 Becton Drive
Franklin Lakes, NJ 07417
www.bd.com

Technical Services: 800.631.0174

*** Invert gently, do not shake**

Printed in USA 08/00 VS5229-3

Courtesy of BD Vacutainer Systems, *Preanalytical Solutions*

INDEX

A

B

C

F

G

H

I

M

N

O

P

T

U

V

W

Y